AF685025

Jim Hom, PhD
Robert L. Denney, PsyD
Editors

Detection of Response Bias in Forensic Neuropsychology

Detection of Response Bias in Forensic Neuropsychology has been co-published simultaneously as *Journal of Forensic Neuropsychology*, Volume 2, Numbers 3/4 and Volume 3, Numbers 1/2 2002.

Pre-publication REVIEWS, COMMENTARIES, EVALUATIONS . . .

"A MUST-BUY FOR EVERY FORENSIC NEUROPSYCHOLOGIST. . . . Fills a critical need . . . no other contemporary single source covers as wide a selection of the most well validated measures used for the detection of response bias. This book includes coverage of virtually all of the well researched methods of detecting response bias available. . . . A GREAT BOOK that every forensic neuropsychologist needs in his or her professional library."

Arthur MacNeill Horton, Jr., EdD, ABPP, ABPN
Chair
Coalition of Clinical Practitioners in Neuropsychology (CCPN)
Past-President
American Board of Professional Neuropsychology
Director
Neuropsychology Clinic, Psych Associates, Towson, Maryland

More pre-publication
REVIEWS, COMMENTARIES, EVALUATIONS . . .

"A MILESTONE in the rapidly expanding clinical domain of forensic neuropsychology. A TIMELY AND SERIOUS BOOK for serious forensic neuropsychologists. Improve both your legal and clinical skills: study this book carefully. THE STATE OF THE ART for evaluating response bias, lack of motivation, and exaggeration of symptom complaints. The authors of the most widely used tests and procedures for detecting response bias present their own strategies and opinions. Included are Rey's methods for detecting malingering, the Portland Digit Recognition Tests, the Test of Memory Malingering, Warrington's Recognitions Memory Test, and the Halstead-Reitan Battery among many others. You will gain in-depth knowledge of these procedures, which will be invaluable for your presentations as an expert witness."

James C. Reed, PhD
Chief Psychologist
St. Luke's Hospital
New Bedford, Massachusetts

"TIMELY . . . will undoubtedly become A VITAL PRACTICE RESOURCE for neuropsychologists evaluating patients in compensation-seeking circumstances. Clinical psychologists will also likely find the material tremendously helpful. Forensic psychologists may well find this text of great benefit as well. For all clinicians who use motivational tests in forensic cases, the sections in each chapter specifically addressing Daubert admissibility issues will be invaluable. Overall, it is difficult to imagine that any clinician engaged in forensic practice involving cognitive or neuropsychological issues will be able to pass up this text."

David T. R. Berry, PhD
Professor of Psychology
University of Kentucky

The Haworth Medical Press
An Imprint of The Haworth Press, Inc.

Detection of Response Bias in Forensic Neuropsychology

Detection of Response Bias in Forensic Neuropsychology has been co-published simultaneously as *Journal of Forensic Neuropsychology*, Volume 2, Numbers 3/4 and Volume 3, Numbers 1/2 2002.

The *Journal of Forensic Neuropsychology* Monographic "Separates"

Below is a list of "separates," which in serials librarianship means a special issue simultaneously published as a special journal issue or double-issue *and* as a "separate" hardbound monograph. (This is a format which we also call a "DocuSerial.")

"Separates" are published because specialized libraries or professionals may wish to purchase a specific thematic issue by itself in a format which can be separately cataloged and shelved, as opposed to purchasing the journal on an on-going basis. Faculty members may also more easily consider a "separate" for classroom adoption.

"Separates" are carefully classified separately with the major book jobbers so that the journal tie-in can be noted on new book order slips to avoid duplicate purchasing.

You may wish to visit Haworth's website at . . .

http://www.HaworthPress.com

. . . to search our online catalog for complete tables of contents of these separates and related publications.

You may also call 1-800-HAWORTH (outside US/Canada: 607-722-5857), or Fax: 1-800-895-0582 (outside US/Canada: 607-771-0012), or e-mail at:

getinfo@haworthpressinc.com

Detection of Response Bias in Forensic Neuropsychology, edited by Jim Hom, PhD, and Robert L. Denney, PsyD (Vol. 2, No. 3/4 & Vol. 3, No. 1/2, 2002). *A guide to techniques and strategies for determining patient compliance during neuropsychological testing.*

Detection of Response Bias in Forensic Neuropsychology

Jim Hom, PhD
Robert L. Denney, PsyD
Editors

Detection of Response Bias in Forensic Neuropsychology has been co-published simultaneously as *Journal of Forensic Neuropsychology*, Volume 2, Numbers 3/4 and Volume 3, Numbers 1/2 2002.

HMP

The Haworth Medical Press
An Imprint of
The Haworth Press, Inc.
New York • London • Oxford

Published by

The Haworth Medical Press®, 10 Alice Street, Binghamton, NY 13904-1580 USA

The Haworth Medical Press® is an imprint of The Haworth Press, Inc., 10 Alice Street, Binghamton, NY 13904-1580 USA.

Detection of Response Bias in Forensic Neuropsychology has been co-published simultaneously as *Journal of Forensic Neuropsychology*, Volume 2, Numbers 3/4 and Volume 3, Numbers 1/2 2002.

© 2002 by The Haworth Press, Inc. All rights reserved. No part of this work may be reproduced or utilized in any form or by any means, electronic or mechanical, including photocopying, microfilm and recording, or by any information storage and retrieval system, without permission in writing from the publisher. Printed in the United States of America.

The development, preparation, and publication of this work has been undertaken with great care. However, the publisher, employees, editors, and agents of The Haworth Press and all imprints of The Haworth Press, Inc., including The Haworth Medical Press® and Pharmaceutical Products Press®, are not responsible for any errors contained herein or for consequences that may ensue from use of materials or information contained in this work. Opinions expressed by the author(s) are not necessarily those of The Haworth Press, Inc. With regard to case studies, identities and circumstances of individuals discussed herein have been changed to protect confidentiality. Any resemblance to actual persons, living or dead, is entirely coincidental.

Cover design by Brooke Stiles

Library of Congress Cataloging-in-Publication Data

Detection of response bias in forensic neuropsychology / Jim Hom, Robert L. Denney, editors.
p. cm.
"Detection of response bias in forensic neuropsychology has been co-published simultaneously as Journal of forensic neuropsychology, volume 2, numbers, 3/4 and volume 3, numbers 1/2 2002."
Includes bibliographical references and index.
ISBN 0-7890-2060-2 (hard : alk. paper)–ISBN 0-7890-2061-0 (soft : alk. paper)
1. Malingering–Diagnosis. 2. Forensic neuropsychology. 3. Neuropsychological tests–Evaluation. I. Hom, Jim. II. Denney, Robert L. III. Journal of forensic neuropsychology.
RA1146 .D48 2003
614'.1–dc21

2002153970

Indexing, Abstracting & Website/Internet Coverage

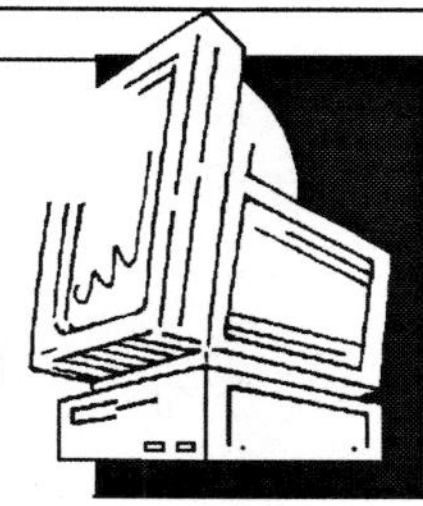

This section provides you with a list of major indexing & abstracting services. That is to say, each service began covering this periodical during the year noted in the right column. Most Websites which are listed below have indicated that they will either post, disseminate, compile, archive, cite or alert their own Website users with research-based content from this work. (This list is as current as the copyright date of this publication.)

Abstracting, Website/Indexing Coverage . . . . Year When Coverage Began

- *CNPIEC Reference Guide: Chinese National Directory of Foreign Periodicals* **1999**
- *Criminal Justice Abstracts* **1999**
- *EMBASE/Excerpta Medica Secondary Publishing Division <URL:http://www.elsevier.nl>* **1999**
- *e-psyche, LLC <www.e-psyche.net>* **2001**
- *Family Violence & Sexual Assault Bulletin* **1999**
- *FINDEX <www.publist.com>* **1999**
- *FRANCIS.INIST/CNRS <www.inist.fr>* **1999**
- *Journal of Clinical Forensic Medicine "Abstracts Section"* **1999**
- *Library and Information Science Annual (LISCA) <www.lu.com>* **1999**
- *PASCAL c/o Institute de L'Information Scientifique et Technique <http://www.inist.fr>* **1999**

(continued)

- ***Psychological Abstracts (PsycINFO)*** **2001**
- ***Published International Literature On Traumatic Stress (The PILOTS Database) <www.ncptsd.org>*** **1999**
- ***Referativnyi Zhurnal (All-Russian Institute of Scientific and Technical Information–in Russian)*** **1999**

Special Bibliographic Notes related to special journal issues (separates) and indexing/abstracting:

- indexing/abstracting services in this list will also cover material in any "separate" that is co-published simultaneously with Haworth's special thematic journal issue or DocuSerial. Indexing/abstracting usually covers material at the article/chapter level.
- monographic co-editions are intended for either non-subscribers or libraries which intend to purchase a second copy for their circulating collections.
- monographic co-editions are reported to all jobbers/wholesalers/approval plans. The source journal is listed as the "series" to assist the prevention of duplicate purchasing in the same manner utilized for books-in-series.
- to facilitate user/access services all indexing/abstracting services are encouraged to utilize the co-indexing entry note indicated at the bottom of the first page of each article/chapter/contribution.
- this is intended to assist a library user of any reference tool (whether print, electronic, online, or CD-ROM) to locate the monographic version if the library has purchased this version but not a subscription to the source journal.
- individual articles/chapters in any Haworth publication are also available through the Haworth Document Delivery Service (HDDS).

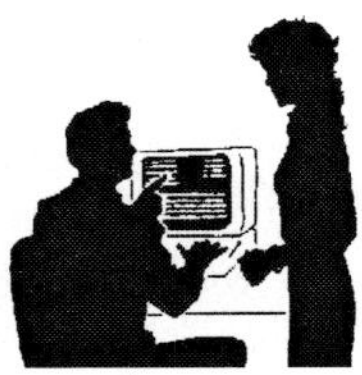

Detection of Response Bias in Forensic Neuropsychology

CONTENTS

ABOUT THE EDITORS

Jim Hom, PhD, is President of The Neuropsychology Center, a clinical services and training facility in Dallas, Texas. He is also a member of the clinical faculty of the Department of Neurology at the University of Texas Southwestern Medical Center in Dallas. He is a Diplomate of the American Board of Professional Neuropsychology and a Fellow in the National Academy of Neuropsychology. He is the Founding Editor of the *Journal of Forensic Neuropsychology* and serves on the editorial boards of several other neuropsychology journals. Dr. Hom has numerous scientific publications in the area of clinical neuropsychology to his credit. He served as President of the National Academy of Neuropsychology in 2002 and has served on the boards of several professional associations, including Division 40 of the American Psychological Association, the American Board of Professional Neuropsychology, and the Coalition of Clinical Practitioners in Neuropsychology. He has more than 20 years of experience in the fields of forensic and clinical neuropsychology.

Robert L. Denney, PsyD, is a forensic psychologist and neuropsychologist at the U.S. Medical Center for Federal Prisoners in Springfield, Missouri. Dr. Denney is Associate Professor and Director of Neuropsychology at the Forest Institute of Professional Psychology in Springfield. He is board certified in forensic psychology by the American Board of Professional Psychology and in neuropsychology by the American Board of Professional Neuropsychology. He has published in the scientific literature on such topics as professional licensure, neuropsychological evaluation of criminal defendants, and malingering of memory disorders, and in such journals as *Archives of Clinical Neuropsychology*, *The Clinical Neuropsychologist*, *Journal of Head Trauma Rehabilitation*, and *Professional Psychology: Research and Practice*. He has also presented throughout the United States on neurolitigation, brain injury, malingering, and admissibility of scientific evidence. He is on the editorial board of the *Journal of Forensic Neuropsychology*.

∞ ALL HAWORTH MEDICAL PRESS BOOKS
AND JOURNALS ARE PRINTED
ON CERTIFIED ACID-FREE PAPER

Preface

The role of a clinical neuropsychologist is to determine the nature of neurocognitive impairment. More often than not, in the forensic setting, the clinical neuropsychologist is asked specifically to determine the relationship of the impairment to brain-related function and causative factors. To this end, clinical neuropsychologists utilize neuropsychological tests. However, as aptly pointed out frequently by counsel, neuropsychological testing is dependent on motivated patient compliance. In fact, most neuropsychological tests assume cooperation and motivation on the part of the patient. With such assumptions met, neuropsychological testing can provide objective performance-related information regarding the status of an individual's brain-related function.

While clinical neuropsychology has this potential, its bane is the requirement for motivated patient compliance. The tacit assumption that the patient is putting forth his/her best effort may not hold in forensic settings, in particular. Frequently, powerful forces or factors can operate that affect the patient's motivation and change his/her behavior during testing, to the point of affecting the accuracy of test performances. It is beyond the scope of this work to address the factors or motivations which may be involved in such situations. Nonetheless, patients are often motivated to prove that they have "real" impairments. The adversarial nature of litigation further magnifies this motivation. The clinical neuropsychologist is left in the position of not only determining neurocognitive function and differential diagnosis, but also having to consider the possible response bias of the patient.

Over the last decade, there has been a growing awareness of the need to consider possible confounding factors in evaluating patients' performances. Negative response bias, symptom validity, exaggeration,

[Haworth indexing entry note]: "Preface." Hom, Jim, and Robert L. Denney. Published in *Detection of Response Bias in Forensic Neuropsychology* (ed: Jim Hom, and Robert L. Denney) The Haworth Medical Press, an imprint of The Haworth Press, Inc., 2002, pp. xi-xvi. Single or multiple copies of this article are available for a fee from The Haworth Document Delivery Service [1-800-HAWORTH, 9:00 a.m. - 5:00 p.m. (EST). E-mail address: getinfo@haworthpressinc.com].

© 2002 by The Haworth Press, Inc. All rights reserved.

malingering, and effort testing all relate to the concept of identifying test results that are not a valid reflection of the patient's abilities. Differentiating willful attempts to exaggerate disability for secondary gain (malingering) from willful exaggeration for primary gain (factitious disorder), non-willful exaggeration (conversion or other psychiatric disorder), or simply poor motivation is a complicated process. As the authors in this book all emphasize, the differentiation must be based on the entire context of the evaluation. Given the complicated nature of this differentiation, we prefer the broad term "response bias" to refer to the various types of possible invalid patient responses. According to the Merriam-Webster dictionary, *bias* is "an inclination of temperament or outlook; especially, a personal and sometimes unreasoned judgment; systematic error introduced into sampling or testing by selecting or encouraging one outcome or answer over others." This definition captures the essence of the problem we face as clinical neuropsychologists in attempting to complete valid assessments.

The goal of this monograph is to have the developers and researchers of the major response bias detection strategies present a review of their methods. Our hope in providing a venue for these authors to review their own work was to allow them the opportunity to lay out those unique insights that, oftentimes, reside only with the test creators and primary clinical researchers. Also, we wanted to provide the authors with a forum to discuss their strategies in regard to each method's scientific basis. We also asked them to address their method's performance in light of many jurisdictions adopting a tighter judicial review of expert witness testimony under the 1993 U.S. Supreme Court decision in *Daubert v. Merrell Dow Pharmaceuticals* (509 U.S. 579). We are excited about the results. Each author's area of research has broadened the field's understanding of the detection of response bias by making unique contributions. Given the productivity and contribution of these authors, we believe the field of neuropsychology will view response bias assessment in forensic settings differently within the next five years. Their contributions will quite likely affect the evolution of this developing field.

Detection of Response Bias in Forensic Neuropsychology is loosely organized into two sections. The first portion deals with techniques specifically designed to identify response bias, and the second deals with characteristics of response bias identification within established psychological and neuropsychological measures. Free-standing tests of response bias are designed for use in conjunction with other psychological and neuropsychological measures as markers to identify negative response bias. For the most part, they have little clinical utility beyond the response bias question (notable exceptions are the Word Memory Test, Warrington Recognition Test, and to a lesser extent, Validity Indicator Profile). The tests need to be included in a clinical battery in such a manner as to make them appear a part of the routine battery. In this regard, it is best to think through carefully where the tests are placed in a battery. Although not yet clarified empirically, it seems prudent to place tests on which even severely impaired individuals perform well (so called "floor effect tests") before much more clinically difficult tasks. Placing such floor effect tests after more difficult clinical measures would seem to decrease their effectiveness. On the other hand, it is clearly appropriate to intersperse more than one response bias measure throughout a lengthy forensic evaluation. It is ultimately up to the evaluator to decide where and how to place multiple response bias measures within a larger battery. The latter portion of this volume deals with response bias indicators inherent within established clinical measures. The clear benefit of using these strategies is that they do not require additional evaluator administration time, they are typically interspersed throughout an entire evaluation, and they have very little face validity as response bias measures. Although they have these benefits, they have a cost as well. Because they are based upon established clinical measures, they appear more susceptible to effects of genuine neurocognitive impairment. Nearly all the authors address this issue by providing caveats when dealing with severely brain injured or those subjects with extreme ages.

Frederick starts the volume off with a review of Rey's tests to detect malingering: the 15-Item Memory Test, the Word Recognition Test, and the Dot Counting Test. Frederick provides us with particularly interesting and unique insights because he was able to visit André Rey's family in France and acquire Rey's original works on these tests. He provides a tremendous service to the field by providing translations and clarity regarding several points related to their administration and interpretation.

Binder presents information on the Portland Digit Recognition Test, and Allen, Iverson, and Green address the Computerized Assessment of Response Bias (CARB). Both of these tests are adaptations of the original Digit Memory Test by Hiscock and Hiscock (1989). In addition to below random responding, these authors describe the more recent trend of using normative based cut-offs to improve test sensitivity. Thompson describes the Victoria Symptom Validity Test (VSVT), another test patterned after the Digit Memory Test. Like the CARB, it is computer administered and scored which allows identification of response latencies, but the VSVT also incorporates two tiers of item difficulty to enhance test sensitivity. Tombaugh discusses another forced-choice, two alternative test, the Test of Memory Malingering. Rather than digits, the TOMM uses line drawn pictures as well as norm referenced cut-offs. Green, Lees-Haley, and Allen present the Word Memory Test (WMT). The WMT uses words rather than digits or pictures and actually presents the information in a verbal learning task as well as a multi-trial two alternative, forced-choice procedure that uses norm based cut-offs. The WMT has the added benefit of a clinically valuable verbal memory test. Frederick reviews the Validity Indicator Profile (VIP), another two alternative, forced-choice procedure, but one that uses item variability to identify invalid results through performance curve analysis. The VIP has verbal and non-verbal subtests. It is unique in that it presents as a general measure of cognitive ability rather than a test of memory, as with each of the preceding tests.

The remaining papers deal with response bias strategies developed for already established clinical tests. Millis reviews the Warrington Recognition Memory Test, a test with verbal and visual subtests. Although originally designed for clinical use to identify memory impairment, its forced-choice, two alternative format allowed for its use in detection of response bias. In this regard, it is used in a similar fashion as the tests listed above. Lees-Haley, Iverson, Lange, Fox, and Allen review the various scales within the MMPI-2 to detect response bias as related to emotional/psychiatric, neurocognitive, and somatic complaints. Mittenberg, Aguila-Puentes, Patton, Canyock, and Heilbronner present various formulas for use with the Halstead-Reitan Battery, WAIS-R/III and WMS-R in differentiating valid traumatic brain injury results from invalid performances. Sweet and King review strategies for detecting rare response sets with the Category Test in evaluating traumatic brain injury. Lastly, Reitan and Wolfson address intra-individual and test-retest inconsistencies that suggest unreliable patient performance on the Halstead-Reitan Battery. A unique characteristic of their method is that it uses the patient's own test responses, like a control, as the basis for determining validity of subsequent performances.

In addition to asking the authors to provide their own insights regarding each strategy's utility in clinical practice, we asked the authors to address each procedure's performance in light of the scientific admissibility expectations presented in *Daubert*. Prior to 1993, courts in the United States used the *Frye* standard in evaluating the scientific merits of expert testimony. This standard was termed the "general acceptance test" because courts evaluated the merits of scientific theories and procedures espoused by expert witnesses on whether or not the theory or procedure had gained general acceptance within its respective field. In 1993, however, the U. S. Supreme Court reinterpreted scientific admissibility issues in light of the revised *Federal Rule of Evidence* 702 which states, "If scientific, technical, or other specialized knowledge will assist the trier of fact to understand the evidence or to determine a fact in issue, a witness qualified as an expert by knowledge, skill, experience, training, or education, may testify thereto in the form of an opinion or otherwise." In essence, *Daubert* and its progeny (*General Electric Co. v. Joiner*, 1997; *Kumho Tire Co. v. Patrick Carmichael*, 1999) outline that trial judges have great latitude and discretion as "gatekeepers" to allow or disallow admission of expert witness testimony. In fact, the Court intimated it is the trial judge's duty to determine if the "reasoning or methodology underlying the testimony is scientifically valid, and whether that reasoning or methodology can be linked to facts of the case." (*Daubert* at 593) *Daubert* specified the court's evaluation was to be a flexible one and tailored to the specific science at issue. Although flexible, the Court, however, did provide a short list of factors to aid the trial judges in their analysis. These factors included these questions:

1. Has the theory or technique been tested or is subject to being tested?
2. Has the theory or technique been subjected to peer review and publication?
3. What is the known or potential rate of error in applying the particular scientific theory or technique? and
4. To what extent has the theory or technique received general acceptance in the relevant scientific community?

Each set of authors addressed these questions in their own manner. We think it important for practicing neuropsychologists to become aware of these issues as they relate to response bias detection strategies just as they are important for neuropsychological and psychological measures in general.

We would like to highlight two themes that run throughout these series of papers. Identification of response bias is a contextual issue requiring clinical judgment regarding a wide variety of facts surrounding a clinical case, not just isolated test scores. And lastly, every author, in some fashion, pointed out that the "state of the art" was to include multiple measures of response bias, ideally spread throughout an assessment battery, to best identify invalid response styles. We think these two points represent a logical, scientific approach to performing neuropsychological assessment in the forensic arena.

Finally, we must point out that, given the information provided in this book, it is clear that the practicing clinical neuropsychologist can no longer simply assume that all his/her patients are putting forth valid effort. Rather, steps must be taken to assess directly motivation, effort, bias, and other such factors. More and more commonly, forensic neuropsychologists are faced not only with identifying neuropsychological impairment but also with the question of whether they addressed the issues of response bias in their evaluation. Hopefully, the information in this volume will aid in this regard.

We would like to thank all the contributors to this work for their time and willingness in providing their unique insights and commentary on their work. It is clear that their research has provided valuable information to the field of forensic neuropsychology. A special acknowledgement goes to Susan Wilfong for her administrative and clerical assistance in putting the book together. Finally, we express special appreciation to Dr. Janice Nici for her dedicated and time-consuming editorial assistance and organizational talents in handling the nitty-gritty details and keeping us on track during all stages of preparation.

Jim Hom, PhD
Robert L. Denney, PsyD

REFERENCES

Daubert v. Merrell Dow Pharmaceuticals, Inc., 509 U.S. 579 (1993).

Frye v. United States, 293 F. 1013 (D.C. Cir. 1923).

General Electric Co. v. Joiner, 522 U.S. 136 (1997).

Hiscock, M., & Hiscock, C. K. (1989). Refining the forced-choice method of r the detection of malingering. *Journal of Clinical and Experimental Neuropsychology*, *11*, 967-974.

Kumho Tire Co. v. Patrick Carmichael, 119 S. Ct. 1167 (1999).

A Review of Rey's Strategies for Detecting Malingered Neuropsychological Impairment

Richard I. Frederick

U.S. Medical Center for Federal Prisoners

SUMMARY. André Rey was a pioneer in clinical psychology, child clinical psychology, and neuropsychology. His contributions to the understanding of brain-behavior relationships were novel, creative, and highly regarded. Rey developed many eponymous tests and procedures. Three are relatively well known in American neuropsychological literature as "tests of malingering": The Rey 15-Item Memory Test (RMT), the Rey Word Recognition Test (WRT), and the Rey Dot Counting Test (DCT), referred to collectively in this paper as the "Rey malingering tests." By citing his original work, this article reports Rey's method of assessing the validity of clinical presentation, his instructional sets for each test, and his process of interpreting test results. Additionally, this

---

Richard I. Frederick is affiliated with the U.S. Medical Center for Federal Prisoners, Springfield, MO.

Address correspondence to: Richard I. Frederick, PhD, Department of Psychology, U.S. Medical Center for Federal Prisoners, Springfield, MO 65807 (E-mail: richardfrederick@yahoo.com).

The author thanks Teresinha Rey and André-Louis Rey for their generous assistance and hospitality in discussing André Rey's work. Some information about Rey's personal history comes from discussions they and the author had on May 21 and 22, 1998. The translations and photograph in the article are used with their permission. The author also thanks Carlos Tomelleri and Thomas Fullerton for their translations of Rey's writings.

The conclusions and opinions reported in this article do not necessarily represent the views of the Federal Bureau of Prisons or the U.S. Department of Justice.

[Haworth co-indexing entry note]: "A Review of Rey's Strategies for Detecting Malingered Neuropsychological Impairment." Frederick, Richard I. Co-published simultaneously in *Journal of Forensic Neuropsychology* (The Haworth Medical Press, an imprint of The Haworth Press, Inc.) Vol. 2, No. 3/4, 2002, pp. 1-25; and: *Detection of Response Bias in Forensic Neuropsychology* (ed: Jim Hom, and Robert L. Denney) The Haworth Medical Press, an imprint of The Haworth Press, Inc., 2002, pp. 1-25. Single or multiple copies of this article are available for a fee from The Haworth Document Delivery Service [1-800-HAWORTH, 9:00 a.m. - 5:00 p.m. (EST). E-mail address: getinfo@haworthpressinc.com].

© 2002 by The Haworth Press, Inc. All rights reserved.

article reviews published research regarding the efficacy of the Rey malingering tests as they have been used in this country. Most instructional sets and interpretive strategies generally have not followed Rey, but have followed those represented as Rey's by Lezak (1983, 1995). *[Article copies available for a fee from The Haworth Document Delivery Service: 1-800-HAWORTH. E-mail address: <getinfo@haworthpressinc.com> Website: <http://www.HaworthPress.com> © 2002 by The Haworth Press, Inc. All rights reserved.]*

KEYWORDS. Malingering, neuropsychological assessment, psychological evidence, André Rey

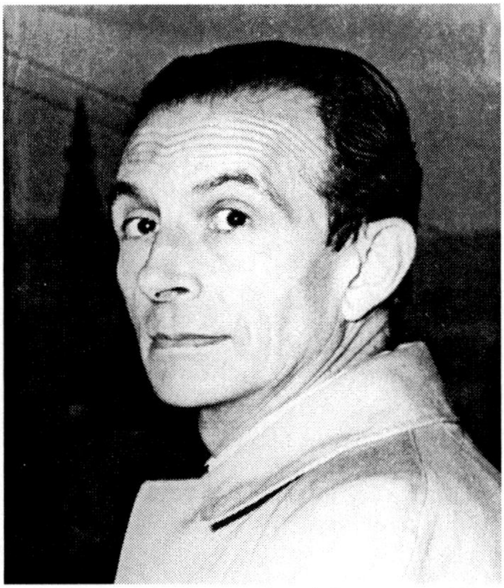

André Rey at the International Congress of Pyschology, Rome, Italy, 1958. Photo courtesy of Teresinha Rey.

André Rey was born in 1906 in Lausanne, Switzerland. His first published paper concerned recent developments in French psychology and philosophy (Rey, 1928). In 1929, he went to Geneva to work with Edouard Claparède, a physician and psychologist, who founded the Institute of Educational Sciences and initiated clinical psychology in Switzerland (Kaschel, Goldenberg, Goldstein, Risberg, Laaksonen, Gaillard, Perret, Tissot, & Oktem-Tanor, 1994). The Institute was linked to the clinical psychology laboratory in the neurology service at Geneva Hospital (l'Hôpital Cantoral de Genève). The objectives of the laboratory were to identify the extent of cognitive deterioration in traumatic brain injury and alcoholism (Kaschel et al., 1994). In 1934, Rey completed his doctoral dissertation, which concerned the assessment of practical intelligence of children. His experiments evaluated the methods by which children from ages 4 to 8 could solve practical problems. For example, he studied how children could obtain by indirect means a piece of candy suspended by a string (Lambercier & Rey, 1935; Winstch, 1935). In 1936, he received a Rockefeller scholarship and went to Harvard University to work with Karl Lashley for two years. His work included improving some of Lashley's methodology for experimentation with animals (Rey, 1938).

Upon his return to Geneva, he resumed his work at the Institute. The problems he addressed through clinical practice were methods of identifying subtle neuropsychological signs, neuroreception, muscular strength and tonus, constructional praxia, visual perception, articulation of language, motor coordination, balance, memory and learning, and concentration. He worked with developmentally delayed children and with patients with different sorts of brain pathology. When Claparède died in 1940, Rey assumed the position as director of the psychology laboratory. He was professor of applied psychology in the Institute of Educational Sciences from 1949 onwards.

In 1954 and 1955, he studied the adaptability of Jewish children from North Africa to live in Palestine, developing language-free general intellectual measures (Rey, 1957). In 1956, he went to Brazil at the request of its government to develop a psychology curriculum at Belo Horizonte. During his stay there, he met his future wife, Teresinha, who went a little later to Geneva for further studies and worked as a psychologist, evaluating and treating children with physical and mental disabilities in partnership with Rey. In 1958, he was named Lecturer for Clinical Psychology for the Faculty of Medicine at Geneva Hospital. In 1958, he began a continuing visiting professorship of psychology in Lyons, France. He had a full private clinical practice from 1938 until 1965. Rey was an advanced amateur entomologist and botanist (he served as president of the Society of Physical and Natural History in Geneva) and published works on the behavior of spiders and caterpillars.

From 1928 until his death in 1965, he published more than 170 articles and books concerning animal psychology, experimental psychology, clinical techniques, test development, clinical interviewing, and diagnostic tools. His works include investigations of elementary brain functions (development of perception: visual, tactual, gustatory; motor coordination, spatial localization, sensory-motor accommodation), more complex brain functions (mental imagery, development of mental processes, and attention), attention and learning (acquisition of learning, associative learning, comparison of learning curves between infants and animals), developmental processes (children's abilities, child psychopathology, developmental delays), assessment techniques (personality tests, intellectual assessment, developmental drawing tests, projective drawing tests), effects of trauma on learning, traumatic brain injury and recovery, and professional issues (relationships between psychologists and psychiatrists, education and training of psychologists). His research was typified by analyses of large data bases collected from clinical practice.

In 1967, the Association of the Friends of André Rey (including Georges de Morsier, Paul A. Osterrieth, Robert Dottrens, and Marc Richelle) published a memorial volume: the *Hommage a André Rey*. A group composed of his last assistants, working with Teresinha Rey, published five volumes of previously unpublished tests. Additionally, Teresinha Rey has been organizing and cataloging Rey's works for the University of Geneva, where they will remain available for future researchers.

Rey is perhaps best known in American psychology as the developer of the Rey Auditory Verbal Learning Test (AVLT), the Rey-Osterrieth Complex Figure Test, and for several techniques for assessing feigned neuropsychological impairment (Lezak, 1995). Lezak also noted his skin writing techniques, and Taylor (1959) reported his work concerning assessment of children's maturational skills by human figure drawings (Rey, 1946). Although his contributions are well-known throughout Europe, only a small body of his work is known in the United States. This article reviews Rey's work particularly with respect to the evaluation of feigned neuropsychological impairment.

GENERAL CAVEATS ON MALINGERING DETECTION BY REY

Rey developed interest in malingering detection partly in response to accusations by insurance companies that most, if not all, claimants were probably only feigning impairment. His techniques were not limited to the malingering tests described in this paper. He developed many techniques and procedures, most of which depended primarily upon a performance curve analysis; that is, a comparison of achievements across a range of test difficulties (see Frederick, Crosby, & Wynkoop, 2000; Rogers, Harrell, & Liff, 1993). Neurologist Georges de Morsier, wrote:

> . . . Rey demonstrated that all simulators (the fear of the insurance experts) were immediately discovered by the characteristic nature of the curves. From the initiation of regular collaboration with the clinic (1940), Rey continually perfected and improved these methods of assessing memory and perception, thus allowing one to see

> in a glance from its graphical representation the mental capacity of the patient and the deficiencies acquired since the patient's illness or trauma. (excerpted from *Hommage a André Rey*, 1967; p. 19)

Rey's general approach to assessing malingering included an understanding that some idiosyncratic presentations could mimic malingering, that use of a single sign was insufficient to make effective discriminations between individuals with real impairment and malingerers, and that an understanding of the context of the evaluation and the potential motivations of malingerers was paramount:

> In this case it is a matter of unmasking the individual, remembering that the exaggeration of symptoms may constitute in itself a behavioral disorder and not always a calculated behavior. It is important, first of all, to evaluate the cultural level of the patient, then to characterize his balance of satisfactions and life style, information which often permits us to understand the need or self-interest leading to the patient's exaggeration or simulation. (Rey, 1958; p. 121)

REY FIFTEEN-ITEM MEMORY TEST

The RMT is probably the best known of Rey's procedures. It generally became known in American neuropsychological literature through Muriel Lezak's second edition of *Neuropsychological Assessment* (1983). The first experimental data for the RMT were reported by Goldberg and Miller (1986). Since that time, a large number of articles have appeared, most of which highlight the limitations of the test in distinguishing between malingerers and individuals with significant neuropsychological impairment.

Instructions

Rey's instructions for this test are as follows:

> First of all we ask him to freely express the data retained after listening to a series of 15 words. Let us suppose this immediate response is very weak (3 or 4 words). Next we will present the following 15 signs grouped by three. [Note: see Figure 1]

> We expose them for 30 seconds, then ask the subject to reproduce them without worrying about their order. We insist upon the fact that there are 15 different elements. During the duration of the exposure we state each series so as to rule out any ambiguity: "Capital A, B, C; 1, 2, 3; a, b, c, small letters; a circle, a square, a triangle; one stick, two sticks, three sticks." We allow two minutes for reproducing the data viewed. (Rey, 1958; p. 121-122)

Lezak (1983) modified these instructions substantially, but made no references to administering the test immediately following a 15-item word list (ostensibly for contrast) or, more particularly, following a weak performance on such a test. She identified the period of memorization as only 10 seconds, and added "a 10-or 15-second quiet delay period can be interpolated" (p. 619). The instructional set of Goldberg and Miller (1986) has been the basis for most research since then: "I am going to show you a card with 15 [emphasized] things on it to remember. When I take the card away, I want you to write down as many of the 15 things as you can remember" (p. 794). After 5 seconds, a prompt was given: "Be sure to look at all of them." The stimulus items were removed after a 10-second exposure.

Other researchers have emphasized different aspects of the instructions. Schretlen, Brandt, Krafft, and van Gorp (1991) and Guilmette,

FIGURE 1

A	**B**	**C**
1	**2**	**3**
a	**b**	**c**
○	□	△
|	||	|||

Hart, Giuliano, and Leininger (1994) emphasized there were 15 different items to remember. Arnett, Hammeke, and Schwartz (1995) presented the RMT as "a very difficult memory test" and added "this is a hard [emphasized] test."

Rogers et al. (1993) argued it might be unethical and clinically unnecessary to describe the task as "difficult." Similarly, Bernard and Fowler (1990) considered it counterproductive to tell patients a test was difficult when it is obviously designed to promote recall. These points are well made. It seems clear from Rey's original instructions that he used the test when performance on a reasonably difficult task reflected evidence of poor effort, and he "insisted" there were 15 different elements only to induce the dissimulating patient to relate the task to the previous test. Otherwise, there does not appear to have been any attempt by Rey to make the task seem difficult by instructional set. In research simulation and clinical practice, Frederick, Sarfaty, Johnston, and Powel (1994), Frederick (1997), and Frederick (2000b) maintained the primary instructional set of Lezak (1983); that is, a 10-second exposure and a 10-second interpolated delay, but administered the Rey after the completion of the AVLT, beginning with the transitional statement: "Now I'm going to *show* you 15 things to remember."

Scoring

Rey was interested in the number of items completed and the number of groups completed. Most research on the Rey has focused on counting the number of completed items. Griffin, Normington, and Glassmire (1996) reported a qualitative analysis of the RMT, focusing on whether the rows were completed out of sequence, when characters were modified (e.g., a reversal of "b" to "d") or embellished (e.g., when the sticks were transformed into Roman numerals).

Interpretation

Rey's interpretation follows:

> If the patient is not intellectually weak, if he is not suffering serious mental deterioration, and especially if he is sincere and cooperates faithfully, he will reproduce the 15 signs without difficulty. In fact, there are only 5 data to be retained at the most, automatisms and associations assuring the reproduction of the 10 others. One may tolerate the forgetting of a group, most often the

> sticks and one of the geometric figures. Forgetting two groups is already suspect and forgetting three allows the conclusion of exaggeration and doubtful collaboration by the subject whose intellectual level is normal and who, moreover, takes great care to describe his disorders. When the 15 signs are reproduced correctly, and the patient has remarked, often spontaneously, that the test was easy, or much easier than the preceding one, we will be able to establish in his performance a collaboration sufficient, at least, for us to push further the investigations and we shall be allowed to take into consideration the difficulties presented on the test of the immediate expression of 15 words.
>
> Let us note, moreover, that if on this first test, the result had been normal, it would be in itself an indication of sincerity and of collaboration, and one could immediately concede a certain amount of credit to the complaints expressed, and direct research onto aspects of memory more differentiated than a simple, immediate evocation of words. . . . One will eliminate without difficulty the cases of intellectual debility or of easily identifiable insanity to other signs and results. (Rey, 1958; pp. 122-123)

Despite Rey's caveats, Lezak (1983) reported only, "Anyone who is not significantly deteriorated can recall at least three of the five character sets" (p. 619). This cut-off score (i.e., fewer than 9 items reproduced) was supported by Goldberg and Miller (1986) and Bernard and Fowler (1990), who considered any performance less than nine items predictive of malingering. Frederick et al. (1994) found this cut-off had a 40% sensitivity and 100% specificity for a large sample of simulating malingerers and normal controls. Greiffenstein, Baker, and Gola (1994) reported that cut-off scores of 9 or 10 had sensitivity of 62% for probable malingerers and specificities of 88% and 81% for individuals with bona fide traumatic brain injury.

The cut-off has often been criticized as too nonspecific for persons with true impairment (Hays, Emmons, & Lawson, 1993; Lee, Loring, & Martin, 1992; Schretlen et al., 1991). Lee et al. (1992) recommended using a cut-off score of fewer than 8 items reproduced, despite only a small gain in specificity for doing so (95% instead of 93%). Hays et al. (1993) recommended interpretation of RMT scores with respect to measured IQ levels, apparently failing to consider the possibility participants had feigned their IQ test performance. Others have considered even the cut-off score of 8 to be too nonspecific (Arnett et al., 1995; Guilmette et al., 1994). Arnett et al. (1995) recommended a cut-off score of fewer than two complete rows. Simon (1994) recommended against the use of less than three rows, finding it too nonspecific (57%) for his control group of severely ill insanity acquittees, although Back, Boone, Edwards, Parks, Burgoyne, and Silver (1996) found the false positive rate (using a cut-off of fewer than 9 items) for 30 patients with schizophrenia was only 13%.

Other researchers have recommended higher cut-off scores, concluding a cut-off of less than 9 was too insensitive (Bernard, Houston, & Natoli, 1993). Greiffenstein, Baker, and Gola (1996) reported that a cut-off score of fewer than 10 items maintained both high specificity and sensitivity. DiCarlo, Gfeller, and Drury (1996) recommend a cutting score of fewer than 14 items(!). Iverson and Franzen (1996; see also Arnett & Franzen, 1997) modified the test to a 16-item test, eliminating the geometric figures, hoping to make the test more sensitive to malingering. The procedure has also been modified by Griffin, Glassmire, Henderson, and McCann (1997) in an attempt to increase sensitivity and specificity. Frederick (2000b) compared a number of the reported sensitivities and specificities for many of these studies.

Rey would seem to readily concede that the RMT is likely to be sensitive to significant mental, neuropsychological, or intellectual impairment. His own caveats include: "*If the patient is not intellectually weak, if he is not suffering serious mental deterioration* . . ." and "Forgetting two groups is already suspect and forgetting three allows the conclusion of exaggeration and doubtful collaboration by the subject *whose intellectual level is normal* and who, moreover, takes great care to describe his disorders" (emphasis added). In support of these contentions, Frederick (2000b) used a variety of methods to estimate that the cut-off of fewer than 9 items was moderately sensitive (58% to 89%) and highly specific (96% to 98%) in a criminal forensic setting with a reasonably low base rate of significant neuropsychological injury or impairment. Analysis using receiver operating characteristic curves for the sample of 723 criminal defendants yielded values for the area under the curve of 0.94 to 0.98, meaning that randomly drawing an RMT score from a pure sample of malingerers would be lower (i.e., fewer items reproduced) than a randomly drawn RMT score from a pure sample of non-malingering criminal defendants 94% to 98% of the time.

Rey's own description of the RMT is as "a very simple maneuver," using it as an example in his discussion perhaps only to avoid detailed descriptions of more elaborate procedures whose "details . . . it is preferable not to disclose."[1] (Indeed, Frederick et al., 1994, found the RMT's sensitivity dropped to 5% when simulating malingerers received only minor coaching.) I suspect Rey would be astonished to find his "simple maneuver" had been elevated to the status of a primary detection strategy and then criticized for its presumptuousness.

REY DOT COUNTING TEST

The DCT and WRT have been evaluated far less than the RMT, but they were his earliest examples of applying malingering detection methodology. The following passage regarding the DCT is from a journal article published in 1941:

> Investigating the disordered character of responses:
>
> Tests to determine sensory thresholds can be utilized for this purpose. Without the subject being able to notice, the intensity of the stimulus is varied in an irregular fashion. The malingerer, sometimes some psychopaths, furnish responses which do not exhibit any relationship between the intensity of the stimulus and that of the perception. For example, determination of tactile threshold with the Weber compass, a study of auditive perception with the acumetric inductor of Foy, etc. The same principle can be applied to more complex psychological operations. For instance, we will present to a subject, in an irregular order, tasks of increasing difficulty. If the times of execution are proportional to the difficulty of the tasks, we are in the presence of a normal or abnormal performance depending on the magnitude of these execution times and in such case, this is not suspect. If this progression fails to occur, if we register gross irregularities, the performance is suspect, or at least it poses a problem that needs to be elucidated.
>
> An example of a test of this type follows: Six cards are presented successively to the subject, each one containing a certain number of dots distributed irregularly. The subject has to count the dots as rapidly as possible without using his finger. The time that transpires between the instant of the presentation and the response is noted.
>
> The cards, numbered one through six, contain respectively seven, 11, 15, 19, 23 and 27 dots. (Each dot is one square millimeter and they are equidistant by .5 centimeters.) The cards are presented in the following order: two, four, three, five, six, one. The establishment of each total (the dot count) necessitates a certain effort of attention that will require a longer time in proportion to the

number of dots counted. If the subject works in earnest we will find a progression of times as we arrange the responses according to the increasing number of dots.

The following table allows one to form an exact idea of the speed of the responses and the progression of times among adult normal individuals:

Percentile:		100	75	50	25	0
Card 1:	7 dots	1 sec	2 sec	4 sec	5 sec	11 sec
2:	11	2	3	4	5	17
3:	15	3	4	6	7	17
4:	19	4	6	7	9	19
5:	23	5	8	10	12	30
6:	27	6	9	11	16	30

The 50th percentile column shows typical results of average individuals, percentiles 100 and 75 columns of fast individuals, and the 25 percentile column those of slow individuals. The zero column displays pathological results originating in subjects who suffer from traumatic encephalopathy (sequelae of head injury).

The examination of these figures allows interesting determinations.

A. The progression is more sharp and regular when we are dealing with faster individuals who have made an effort to perform well.

B. The progression is less regular among individuals who are slower or who suffer from attention deficits. This however is a relative irregularity for which our table furnishes the tolerance limit. If the irregularity would become more pronounced it would give rise to question about the good will and good faith of the subject. We can, however, tolerate a strongly aberrant result in the midst of the progression. Actually, an accident can happen, or a scrupulous individual may repeat the count of the groups of dots. One must take into consideration errors whose distribution corresponds to indications furnished by the time measures. An error in this account is less suspect if it occurs in a group where the dots are more numerous. Finally, in the presence of suspect performances, it is always useful to repeat these tests several times.

It needs to be added that the principle of the multi-sense character of a single test needs to be applied to the tracking down of malingering as it applies to psychological diagnosis in general. In the psychological plane, a single suspect result raises a hypothesis and orients research; it does not create a certainty.

Use of tests of different degrees of difficulty combined with changes of attitude of the examiner.

This is the group of procedures that is most important and most efficacious to investigate malingering and absence of effort. Let us suppose the psychologist has available several tests of the same type for which it has been established that differences in performance are the rule. In that manner, Test B must produce among all conscientious individuals quantitatively superior results (timewise) compared to Test A.

We will begin by presenting the easy test (A) after patiently having listened to the patient's complaints. We will let him work freely and we will observe him with benevolence. If the result is poor and there is otherwise reason to suspect the good will of the subject we will then proceed to Test B, which is the more difficult one. At this moment we will change our attitude. We will declare to the patient we are afraid he has abused the benevolence that we have shown him, that the result he has furnished is suspect, and that from this point on we expect a more conscientious performance from him. We then give him Test B. If, with this more difficult test, his performance is superior or equal to that produced on the easier test then this is an indication that confirms the presence of an initial tendency to not make much of an effort.

We have already proposed a great number of tests that allow us to realize the maneuver we have just described. For example, here are two procedures which are perhaps new and will augment a stock of useful procedures. Let us return to the test of groups of dots. It will serve as Test B difficult. Let's imagine presently a Test A of the same type but much easier. Instead of using irregular groups, we are going to distribute the dots in geometric groups. The total number will be much easier to establish and consequently responses will be faster. On six cards we will distribute groups numbering respectively 8, 12, 16, 20, 24, and 28 dots. Each group will be composed of the following groups–8 would be two squares of four, 12 would be two squares of five plus two separate dots, 16 would be four diamonds of four, 20 would be four groups of five (square of four dots with one dot in the middle), 24 would be four groups of six (rectangle of six dots), 28 would be four groups of five plus two groups of four. The cards numbered from one to six are presented in the following order: 2, 4, 3, 5, 6, 1. This test elicits a psychological mechanism which is different from that of the first test. To obtain the total number of dots in the irregular groupings it is necessary to count dots one by one; attention plays a principal role. Whenever the dots are grouped the numerical value of each group is perceived almost instantaneously and it is sufficient to make an elementary addition or multiplication to obtain the total. (In giving instructions one must insist that the subject count as fast as possible and using the quickest means.) The number of dots in this case does not play more than an insignificant role and the progression of times of response is very weak. Following is a table that gives an idea of the rapidity of response among normal adults. We will notice the weak dispersion of the results.

Percentile:		100	75	50	25	0
Card 1:	8 dots	.5 sec	1 sec	1 sec	2 sec	3 sec
	12	1	2	2	2	3
	16	1	2	2	4	5
	20	1	1	2	4	5
	24	2	2	2	5	6
	28	2	2	3	5	7

Test A is clearly easier than the previous test (B) and we should have a total time for (A) which is less than the total time for (B). We can then utilize the system of test AB according to the procedure described above. These are examples of normal reaction.

Adult Subjects (comparison of total times for the six cards of each series)

	Test A (Easy) Grouped dots	Test B (Difficult) Irregularly distributed dots	Difference B − A
Subject X	9 sec	31 sec	+22
Subject Y	11	31	+20
Subject Z	12	33	+21

The following are examples of pathological reactions or responses that do not elicit suspicion:

Traumatic Encephalopathy, chronic case, the accident happened approximately two years ago.

	A	B	Difference B − A
Subject L	21 sec	37 sec	+16
Subject M	22	38	+16
Subject N	24	69	+45

In these three cases, the slowness of response is explained by slowness of mentation and troubles of attention and perception. It is proportional to the degree of difficulty of the tests.

Here is an example of a suspect result:

	A	B	Difference B − A
Subject D	57 sec	42 sec	−15

The subject spends more time with the easy test than with the difficult test. He has counted the dots of the figures in test A instead of evaluating the groups and proceeding arithmetically. This is a case of idiopathic feeble-mindedness (Rey, 1941; pp. 312-316).

Instructions

In this passage, Rey described two separate procedures using the dots. One uses the "irregularly distributed" dots or "ungrouped" dots, as they are commonly referred to. Rey directed patients to count the dots as quickly as possible by the fastest means possible. The other procedure involves both sets of dots, but the grouped dots are presented first, and a "shift of attitude" constituted a principal aspect of the administration. Lezak (1983) reported the procedure as either an ungrouped administration or one in which grouped dots were presented after the ungrouped dots. The combined presentation with no shift of attitude seems to have been the standard form of administration in research since then (Binks, Gouvier, & Waters, 1997; Frederick et al., 1994; Lee, Boone, et al., 2000; Paul, Franzen, Cohen, & Fremouw, 1992; Rose, Hall, & Szalda-Petree, 1998), but Frederick (1997) included instructions to not count out loud or by using one's fingers (to minimize counting strategies that would likely slow down the speed of counting).

Scoring

Frederick et al. (1994) used only a comparison of counting times for the grouped and ungrouped dots, identifying positive findings as any occurrence of ungrouped counting time faster than grouped counting time. Paul et al. (1992) and Lee et al. (2000) also scored the number of counting errors for ungrouped and grouped dots, and for all dots. Rose et al. (1998) and Binks et al. (1997) included counts of the number of deviations from linearity for ungrouped and grouped sets of dots. Frederick (1997) proposed a scoring method which transformed information about counting times and counting errors (total of absolute errors from correct number of dots per card) into a single score.

Interpretation

The DCT has not generally been found to be very sensitive to the presence of malingering. Frederick et al. (1994) found the presence of faster time to count ungrouped dots had only a 5% sensitivity among simulating malingerers. Rose et al. (1998) did not find any useful aspect of the DCT in the detection of malingering. Paul et al. (1992) generated a number of measures to discriminate successfully between simulators and controls, but they did not cross validate their cut-off scores. Binks et al. (1997) determined that the score which best discriminated between simulators and non-simulators was the total number of counting errors across all 12 cards, but no cut-off score was reported.

Rey's approach to the DCT, *performance curve analysis*, has been described by Rogers et al. (1993) and investigated by Frederick and Foster (1991), Frederick et al. (1994), Frederick (1997), Frederick and Crosby (2000), Frederick, Crosby, and Wykoop (2000), Gudjonsson and Shackleton (1986), and McKinzey, Podd, Krehbel, and Raven (1999). It is likely performance curve analysis has proven inadequate for DCT only because there are so few instances to compare. As a consequence, single arithmetic errors or recounting by the diligent patient significantly disrupt the linearity of the performance curve. Other tests which incorporate a performance curve analysis strategy, such as the Validity Indicator Profile (VIP; see Frederick, Crosby, & Wynkoop, 2000), generate the performance curve by smoothing a large number of data points (i.e., by "hanning"), so that single instances of error do not substantially alter the general shape of the performance curve.

REY WORD RECOGNITION TEST

The previous passage continues with a discussion of how the procedure of comparing easy and difficult tasks applies to the WRT:

> Let's go on to another example. It refers to a procedure which exploits the normal correlations between evocative memory and recognition memory. The easy test (A) will consist of recognizing words which are heard mixed with unknown words. We show the subject the five columns of words in the following table. We turn the page before he has been able to examine them one-by-one. We announce to him that we are going to read a certain number of words and that these words will be found in the columns shown previously, mixed with other unknown words. Instructions finished, the subject must take the paper and underline all the words that he remembers.
>
> Series of 30 words containing 15 words to recognize:

goodbye	tomorrow	tub	herb	lightning
half	toy	grain	boot	knee
gift	wool	pike	ash	hair
chamois	force	entrance	local	fly
morning	fashion	concert	filet	fault
airplane	shoe polish	biscuit	corridor	countryman

> Series of 15 words to read (one per second): *half, chamois, morning, toy, wool, shoe polish, grain, pike, herb, ash, local, corridor, knee, fault, countryman.*
>
> After the reading we introduce a pause of five seconds and then we present the page carrying the five columns. We allow two minutes for the subject to underline the words. If the result is poor and if there is reason otherwise to suspect or to distrust, we will proceed to test B which is more difficult. It is a good idea to introduce a pause of ten minutes between the two tests. Before starting test B, we will have emphasized the poor performance on A and required more conscientious effort on the new work.

Test B consists of recalling as many words as possible after one hearing of the series. Reading series is as follows: *drum, curtain, belt, coffee, school, relative, sun, garden, cap, countryman, mustache, turkey, color, house, stream.* We introduce a pause of five seconds after the last word is read. The free recall period lasts two minutes. The following is a table of the results:

Percentile:	100	75	50	25	0
Recall:					
Educated Adult Subjects (high school education)	14	10	8	7	5
Less Educated Subjects (elementary education)	10	7	6	4	2
Recognition:					
Educated	15	15	14	12	8
Less educated	14	12	10	7	5

If we examine these figures, we realize that in general more words are recognized than recalled whatever the intrinsic value of memory may be. Just suppose that the patient at the time of test A has not recognized more than three words which is a clearly pathological result, but he is able to recall four during test B, which is more difficult. Let's suppose that all question of incomprehension or technical error is eliminated, that there is no alexia and that there has not been any transient malaise or discomfort. If all of these conditions are fulfilled, we are in the presence either of an individual of a particular mnestic type which would be quite rare, or an individual who does not make an effort or who is trying to fool us. In the first case, the type must remain constant and we will reencounter it in repeating the test in an equivalent form and in pushing further the comparative study of mechanisms of recall and recognition. In the second case, retesting will not put in evidence any systematic difference; we shall be increasingly diffident, and very soon we will be able to attempt to put the subject in the presence of facts and figures. His reaction will then be quite interesting (Rey, 1941; pp. 316-318).

Instructions

Lezak (1983, 1995) and Greiffenstein et al. (1994) followed the instructional set in generally the same fashion as Rey; that is, the 15-word list is presented for memorization and then a 30-word list is presented on a sheet of paper. The patient circles the words which were presented for memorization. Frederick et al. (1994), Frederick (1997), Frederick (2000a), and Greiffenstein et al. (1996) modified the instructional set by eliminating the presentation of the sheet of words, instead presenting the 30-word recognition list orally, directing participants to quickly determine if each word had been on the 15-word memorization list (a two-alternative forced-choice technique; see Frederick, 1997, for a detailed description of accompanying instructions and practice items).

Scoring and Interpretation

Generally, scoring has proceeded in the same way as described by Rey: a comparison of total recognized words to total recalled words (on the first trial). Frederick et al. (1994) found this method was about 4% sensitive and about 97% specific (but Greiffenstein et al., 1996, reported a much higher sensitivity of 58%, with specificity of 88%). Greiffenstein et al. (1996) examined various methods of deriving a useful cut-off score; the preferred score is calculated by adding correct recognitions to correct rejections. This *accuracy score* demonstrated a sensitivity of 80% and specificity of 85% in discriminating between probable malingerers and patients with traumatic brain injury. Frederick (2000a) computed a *memory comparison score* which was derived by first totaling the number of correctly recognized words and then subtracting the number of incorrectly recognized words, and then by subtracting the number of correctly recalled words (out of 15) from the first trial of the AVLT. Frederick (2000a) reported that values greater than or equal to 0 were consistent with other evidence of compliance, and values less than 0 were strongly associated with other indications of malingering.

DAUBERT ISSUES

RMT. I agree with Vallabhajosula and van Gorp (2001) that the RMT does not enjoy general acceptance among neuropsychologists or forensic psychologists as a *primary detection strategy*. Published error rates for various cut-off scores for the RMT vary greatly, and probably reflect the limitations of research design (Frederick, 2000b). Although I do not believe the RMT meets *Daubert* criteria for acceptability as evidence as a primary detection strategy, I certainly see no problem with including the test as part of an overall strategy to evaluate the believability of performance in the way described by Rey.

DCT. I conclude the DCT does not meet *Daubert* criteria for acceptability as evidence regarding malingered cognitive impairment. It does not enjoy general acceptance as a procedure to investigate malingering, and it does not have a research literature supporting any of the potential scoring routines which have been investigated for it.

WRT. I do believe the process of evaluating memory disorders by comparing recall and recognition memory (e.g., by use of the WRT and AVLT) meets *Daubert* criteria. The processes described (by Frederick, 2000; Greiffenstein et al., 1994, 1996) in peer-reviewed journals consistently show good sensitivity and specificity (see also Haines & Norris, 2001, for differences among patient groups and different types of malingering groups). The problem with comparison of recognition and recall memory performances tends to be that the process is not sensitive to malingering, but accounting for false positive recognitions seems to raise the sensitivity substantially, with only a minimal decrement in specificity. The practice is logically coherent, and probably has enjoyed general acceptance as a strategy since Lezak's description of the process in 1983, if not earlier.

USING THE REY MALINGERING TESTS

Using the Tests for Research Purposes

I have used the Rey tests to conduct research on malingering detection for the past 10 years. I have constructed criterion groups based on Rey test performance (e.g., Frederick, 1997). Given that most of the clinical patients I have sampled to form criterion groups did not have severe neuropsychological impairment or mental retardation, it seemed likely that positive scores on two or three Rey malingering tests were predictive of malingering, given the generally high specificity of the tests. On the other hand, given the generally low estimates of sensitivity for the tests, it seemed likely that "negative" criterion groups (inclusion rule: "no positive scores" on the tests) would probably be significantly contaminated by malingerers who were not so obvious as to perform too badly on the Rey tests. A consequence of this is that the test or technique being validated will appear to have lower specificity than it actually does. I have discussed this problem at length in Frederick (2000b) and argued that the RMT probably has excellent discriminatory power in a forensic criminal setting in which there is a low base rate of significant neuropsychological impairment.

Currently, my preference is to use the Rey malingering tests as dependent variables. Not only does this forestall any criticism for using them to establish criterion groups, I have found they reliably demonstrate significant mean separations (e.g., Cohen's $d \geq 1.0$) for criterion groups that appear to be substantially different with respect to an intention to perform well on collaterally administered cognitive tests (Frederick, 2000b).

Using the Tests Clinically

I would encourage any forensic evaluator to routinely administer the RMT in the manner Rey described (i.e., after a 15-word recall task), but perhaps using a modified form of Lezak's instructional set, for example, as suggested by Frederick (1997). Just as an illustration, consider the data in Table 1. These data are from 686 criminal defendants who completed the AVLT, the RMT, and the VIP. I have previously described the sample from which they are taken in Frederick, Crosby, and Wynkoop (2000), and Frederick (2000a, 2000b). Classifications of Irrelevant and Malingering on the VIP reflect an intention to respond incor-

TABLE 1. Cross-Classification of Categorizations on the Validity Indicator Profile (VIP), the Rey 15-Item Memory Test (RMT), and the Rey Auditory Verbal Learning Test (AVLT)

			VIP Classification			
			Motivated to Perform Well		Motivated to Perform Poorly	
			Compliant	Careless	Irrelevant	Malingering
AVLT	RMT	*n*				
> 4 items	> 8 items	395	70.6%	24.9%	6.1%	0.5%
< 5 items	> 8 items	224	51.3%	38.8%	9.4%	0.4%
> 4 items	< 9 items	14	0.0%	50.0%	35.7%	14.3%
< 5 items	< 9 items	53	13.2%	28.3%	45.3%	13.2%

Note. $N = 686$. Participants are all criminal defendants. AVLT is the number of words recalled correctly on the first trial. RMT is the number of items reproduce. VIP classifications refer to its best classification of approach to testing without any additional contextual information. The classifications here refer to performance on the VIP nonverbal subtest only.

rectly. These data support Rey's view that the RMT might amplify the meaning of poor performance on the AVLT. It is easily observed that the rate at which defendants are classified as "motivated to perform poorly," is correlated with their joint performance on the 15-word recall list and the RMT. Most notably, when "weak" performances on the first trial of the word-recall task are followed by acceptable performances on the RMT, the rate at which defendants are classified as motivated to perform poorly is only 9.8% (and 51.3% are classified as Compliant), but when "weak" performances are followed by unacceptable performances on the RMT, the rate of classification as motivated to perform poorly is 58.5%.

In this light, I routinely tell others that I find the RMT to be one of the most useful malingering techniques available: it's free. You can generate your own copy wherever you are; you need just a pencil and two pieces of paper. It takes a minute to administer. It is scored instantaneously. A positive score is generally meaningful and should lead to further investigation of why the performance is so poor. What are the pitfalls? A negative score generally means little, because the task demand is low (Faust & Auckley, 1998), because the test may not have face validity (thus, easily discerned to be an artifice), and because minimal coaching allows successful completion for the malingerer (Frederick et al., 1994). Positive scores may reflect significant neuropsychological impairment (e.g., see Schretlen et al., 1991). As noted by Vallabhajosula and van Gorp (2001), a successful malingering test "should be sensitive to faking but insensitive to genuine memory disorders," and the RMT does not appear to have fulfilled these criteria. Consequently, the RMT remains a useful procedure to investigate suspicious presentations, but it does not appear to have the capacity to be used reliably as a sole detection strategy for malingered cognitive impairment.

On the other hand, the WRT, and especially the process of comparing recall to recognition memory, has been demonstrated to be especially effective at identifying malingered cognitive impairment (Frederick, 2000; Greiffenstein et al., 1994, 1996; Haines & Norris, 2001). These studies typically modified Rey's approach by considering misrecognition errors in comparisons of recall and recognition memory. The DCT has not been shown to be an especially effective method of investigating malingered cognitive impairment, although Rey's strategy, performance curve analysis, has proven especially effective (Frederick, Crosby, & Wynkoop, 2000). It is likely the DCT could be improved with additional trials; six trials may be insufficient for reliable measurement of intention.

The caveats for the use of any procedure to evaluate malingered cognitive impairment are best summed up in the clinical wisdom of Rey:

> We see how it is possible to suspect the exaggeration and the simulation by using appropriately a battery of tests. It is sufficient to know the degree of intrinsic difficulty of each test well. However, the tests must be numerous in order to accumulate the suspicious signs: We will not be able to arrive at a conclusion on a single sign. Besides, it is always necessary to attribute these signs to the particular problem of the individual, to the traits of his personality, and to establish clearly what interests he may have in simulating disorders of a psychological nature. (Rey, 1958; p. 123)

NOTE

Mme. Rey described to me many elaborate procedures Rey used for the assessment of feigning which have not been reported in American neuropsychological literature. Each essentially comprises a series of tasks which seem difficult but are not. Rey apparently plotted performance curves to demonstrate inconsistencies between performance accuracy and true difficulty levels.

REFERENCES

Arnett, P. A., & Franzen, M. D. (1997). Performance of substance abusers with memory deficits on measures of malingering. *Archives of Clinical Neuropsychology, 12*, 513-518.

Arnett, P. A., Hammeke, T. A., & Schwartz, L. (1995). Quantitative and qualitative performance on Rey's 15-Item Test in neurological patients and dissimulators. *The Clinical Neuropsychologist, 9*, 17-26.

Association des amis d'André Rey (1967). *Hommage a André Rey*. Brussells: Dessart.

Back, C., Boone, K. B., Edwards, C., Parks, C., Burgoyne, K., & Silver, B. (1996). The performance of schizophrenics on three cognitive tests of malingering, Rey 15-Item Memory Test, Rey Dot Counting, and Hiscock Forced-Choice Method. *Assessment, 3*, 449-457.

Bernard, L. C., Houston, W., & Natoli, L. (1993). Malingering on neuropsychological memory tests: Potential objective indicators. *Journal of Clinical Psychology, 49*, 45-53.

Bernard, L. C., & Fowler, W. (1990). Assessing the validity of memory complaints: Performance on brain-damaged and normal individuals on Rey's task to detect malingering. *Journal of Clinical Psychology, 49*, 432-436.

Binks, P. G., Gouvier, W. D., & Waters, W. F. (1997). Malingering detection with the Dot Counting Test. *Archives of Clinical Neuropsychology, 12*, 41-46.

DiCarlo, M. A., Gfeller, J. D., & Drury, J. A. (1996, October). Assessing feigned cognitive impairment with Rey's 15-Item Memory Test: Is this task easy or what? Poster presented at the Annual Meeting of the National Academy of Neuropsychology, New Orleans, LA.

Faust, D., & Auckley, M. A. (1998). Did you think it was going to be easy? Some methodological suggestions for the investigation and development of malingering detection techniques. In C. R. Reynolds (Ed.). *Detection of Malingering During Head Injury Litigation* (pp. 1-54). New York: Plenum.

Frederick, R. I. (1997). *Validity Indicator Profile.* Minnetonka, MN: NCS Assessments, Inc.

Frederick, R. I. (2000a). A personal floor effect strategy to evaluate the validity of performance on memory tests. *Journal of Clinical and Experimental Neuropsychology, 22*, 720-730.

Frederick, R. I. (2000b). Mixed group validation: A method to address the limitations of criterion group validation in research on malingering detection. *Behavioral Sciences and the Law, 18*, 693-718.

Frederick, R. I., Crosby, R., & Wynkoop, T. F. (2000). Performance curve classification of invalid responding on the Validity Indicator Profile. *Archives of Clinical Neuropsychology, 15*, 281-300.

Frederick, R. I., Sarfaty, S.D., Johnston, J.D., & Powel, J. (1994). Validation of a detector of response bias on a forced-choice test of nonverbal ability. *Neuropsychology, 8*, 118-125.

Goldberg, J. O., & Miller, H. R. (1986). Performance of psychiatric inpatients and intellectually deficient individuals on a task that assesses the validity of memory complaints. *Journal of Clinical Psychology, 42*, 792-795.

Greiffenstein, M. F., Baker, W. J., & Gola, T. (1994). Validation of malingered amnesia measures in a large clinical sample. *Psychological Assessment, 6*, 218-224.

Greiffenstein, M. F., Baker, W. J., & Gola, T. (1996). Comparison of multiple scoring methods for Rey's malingered amnesia measures. *Archives of Clinical Neuropsychology, 11*, 283-293.

Griffin, G. A. E., Glassmire, D. M., Henderson, E. A., & McCann, C. (1997). Rey II: Redesigning the Rey Screening Test of Malingering. *Journal of Clinical Psychology, 53*, 757-766.

Griffin, G. A. E., Normington, J., & Glassmire, D. (1996). Qualitative dimensions in scoring the Rey Visual Memory Test of Malingering. *Psychological Assessment, 4*, 383-387.

Gudjonsson, G. H., & Shackleton, H. (1986). The pattern of scores on Raven's Matrices during "faking bad" and "non-faking" performance. *British Journal of Clinical Psychology, 25*, 35-41.

Guilmette, T. J., Hart, K. J., Giuliano, A. J., & Leininger, B. E. (1994). Detecting simulated memory impairment: Comparison of the Rey Fifteen-Item Test and the Hiscock Forced-Choice Procedure. *The Clinical Neuropsychologist, 8*, 283-294.

Haines, M. E., & Norris, M. P. (2001). Comparing student and patient simulated malingerers' performance on standard neuropsychological measures to detect feigned cognitive deficits. *The Clinical Neuropsychologist, 15*, 171-182.

Hays, J. R., Emmons, J., & Lawson, K. A. (1993). Psychiatric norms for the Rey 15-Item Visual Memory Test. *Perceptual and Motor Skills, 76*, 1331-1334.

Iverson, G. L., & Franzen, M. D. (1996). Using multiple objective memory procedures to detect simulated malingering. *Journal of Clinical and Experimental Neuropsychology, 18*, 38-51.

Kaschel, R., Goldenberg, G., Goldstein, L. H., Risberg, J., Laaksonen, R., Gaillard, F., Perret, E., Tissot, R., & Oktem-Tanor, O. (1994). *Neuropsychology in Europe: A partial account of history and perspectives.* Paris: Approche Neuropsychologique des Apprentissages Chez L'Enfant.

Lambercier, M., & Rey, A. (1935). Contribution a l'etude de l'intelligence pratique chez l'enfant [Contribution to the study of practical intelligence in children]. *Archives de Psychologie, 25*, 1-59.

Lee, A., Boone, K. B., Lesser, I., Wohl, M., Wilkins, S., & Parks, C. (2000). Performance of older depressed patients on two cognitive malingering tests: False positive rates for the Rey 15-Item Memorization and Dot Counting Tests. *The Clinical Neuropsychologist, 14*, 303-308.

Lee, G. P., Loring, D. W., & Martin, R. C. (1992). Rey's 15-Item Visual Memory Test for the detection of malingering: Normative observations on patients with neurological disorders. *Psychological Assessment, 4*, 43-46.

Lezak, M. D. (1983). *Neuropsychological assessment.* (2d ed.). New York: Oxford.

Lezak, M. D. (1995). *Neuropsychological assessment.* (3d ed.). New York: Oxford.

McKinzey, R. K., Podd, M. H., Krehbel, M. A., & Raven, J. (1999). Detection of malingering on Raven's Standard Progressive Matrices: A cross-validation. *British Journal of Clinical Psychology, 38*, 435-439.

Paul, D., Franzen, M. D., Cohen, S. H., & Fremouw, W. (1992). An investigation into the reliability and validity of two tests used in the detection of dissimulation. *International Journal of Clinical Neuropsychology, 14*, 1-9.

Rey, A. (1928). French philosophy in 1926 and 1927. *Philosophical Review, 37*, 527-556.

Rey, A. (1938). Le destruction progressive du cortex cérébral chez le rat et ses effets immédiats [The progressive destruction of the cerebral cortex in the rat and its immediate effects]. *Archives de Psychologie, 27*, 1-88.

Rey, A. (1941). L'examen psychologique dans les cas d'encéphalopathie traumatique [The psychological examination in cases of traumatic encephalopathy]. *Archives de Psychologie, 28*, 286-340.

Rey, A. (1946). Epreuves de dessin: témoins du développement mental [Drawing tests as evidence of mental development]. *Archives de Psychologie, 31*, 369-380.

Rey, A. (1957). *Enfants Juifs Nord-Africains: Essai psycho-pédagogique a l'intention des educateurs* [*North-African Jewish children: Psycho-pedagogic essay for the use of educators*]. Tel-Aviv: Departement pour l'Aliyah des Jeunes de l'Agence Juive.

Rey, A. (1958). *L'examen clinique en psychologie* [*The psychological examination*]. Paris: Presses Universitaires de France.

Rogers, R., Harrell, E. H., & Liff, C. D. (1993). Feigning neuropsychological impairment: A critical review of methodological and clinical considerations. *Clinical Psychology Review, 13*, 255-274.

Rose, F. E., Hall, S., & Szalda-Petree, A. D. (1998). A comparison of four tests of malingering and the effects of coaching. *Archives of Clinical Neuropsychology, 13*, 349-363.

Schretlen, D., Brandt, J., Krafft, L., & van Gorp, W. (1991). Some caveats in using the Rey 15-Item Memory Test to detect malingered amnesia. *Psychological Assessment, 3*, 667-672.

Simon, M. J. (1994). The use of the Rey Memory Test to assess malingering in criminal defendants. *Journal of Clinical Psychology, 50*, 667-672.

Taylor, E. M. (1959). *The appraisal of children with cerebral deficits*. Cambridge, MA: Harvard University Press.

Vallabhajosula, B., & van Gorp, W. G. (2001). Post-*Daubert* admissibility of scientific evidence on malingering of cognitive deficits. *Journal of American Academy of Psychiatry and Law, 29*, 207-215.

Wintsch, J. (1935). A propos d'une etude sur l'intelligence pratique chez l'enfant [A study of practical intelligence in children]. *Zeitschrift fuer Kinderpsychiatrie, 2*, 146-149.

The Portland Digit Recognition Test: A Review of Validation Data and Clinical Use

Laurence M. Binder

Independent Practice

SUMMARY. The Portland Digit Recognition Test (PDRT) is a valid measure of motivation to perform poorly on memory tests that is useful in forensic evaluations. Validation data and clinical use are described. The PDRT meets standards of the *Daubert* decision for the admissibility of scientific data into the courtroom by expert witnesses. The PDRT has been tested in scientific studies, results of scientific studies have appeared in peer-reviewed journals, the error rate is known, and it is well accepted in the scientific community according to published articles. A survey showed that 27% of forensic neuropsychologists reported using the PDRT consistently (Essig, Mittenberg, Petersen et al., 2001). Cutoff scores are available with 100 percent specificity, and these cutoff scores have moderate sensitivity for detection of poor motivation. The strongest psychometric evidence of faking a memory deficit occurs when a forced choice test result is significantly worse than chance. Data indicate that worse than chance results occur regularly on the PDRT. *[Article copies available for a fee from The Haworth Document Delivery Service: 1-800-HAWORTH. E-mail address: <getinfo@haworthpressinc.com> Website: <http://www.HaworthPress.com> © 2002 by The Haworth Press, Inc. All rights reserved.]*

Laurence M. Binder is in independent practice, Beaverton, OR.

Address correspondence to: Laurence M. Binder, 4900 SW Griffith Drive, Suite 244, Beaverton, OR 97005 (E-mail: Larry_binder@email.msn.com).

[Haworth co-indexing entry note]: "The Portland Digit Recognition Test: A Review of Validation Data and Clinical Use." Binder, Laurence M. Co-published simultaneously in *Journal of Forensic Neuropsychology* (The Haworth Medical Press, an imprint of The Haworth Press, Inc.) Vol. 2, No. 3/4, 2002, pp. 27-41; and: *Detection of Response Bias in Forensic Neuropsychology* (ed: Jim Hom, and Robert L. Denney) The Haworth Medical Press, an imprint of The Haworth Press, Inc., 2002, pp. 27-41. Single or multiple copies of this article are available for a fee from The Haworth Document Delivery Service [1-800-HAWORTH, 9:00 a.m. - 5:00 p.m. (EST). E-mail address: getinfo@haworthpressinc.com].

© 2002 by The Haworth Press, Inc. All rights reserved.

KEYWORDS. Malingering, brain injuries

Forced-choice testing, also known as symptom validity testing, was first used for the evaluation of functional vision loss (Brady & Lind, 1961). Later, it was suggested as a method for the assessment of exaggeration of neuropsychological disabilities (Pankratz, 1979; 1983). The first case study documenting motivation to exaggerate impairment with a forced-choice measure of memory employed a recognition memory task with presentations of a pen or a pencil (Binder & Pankratz, 1987). The first digit recognition task employed increasing levels of difficulty as the test progressed, an important innovation (Hiscock & Hiscock, 1989). The Portland Digit Recognition Test (PDRT) was a modification of the Hiscock procedure (Binder, 1990; Binder & Willis, 1991).

DESCRIPTION

The test will be described here only in general in an effort to protect its security. The 72 *recognition* memory items of the PDRT include 36 items classified as easy with shorter delays and 36 items classified as hard with longer delays. Examinees must perform an interpolated task between presentation of the item to be remembered and presentation of the recognition probe. The PDRT is administered by an examiner. An experimental, unpublished, computerized version (Rose, Hall, Szalda-Petree et al., 1998) and shorter versions (Greiffenstein, Baker, & Gola, 1994) also exist. These alternative versions are not the same test, and the limited available data on their validity will not be discussed in any detail.

The entire test requires 40 minutes for a typical, reasonably efficient examinee. Some examinees take longer. The length of the test is justifiable for an examinee who is exaggerating impairment, but it is too long for the majority of examinees who were passing the test. Therefore, an abbreviated form has been developed that reduces administration time to about 20 minutes for those examinees who are performing well (Binder, 1993b).

RELIABILITY AND VALIDITY STUDIES

The PDRT has split-half reliability of .92 on nonpatient controls and .82 on patients with brain dysfunction (Binder & Willis, 1991). The standard error of measurement for the 30-second items is 1.35.

Like any forced-choice test, a result from the PDRT can be statistically evaluated with the z approximation of the binomial theorem. Performance significantly worse than chance indicates that the examinee deliberately provided wrong answers.

The initial validation study (Binder & Willis, 1991) compared six groups of adults: nonpatient simulators, nonpatient controls, patients with affective disorders not seeking compensation, patients with brain dysfunction not seeking compensation, patients with well-documented brain dysfunction seeking financial compensation, and mild head trauma patients seeking compensation. Three of the six groups had no inducement to perform poorly, two of the groups had real-life incentives in the form of personal injury and workers compensation claims, and the simulators were asked to pretend that they were faking brain injury. This study did not include a clinical group of patients diagnosed as malingerers. The mild head trauma group was an unselected, consecutive series of referrals to my independent practice who frequently showed no evidence of poor motivation on testing. The four groups of patients were equated on age, education, and gender distribution. The majority of the brain dysfunction not seeking compensation group had suffered moderate or severe traumatic brain injury (TBI) or medically intractable epilepsy verified by intensive EEG monitoring. This group of patients with brain dysfunction provided the most relevant comparison data for an individual examinee seeking financial compensation, because the members of the group were both motivationally normal in a financial sense and also genuinely cognitively impaired.

The data showed that the brain dysfunction not seeking compensation group was significantly superior to all three compensation-seeking groups in total PDRT score. The patients with affective disorders who were not seeking compensation did not differ from the patients with brain dysfunction not seeking compensation, but they were superior to the mild head trauma patients seeking compensation. The nonpatient simulators performed significantly worse than any other group, and the normal controls performed significantly better than all other groups. In summary, the data indicated that PDRT scores were related to the presence of real or pretended financial incentives.

Validation efforts were extended with a comparison of a mild head trauma group with financial incentives, a brain dysfunction group with financial incentives, and a brain dysfunction group without financial incentives (Binder, 1993a). About half of the subjects had been included in the previous validation study (Binder & Willis, 1991). In the second study, the three groups were equated on verbal learning ability as measured by the Rey Auditory-Verbal Learning Test (RAVLT), as well as on gender, age, and education. Despite the groups being equated on RAVLT scores, the mild head trauma patients performed significantly worse on the PDRT than the other two groups, and the group with brain dysfunction who had no financial incentives performed significantly better than the other two groups. The group with brain dysfunction and financial incentives was significantly superior to the mild head trauma group. This study provided additional evidence that the PDRT measured motivation.

The initial validation data led to cutoff scores that were replicated when the brain dysfunction without financial incentive group was first extended and then replicated again when this group was extended to 120 patients (Binder & Kelly, 1996). No patient in the brain dysfunction without financial incentives group scored worse than 19 out of 36 correct on the easy items, 18 out of 36 correct on the hard items, or 39 out of 72 correct on the total score. These cutoff scores increased the sensitivity of the test; examinees who performed below the cutoff scores failed the test even if they did not perform significantly worse than chance. In an unselected, consecutive series of mild head trauma patients seeking compensation (Binder, 1993a), 33% performed below the cutoff scores on either the easy, hard, or total scores. Significantly below chance performance on either the easy, hard, or total scores was found in 17% of this group.

PDRT performance was related to performance on other neuropsychological measures. The PDRT was related to WAIS-R Full Scale IQ in patients with traumatic brain injury, $r = .49$, $p < .001$, and in patients with intractable epilepsy, $r = .55$, $p < .02$. PDRT scores were directly related to total score on the five learning trials of the RAVLT, $r = .39$, $p < .01$ (Binder, 1993a). Low IQ patients were included in the sample, and patients with IQs under 80 averaged 57.4 correct out of a total possible score of 72, or 80% (Binder & Kelly, 1996).

In summary, notwithstanding the association between PDRT scores and neuropsychological performance, the data indicate that the PDRT measures motivation to perform poorly rather than a cognitive ability. PDRT performance was more strongly associated with the presence of financial incentives than the presence of brain dysfunction. After equating for RAVLT scores, persons with well documented brain dysfunction performed better than persons with financial incentives who had a history of mild head trauma. Persons with brain dysfunction and financial incentives performed better than the group with a history of mild head trauma and financial incentives. Patients with a history of TBI and IQ scores under 80 did not fail the PDRT.

Performance on the PDRT in relation to demographic variables has also been studied (Binder & Kelly, 1996; Binder & Willis, 1991). African-Americans and Caucasians did not differ significantly after TBI (Binder & Kelly, 1996). Neither age nor gender was significantly related to PDRT scores, but education had a modest, significant relationship, $r = .25$, $p < .01$.

SENSITIVITY

Sensitivity refers to the proportion of examinees with the condition of interest that are identified correctly by the test. In the case of the PDRT, sensitivity refers to the proportion of malingering patients who are correctly identified. Data indicating that a third of a consecutive clinical series of mild head trauma patients fell below the PDRT cutoff scores (Binder, 1993a) do not directly assess the sensitivity of the test; an unknown proportion of the patients with mild head trauma probably were well motivated. However, it can be assumed from these data that the sensitivity of the PDRT in clinical settings is greater than 33%. In another clinical series of patients assigned to a poor motivation group on the basis of external evidence of malingering, the PDRT total score cutoff of below 39 correct identified 20 of 26 examinees or 77% (Bianchini, Mathias, Greve et al., in press). In a meta-analytic review, it was reported that among normal simulators 39% performed below the established PDRT cutoff scores (Vickery, Berry, Inman et al., 2001). These reviewers aggregated sensitivity data from a 27-item version of the PDRT (Greiffenstein et al., 1994) and from the computerized version (Rose et al., 1998) with data from the regular PDRT.

Data from experimental simulators also provides information on sensitivity. Patients with traumatic brain injuries (TBI) and control participants were asked to simulate deficits on the PDRT in another study (Ju & Varney, 2000). These investigators analyzed a total score cutoff of below 31 correct demonstrating performance significantly worse than chance, and they reported that 23% of their simulators fell in this range. In the same series approximately 56% performed worse than the total score cutoff of 39 correct, according to data provided in a table. In another investigation of nonpatient simulators, the total score cutoff correctly detected 39%, almost half of who had been warned that the test battery would include measures to detect incomplete effort (Gunstad & Suhr, 2001).

It is clear from these studies that the PDRT will fail to identify some examinees who are motivationally impaired using the original cutoff scores. Its sensitivity ranged from 39% with nonpatient simulators to 56% with TBI patients instructed to simulate to 77% with patients with external evidence of malingering. Sensitivity rates might have been slightly higher had these investigators used cutoffs on the easy, hard, and total scores in combination. Sensitivity rate clearly is sample dependent, considering the differences between the clinical series (Bianchini et al., in press) and the simulation studies reported here. It is not surprising that student simulator studies will show lower rates of sensitivity than clinical malingerers (Haines & Norris, 2001), although the explanation for this phenomenon is unclear.

Sensitivity can be increased at the expense of specificity. The studies summarized above utilized cutoff scores that were 100% specific; no person with brain dysfunction who lacked financial incentives performed below these cutoffs. In order to increase the sensitivity of the test, we first reported all scores from our group of 120 patients with brain dysfunction without financial incentives, and then recommended consideration of higher cutoff scores (Binder & Kelly, 1996). For example, total scores below 46 occurred in only five cases (4%). Scores below 44 occurred in only two cases (2%). We recommended that clinicians consider use of these higher cutoff scores (Binder & Kelly, 1996). A paper now is in preparation examining the accuracy of the PDRT when cutoff scores with specificity below 100% are used.

Shorter versions of the PDRT that have been used by some clinicians will not be as sensitive as the full 72 item version. Some clinicians choose to administer only the 36 easy items, but this procedure is unwise, because sensitivity of the PDRT is greater on the hard than on the easy items (Binder, 1993a). More frequent performances below the cutoffs and more frequent significantly below chance performances occurred in the hard than in the easy items in this study. Versions with fewer items also are problematic, because they are less likely to yield results that are significantly worse than chance. For example, a score of 30 of 72 correct is significant at the .10 level, but a proportionately equal score of 15 of 36 correct is significant at the .21 level.

SPECIFICITY

Specificity refers to the proportion of examinees that do not have the condition of interest who are correctly classified. In the case of the

PDRT, specificity refers to the accuracy of the test among examinees who are not malingerers. The original cutoff scores are 100% specific. As noted above, the original sample of patients with brain dysfunction without financial incentives (Binder & Willis, 1991) yielded cutoff scores that were replicated on two occasions when the sample was extended (Binder, 1993; Binder & Kelly, 1996). This group included a majority of patients with well-documented moderate to severe TBIs, and most of the remainder had medically intractable epilepsy documented by intensive EEG monitoring. The remainder had a variety of other neurologic conditions. The original cutoff scores were 100% specific each time the sample size was extended.

ADDITIONAL LITERATURE

The PDRT has been endorsed by other authors as a valid test instrument for the assessment of motivation to perform poorly. It was judged to be one of the two best forced-choice tests in one review (Etcoff & Kampfer, 1996). Another review described the test as a "valid" measure of motivation to perform poorly (Golden & Grief, 1998, p. 137). The PDRT was used as one of the clinical measures in a validation study of a forerunner of the Validity Indicator Profile (Frederick, Sarfaty, Johnston et al., 1994). The PDRT was used to document motivational impairment in a series of case studies of women suing for damages associated with alleged silicone breast implant illness (Youngjohn, Spector, & Mapou, 1997). In a review that considered all versions of the PDRT, including a 27-item version and a computerized version, the authors concluded that the PDRT demonstrated moderate sensitivity and high specificity (Vickery et al., 2001).

Lezak (1995) criticized the test in her non-peer reviewed textbook. In her opinion, the interpolated task requirement of the PDRT made it similar to the Consonant Trigram Test, a test known to be sensitive to traumatic brain injury. When making this criticism, Lezak failed to refer to any data correlating performance on the PDRT and Consonant Trigram Test. She also failed to acknowledge that the PDRT is a measure of recognition memory and the Consonant Trigram Test is a measure of recall and that the difficulty level of recall measures typically exceeds the difficulty level of recognition memory tasks. Lezak's criticism should be regarded as a hypothesis contradicted by the available data showing that the PDRT was not sensitive to brain injury in the absence of external incentives for poor performance. Binder and Kelly (1996) addressed

Lezak's criticism by showing that patients with brain dysfunction performed well on the PDRT in the absence of financial incentives. People with moderate and severe brain injuries, medically intractable epilepsy, and other neurological conditions always performed above the cutoff. Based on these data, Binder and Kelly (1996) argued that scores below the cutoff cannot be explained by brain dysfunction after mild head injury.

The PDRT is one of many forced-choice, digit recognition tests. This family of tests has been reviewed favorably (Etcoff & Kampfer, 1996; Sweet, 2000).

THE PDRT AND DAUBERT

The admissibility of scientific evidence using the *Daubert* criteria hinges on several questions which will be discussed in turn. There is no fixed method set by law or judicial precedent for use of the *Daubert* criteria. The trial judge has the right to decide what testimony to exclude, based on her or his evaluation of the credibility of the testimony in relation to these criteria.

Has the PDRT Been Tested? Has the PDRT Been Subjected to Peer Review in Publication?

In this paper, I have reviewed several studies validating the PDRT in its original format using both clinical groups and experimental simulators (Binder, 1993; Binder & Kelly, 1996; Binder & Willis, 1991; Gunstad & Suhr, 2001; Ju & Varney, 2000; Vickery et al., 2001). Studies reviewed above clearly show that the PDRT has undergone scientific scrutiny through validity studies.

Validation and case studies have been published in various well-regarded peer reviewed neuropsychological journals. A series of case studies with the initial test description first appeared in *The Clinical Neuropsychologist* (Binder, 1990) and other cases also were described in the *Archives of Clinical Neuropsychology* (Binder, 1992a) and again in *The Clinical Neuropsychologist* (Youngjohn et al., 1997). The initial validation data were published in *Psychological Assessment* (Binder & Willis, 1991). An extension of the validation data appeared in the *Journal of Clinical and Experimental Neuropsychology* (Binder, 1993a). Other validation data and details on performance by the sample of 120 patients with brain dysfunction who had no financial incentives were published in *Assessment* (Binder & Kelly, 1996). The PDRT was used to select poorly motivated patients in a validation study of another measure of motivation published in *Neuropsychology* (Frederick et al., 1994). The test was favorably reviewed in *Neuropsychology Review* where Etcoff and Kampfer (1996) concluded that it was one of the two best-validated forced choice measures of motivation. Other studies in *The Clinical Neuropsychologist* examined performance by simulators (Gunstad & Suhr, 2001) and anecdotally described performance by silicone breast implant litigants (Youngjohn et al., 1997). In the *Archives of Clinical Neuropsychology*, a meta-analytic review of studies concluded that the PDRT had moderate sensitivity and high specificity (Vickery et al., 2001). Unfortunately, this meta-analysis lumped together data from the regular version of the test with shorter versions and a computerized version.

What Is the Known or Potential Rate of Error in the Use of the PDRT?

A neuropsychologist who relies on the PDRT to establish that an examinee was well motivated might be attacked during cross examination because the test possesses only moderate sensitivity. Clearly, the neuropsychologist should rely on multiple test observations and historical data before ruling out poor motivation as an explanation for test abnormalities. A test with moderate sensitivity will generate some false negative errors. The PDRT will fail to detect some cases of motivational impairment.

The high specificity of the PDRT is its strength. If the original cutoff scores with 100% specificity are used, then it is reasonable to conclude that all PDRT scores below the cutoffs result from motivational failure. The clinician can be confident in concluding that a patient provided incomplete effort on the PDRT itself whenever the easy, hard, or total score falls below the cutoff. Clinical judgment is required to determine if failure on the PDRT or any other motivational test is the product of malingering. The diagnosis of malingering should be made only after consideration of all available data.

If the PDRT result is significantly worse than chance, the interpretation clearly is unambiguous. Authorities agree that performance on a forced-choice test that is significantly worse than chance indicates that the patient *deliberately* provided wrong answers. In previous work, we used a probability level of $p < .10$ for evaluating significance of a result from an individual through the z approximation of the binomial theorem. Reynolds (1998) argued that the probability level of .05 was too conservative in evaluating the significance of a below chance result, and he suggested that *p* levels of .10 or .15 were more appropriate.

Interpretation of scores with less than 100% specificity for poor effort clearly requires more caution. In such cases, there should be evidence of poor cooperation from other sources before concluding that such an examinee is malingering. As an additional caveat, infrequently there are patients with frank brain injury and financial incentives who fake bad on the PDRT (Binder, 1993a). In these cases, the clinician should conclude that the examination was invalid, and conclusions regarding cognitive abilities should not be drawn from invalid data.

Data reviewed above in the sections on sensitivity and specificity provide the best estimates of error rate. If the original cutoff scores are utilized, the false positive error rates approach zero. In a sample preselected for suspicion of malingering, the false negative error rate, based only on the total score cutoff, is about 23% (Bianchini et al., in press).

To What Extent Has the PDRT Received General Acceptance?

The PDRT has been accepted in the scientific literature and by clinicians for use in their practice. The literature reviewed here indicates that the PDRT has scientific acceptance. More broadly, it is clear that forced choice tests such as the PDRT are useful for the assessment of motivation to perform poorly (Sweet, 2000). There is no dispute in the literature regarding the interpretation of significantly worse than chance performance, and little dispute regarding the interpretation of scores below the cutoffs. Neuropsychologists have reviewed the PDRT favorably (Etcoff & Kampher, 1995; Golden & Grief, 1998).

Test usage and sales are indexes of clinical acceptance. I have sold over 400 copies of the test to practitioners in all 50 states of the United States, several Canadian provinces, and a few other foreign countries. In addition, an unknown number of clinicians are using unauthorized copies of the test. As of December 2001, when this paper was under revision, I was continuing to sell copies of the test. A survey of forensic neuropsychologists reported that 27% typically used the PDRT, an impressive figure (Essig, Mittenberg, Petersen et al., 2001).

Legal testimony by neuropsychologists on PDRT results has been allowed by judges consistently for many years in many jurisdictions. Anecdotal evidence indicates that lawyers have not entered successful objections to such testimony based on *Daubert* or earlier standards for admissibility.

CLINICAL USE OF THE PDRT

The following clinical anecdote is useful because it includes the written opinion of the trier of fact, an attorney-arbitrator. I testified in a personal injury lawsuit that the plaintiff, who had suffered a whiplash injury in a motor vehicle accident, was malingering. My conclusion was based on many data, including the minor nature of the insult to the plaintiff's head, late onset of stuttering two months after the injury, extremely poor test performances including IQ scores below 70 in multiple examinations with two examiners, and failure on multiple measures of motivation including the PDRT.

This lawsuit was tried before a single arbitrator. In his written opinion, the arbitrator referred to the examinee's total score of 32 out of 72 on the PDRT, stating, "It is obvious that someone should get at least half of the answers right . . . Random chance should not result in a score of 32." The arbitrator also reasoned that if the examinee was correct on only 12 of 72 items and guessed at the other 60, then he would have received a score of about 42 correct. The arbitrator rejected the claim of permanent traumatic brain injury, relying in part on the PDRT. Apparently, he found the PDRT more persuasive than other measures of motivation; in his opinion he did not refer to other measures that also were failed.

The most persuasive result on any measure of motivation to perform poorly occurs when a forced choice test yields a score significantly below chance, a result indicating that the examinee deliberately provided wrong answers. Clinicians are more confident when stating that an examinee faked bad, was grossly uncooperative, or malingered if a forced choice test score is significantly below chance. Clinicians rated their confidence level in diagnosing malingering much higher when this test result occurred (Trueblood & Binder, 1997). Case reports of malingering with failure on the PDRT have been published (Binder, 1990; Binder, 1992a,b; Youngjohn et al., 1997).

It seems unlikely that any other currently available test will yield results significantly below chance as frequently in clinical practice as the PDRT. The reader can inspect the other papers in this volume to learn if the frequencies of significantly below chance performance are reported for other measures. PDRT scores frequently are significantly below chance in patients with financial incentives. Seventeen percent of a sample of 103 mild head trauma patients with financial incentives performed significantly worse than chance on at least one section of the PDRT compared with 33% who performed below the cutoff scores

(Binder, 1993a). Twenty-three percent of a group of experimental simulators obtained a total score significantly below chance (Ju & Varney, 2000). Mean PDRT scores by well-motivated patients with brain dysfunction are 80-83% correct (Binder, 1993; Binder & Kelly, 1996). Mean correct for well-motivated patients on other forced-choice tests is over 95% (Guilmette, Hart, & Giulianao, 1993; Inman, Vickery, Berry et al., 1998; Prigatano & Amin, 1993). Hence, errors are several times more common on the PDRT than on the easier forced choice tests. Examinees who wish to malinger without being detected may view other forced choice tests as too easy to perform in worse than chance fashion.

The length of the PDRT and the fact that half of the 36 items include the longest delay interval of 30 seconds contributes to its sensitivity. Examinees are more likely to perform worse than chance or score below cutoffs on the long delay items than the short delay items (Binder, 1993a). As shown above, more items lead to stronger levels of significance when examinees perform worse than chance. Application of the binomial theorem for significance testing can be made to the whole test, the last 54 items with the 18 second and 30 second delays, or the last 36 items with the 30 second delays.

The PDRT is most useful when it is not abbreviated except when performance is good (Binder, 1993b). For example, the PDRT-27 (Greiffenstein et al., 1994) possesses less empirical support than the complete PDRT, and with only 27 items, it is much less likely to yield results that are significantly worse than chance than the PDRT. An idiosyncratic selection of PDRT items is a new test altogether. It is not the PDRT. Unless the author's method of abbreviating the PDRT for examinees with good performance is used (Binder, 1993b), a task utilizing a subset of PDRT items should not be labeled as the PDRT.

It is possible that some malingerers will pass the PDRT and fail another, forced choice test that is easier for well-motivated patients. The easier forced choice tests, for example, the Hiscock Forced Choice Procedure (HFCP; Hiscock & Hiscock, 1989), have higher cutoff scores. A malingerer concerned about avoiding detection might decide that he/she needed to score well above 50% correct on any forced choice test. A score of, for example, 75% correct would pass the PDRT and fail the HFCP. Hypothetically, there is no reason why the same malingerer could not obtain the same score on both tests.

Cautions for interpretation have been discussed in the PDRT manual (Binder, 1993c). The PDRT has not been validated in some populations, including persons with developmental mental retardation and children.

Cutoff scores should be applied with caution in these populations although dramatic intellectual loss (WAIS-R IQ below 80) associated with TBI is not associated with performance below the PDRT cutoffs (Binder & Kelly, 1996).

Performance below the cutoff scores calls into question the validity of the remainder of the neuropsychological examination. A review of additional clinical, historical, and other psychometric data is necessary in order to determine if a diagnosis of malingering is appropriate. If the clinician determines that the examinee was not well motivated in the testing, then the examination is invalid. The possibility of cerebral dysfunction remains, although it may be unlikely in many cases. Qualified clinicians may be able to estimate the probability of cerebral dysfunction despite an invalid examination based on clinical data regarding the severity of head injury.

The major problem with all measures of motivation to perform poorly, including the PDRT, is their moderate sensitivity. Sensitivity can be improved through the use of multiple measures of effort (Orey, Cragar, & Berry, 2000). Anecdotal observations indicate that multiple measures of effort are useful, because one measure may be passed while another measure is failed. Sensitivity can be improved on a single test only at the expense of specificity, and so this step should be undertaken with cautious regard for potential rates of error.

Clearly, the clinician should use a series of the best measures available. Many clinicians appear to rely on grossly insensitive measures such as the standard recall version of Rey's Fifteen Item Test (Frederick et al., 1994; Millis & Kler, 1995) or their own clinical judgment of level of cooperation, often while ignoring historical evidence suggestive of the possibility of malingering. There are no published data showing that a clinician can determine through qualitative observations that poor motivation can be ruled out. Relying on insensitive measures of motivation is as bad as not using any measures of motivation and is tantamount to burying one's head in the sand. The PDRT is one of several well-validated measures of motivation described in this volume.

REFERENCES

Bianchini, K.J., Mathias, C.W., Greve, K.W., Houston, R.J., & Crouch, J.A. (in press). Classification accuracy of the Portland Digit Recognition Test in traumatic brain injury. *The Clinical Neuropsychologist*.

Binder, L.M. (1990). Malingering following minor head trauma. *The Clinical Neuropsychologist*, *4*, 25-36.

Binder, L.M. (1992a). Malingering detected by forced-choice testing of memory and tactile sensation: a case report. *Archives of Clinical Neuropsychology, 7*, 155-163.

Binder, L.M. (1992b). Malingering and deception. In A. Puente & R. McCaffrey (Eds.), *Handbook of Neuropsychological Assessment: A Biopsychosocial Perspective* (pp. 353-374). New York: Plenum.

Binder, L.M. (1993a). Assessment of malingering after mild head trauma with the Portland Digit Recognition Test. *Journal of Clinical and Experimental Neuropsychology, 15*, 170-183.

Binder, L.M. (1993b). An abbreviated form of the Portland Digit Recognition Test. *The Clinical Neuropsychologist, 7*, 104-107.

Binder, L.M. (1993c). *Portland Digit Recognition Test Manual*, 2nd Ed. Beaverton, OR: Author.

Binder, L.M., & Kelly, M.P. (1996). Portland Digit Recognition Test performance by brain dysfunction patients without financial incentives. *Assessment, 3*, 403-409.

Binder, L.M., & Pankratz, L. (1987). Neuropsychological evidence of a factitious memory complaint. *Journal of Clinical and Experimental Neuropsychology, 9*, 167-171.

Binder, L.M., & Willis, S.C. (1991). Assessment of motivation after financially compensable minor head trauma. *Psychological Assessment, 3*, 141-147.

Brady, J.P., & Lind, D.L. (1961). Experimental analysis of hysterical blindness. *Archives of General Psychiatry, 4*, 331-339.

Essig, S.M., Mittenberg, W., Petersen, R.S., Strauman, S., & Cooper, J.T. (2001). Practices in forensic neuropsychology: Perspectives of neuropsychologists and trial attorneys. *Archives of Clinical Neuropsychology, 16*, 271-291.

Etcoff, L.M., & Kampfer, K.M. (1996). Practical guidelines in the use of symptom validity and other psychological tests to measure malingering and symptom exaggeration in traumatic brain injury cases. *Neuropsychology Review, 6*, 171-201.

Frederick, R.I., Sarfaty, S.D., Johnston, J.D., & Powel, J. (1994). Validation of a detector of response bias on a forced-choice test of nonverbal ability. *Neuropsychology, 8*, 118-125.

Golden, C.J., & Grier, C.A. (1998). Detecting malingering on the Luria-Nebraska Neuropsychological Battery. In C.R. Reynolds (Ed.), *Detection of Malingering During Head Injury Litigation* (pp. 133-162). New York: Plenum Press.

Greiffenstein, M., Baker, W.J., & Gola, T. (1994). Validation of malingered amnesia measures with a large clinical sample. *Psychological Assessment, 6*, 218-224.

Guilmette, T.J., Hart, K.J., & Giulianao, A.J. (1993). Malingering detection: The use of a forced-choice method in identifying organic versus simulated memory impairment. *The Clinical Neuropsychologist, 7*, 59-69.

Gunstad, J., & Suhr, J.A. (2001). Efficacy of the full and abbreviated forms of the Portland Digit Recogntion Test: Vulnerability to coaching. *The Clinical Neuropsychologist, 15*, 1-8.

Haines, M.E., & Norris, M.P. (2001). Comparing student and patient simulated malingerers' performance on standard neuropsychological measures to detect feigned cognitive deficits. *The Clinical Neuropsychologist, 15*, 171-182.

Hiscock, M., & Hiscock, C.K. (1989). Refining the forced-choice method for the detection of malingering. *Journal of Clinical and Experimental Neuropsychology, 11*, 967-974.

Inman, T.H., Vickery, C.D., Berry, D.T.R., Lamb, D.G., Edwards, C.L., & Smith, G.T. (1998). Development and initial validation of a new procedure for evaluating adequacy of effort given during neuropsychological testing: The Letter Memory Test. *Psychological Assessment, 10*, 128-139.

Ju, D., & Varney, N.R. (2000). Can head injury patients simulate malingering? *Applied Neuropsychology, 7*, 201-207.

Lezak, M.D. (1997). *Neuropsychological Assessment* (3rd Ed.). New York: Oxford University Press.

Millis, L.R., & Kler, S. (1995). Limitations of the Rey Fifteen-Item Test in the detection of malingering. *The Clinical Neuropsychologist, 9*, 241-244.

Orey S.A., Cragar D.E., & Berry D.T.R. (2000). Effects of two motivational manipulations on the neuropsychological performance of mildly head-injured college students. *Archives of Clinical Neuropsychology, 15*, 335-348.

Pankratz, L. (1979). Symptom validity testing and symptom retraining: Procedures for the assessment and treatment of functional sensory deficits. *Journal of Consulting and Clinical Psychology, 47*, 409-410.

Pankratz, L. (1983). A new technique for the assessment and modification of feigned memory deficit. *Perceptual and Motor Skills, 57*, 367-372.

Pankratz, L., & Binder, L.M. (1997). Malingering on cognitive measures. In R. Rogers (Ed.) *Clinical assessment of malingering and deception* (2nd ed.), (pp. 223-236). New York: Guilford.

Reynolds, C.R. (1998). Common sense, clinicians, and actuarialism in the detection of malingering during head injury litigation. In C.R. Reynolds (Ed.), *Detection of Malingering During Head Injury Litigation* (pp. 261-286). New York: Plenum.

Rose, F.E., Hall, S., Szalda-Petree, A.D., & Bach, P.J. (1998). A comparison of four tests of malingering and the effects of coaching. *Archives of Clinical Neuropsychology, 13*, 349-363.

Sweet, J.J. (2000). Malingering: Differential diagnosis. In J.J. Sweet (Ed.), *Forensic Neuropsychology* (pp. 255-285). Lisse: Swets & Zeitlinger.

Trueblood, W., & Binder, L.M. (1997). Psychologists' accuracy in identifying neuropsychological test protocols of clinical malingerers. *Archives of Clinical Neuropsychology, 12*, 13-27.

Vickery, C.D., Berry, D.T.R., Inman, T.H., Harris, M.J., & Orey, S.A. (2001). Detection of inadequate effort on neuropsychological testing: A meta-analytic review of selected procedures. *Archives of Clinical Neuropsychology, 16*, 45-73.

Youngjohn, J.R., Spector, J., & Mapou, R.L. (1997). Neuropsychological findings in silicone breast-implant complainants: Brain damage, somatization, or compensation neuroses? *The Clinical Neuropsychologist, 11*, 132-141.

The Victoria Symptom Validity Test: An Enhanced Test of Symptom Validity

Garrie B. Thompson III

Independent Practice

SUMMARY. The Victoria Symptom Validity Test (VSVT) is a computer-administered and scored, two-alternative, forced-choice symptom validity test designed to assess the validity of a patient's purported cognitive impairments (Slick, Hopp, Strauss, & Thompson, 1997). The VSVT benefits from numerous enhancements that increase its sensitivity beyond that of other earlier symptom validity tests without increasing its administration time or decreasing its specificity. It also has the ability to generate graphs and reports that can be used to assist the jury and the court in assessing whether a plaintiff's purported cognitive impairments are valid without the requirement of an extensive understanding of binomial probability theory. The VSVT's reliability and validity is inherent in its use of binomial probability theory, which has been used in many other well known symptom validity tests, and recent studies have demonstrated the VSVT's ability to detect response bias or malingering. Therefore, the VSVT likely meets the new *Daubert* standards for the admissibility of scientific evidence presented in a courtroom. Recent studies have also identified empirically validated cut-off scores for the VSVT that may further serve to enhance its sensitivity. *[Article copies available for a fee from The Haworth Document Delivery Service: 1-800-HAWORTH. E-mail address: <getinfo@haworthpressinc.com> Website: <http://www.HaworthPress.com> © 2002 by The Haworth Press, Inc. All rights reserved.]*

Garrie B. Thompson III is in independent practice, Boca Raton, FL.

Address correspondence to: Garrie B. Thompson, PhD, 200 West Palmetto Park Road, Suite 306, Boca Raton, FL 33432 (E-mail: GBTIII@msn.com).

[Haworth co-indexing entry note]: "The Victoria Symptom Validity Test: An Enhanced Test of Symptom Validity." Thompson, Garrie B. III. Co-published simultaneously in *Journal of Forensic Neuropsychology* (The Haworth Medical Press, an imprint of The Haworth Press, Inc.) Vol. 2, No. 3/4, 2002, pp. 43-67; and: *Detection of Response Bias in Forensic Neuropsychology* (ed: Jim Hom, and Robert L. Denney) The Haworth Medical Press, an imprint of The Haworth Press, Inc., 2002, pp. 43-67. Single or multiple copies of this article are available for a fee from The Haworth Document Delivery Service [1-800-HAWORTH, 9:00 a.m. - 5:00 p.m. (EST). E-mail address: getinfo@haworthpressinc.com].

© 2002 by The Haworth Press, Inc. All rights reserved.

KEYWORDS. Victoria Symptom Validity Test, malingering, *Daubert* decision, forced-choice test

The Victoria Symptom Validity Test (VSVT; Slick et al., 1997) is a computer-administered two-alternative forced-choice symptom validity test. The test is designed to assess the validity of a patient's reported cognitive impairments. The VSVT, like many other similar symptom validity tests, involves presenting a number of forced-choice decisions to a patient ostensibly to assess the presence or severity of purported cognitive impairment(s). In the case of the VSVT, the patient is told that the test is assessing memory and that it requires concentration. The test administers a total of 48 items, presented in three blocks of 16 items each. For each item administered, a five-digit study number is first presented on a computer screen during the "Study Trial" and then is immediately followed by the "Retention Interval" during which a blank computer screen is shown. Then a "Recognition Trial" is presented during which two five-digit numbers are presented on the computer screen, one of which was shown initially in the Study Trial, referred to as the study number, and a second number that serves as a foil. The patient is then required to identify which of the two five-digit numbers was shown during the Study Trial by pressing a designated key on the right or left side of a computer's keyboard. Patients are also instructed to make their selection as quickly as they can without making mistakes.

The VSVT utilizes a number of techniques to increase its sensitivity to detecting response bias by increasing the *perceived* difficulty of test items in several ways without increasing the *actual* difficulty of the test. First, the length of the Retention Interval is increased from 5-seconds for the first block of items, to 10-seconds for the second block, to 15-seconds for the third block. With each increase in the length of the Retention Interval, the patient is told that the test may be more difficult in order to enhance the perceived difficulty of the VSVT. However, research has shown that the majority of patients with documented memory impairments and who were not in litigation did not make significantly more errors with increases in the length of the retention intervals (Slick et al., 1997).

To further enhance the perceived difficulty of the VSVT, the 48 items are divided into 24 Easy Items and 24 Difficult Items. The five-digit Easy Items share no common digits with the foil that is presented in the Recognition Trial. In contrast, Difficult Items share all the digits with the foil; however, two of the digits in the foil are transposed to make the Difficult Items appear to be more difficult. However, again, research has shown that, while the Difficult Items give the perception of being more difficult, in reality these items are not significantly more difficult as non-compensation-seeking patients with documented head injuries do not miss significantly more Difficult Items (Slick et al., 1997). The inclusion of the Easy versus Difficult Items feature significantly enhances the sensitivity of the VSVT without increasing the administration time. Other symptom validity tests such as the Portland Digit Recognition Test (PDRT; Binder, 1993) have incorporated distraction techniques such as counting backwards during the retention interval (i.e., the interval between the initial presentation of the target stimulus and the presentation of the recognition trial where the patient is asked to select the target stimulus from one of two possible choices). Although this manipulation was added to increase the sensitivity of the PDRT, the addition of this distraction task was also felt to be problematic as the test took the better part of an hour to administer (Lezak, 1995). In contrast, the VSVT takes approximately 18-25 minutes to administer. It was also felt that patients who may have performed at their best on other tests may become annoyed with the PDRT, either because they felt that it insulted their intelligence or that it was boring and that at some point patients may exhibit less than optimal effort on this test (Lezak, 1995).

The VSVT computer program records the number of Easy and Difficult Items correctly completed, the response latency for each item, and the right or left preference (i.e., the proportion of the right-side responses minus the left-side responses). This right-left preference score serves to alert the clinician to possible visual field cuts or to left neglect, a feature that may further enhance its specificity by identifying valid impairments that could result in scores that might otherwise raise suspicion of response bias or malingering.

The VSVT includes a third classification category to enhance its sensitivity while minimally affecting its specificity. Unlike the traditional symptom validity tests that use a dichotomous classification rule based on more extreme scores, scores that are significantly above or significantly below chance to indicate valid and invalid responding, respectively, the VSVT broadens the categories used to classify a patient's scores to include Valid, Invalid, and Questionable. This allows the clinician to rule out random responding with a higher degree of certainty. When the patient obtains scores that fall significantly above or below chance levels (more extreme scores), they are unequivocally classified as Valid or Invalid, respectively. Scores that occur around chance level performance are highly infrequent among outpatient non-compensation-seeking patients with even moderate to severe head injuries (Slick et al., 1997) and are therefore classified as Questionable.

The VSVT also records the response latencies for each response as research suggests that unusually long response latencies are associated with symptom exaggeration or malingering (Beetar & Williams, 1995; Greiffenstein, Baker, & Gola; 1994). Although the validity of the patient's responses should never be judged solely on the basis of the length of response latencies, this information can be helpful in interpreting less extreme scores that fall in the Questionable range.

In addition to offering computer administration and scoring, the VSVT also prints a six-page report of all calculated values as well as interpretive statements about these values. Additionally, the VSVT allows the clinician to print either 8.5″ × 11″ black and white or color graphs (portrait mode) of the patient's scores as well as useful comparison groups that include the following: Control group, Feigning group, Non-compensation-seeking group, and a Compensation-seeking group. These reference groups consist of a control group of 95 undergraduates from the University of Victoria in British Columbia, 32 non-compensation-seeking neurological patients, 205 compensation-seeking medicolegal patients seen in private practice with varying degrees of head injuries, mostly from motor vehicle accidents, and 43 undergraduate students also from the University of Victoria who were asked to feign cognitive impairments as convincingly as possible (Slick et al., 1997). Graphs of these comparison groups present compelling visual information about the patient's performance and how it directly compares with other relevant groups. These graphs can also allow jurors to make accurate decisions about the patient's performance without requiring them to fully understand the theoretical underpinnings of binomial probability or bayesian statistics. Rather, jurors can examine the graphs visually and determine, for example, whether the patient's scores more closely match the Control group, the Non-compensation-seeking group, the Compensation-seeking group, or the Feigning group.

DOES THE VSVT MEET THE DAUBERT STANDARD?

Through a series of Supreme Court decisions the standard announced by the D.C. Circuit Court in 1923 in *Frye v. United States* has been extended and modified to become what is now referred to as the *Daubert* standard. Under the previous *Frye* "general acceptance" standard, expert testimony based on scientific evidence was admissible if the testimony "... was sufficiently established to have gained general acceptance in the field in which it belongs" (American Psychology-Law Society, 2001, p. 1). The new *Daubert* standard for admissibility for scientific expert testimony has suggested that the following questions would assist the judges in "determining whether a theory or technique is scientific knowledge that will assist the trier of fact (*Daubert*, at 593): (1) Has the theory or technique been tested or is it subject to being tested? (2) Has the theory or technique been subjected to peer review and publication? (3) What is known about the potential rate of error in applying the particular scientific theory or technique? (4) To what extent has the theory or technique received general acceptance in the relevant scientific community?" (American Psychology-Law Society, 2001). The following sections of this article will demonstrate how the VSVT meets the new *Daubert* standard by addressing each of the four questions listed above.

HAS THE THEORY OR TECHNIQUE BEEN TESTED?

As previously discussed, the VSVT is based on binomial probability theory, a theory that has been extensively validated and documented in the scientific literature. Previous authors have noted, "As the binomial theorem is theoretically based it does not require comparison to a normative data base; it is simply a formula of probability" (Denney, 1999, p. 90), and as such, it affirmatively answers the first of the *Daubert* questions. The application of the binomial probability theory to detect response bias or malingering has also been widely discussed in the literature since its inception when Pankratz (1979) developed the Symptom Validity Technique and demonstrated its utility in identifying response bias or malingering.

HAS THE THEORY OR TECHNIQUE BEEN SUBJECTED TO PEER REVIEW AND PUBLICATION?

Numerous symptom validity tests, which employ binomial probability theory in a manner similar to the VSVT, are published in peer-reviewed journals and have enjoyed widespread use in the psychological community. Published tests that have successfully employed binomial probability to assess the validity of symptoms include tests such as the

Hiscock Digit Memory Test (HDMT; Hiscock & Hiscock, 1989), the Portland Digit Recognition Test (PDRT; Binder, 1993), the Test of Memory Malingering (TOMM; Tombaugh, 1996), the Computerized Test of Response Bias (CARB; Allen, Conder, Green, & Cox, 1997), and several others.

Additionally, the VSVT is a published test, has an extensive Professional Manual that documents its reliability, validity, other psychometric properties, as well as its use in the detection of response bias. Furthermore, since the publication of the VSVT, several studies published in peer-reviewed journals have documented its ability to detect response bias or malingering (Bianchini, Mathias, & Greve, 2001; Doss, Chelune, & Naugle, 1999; Grote et al., 2000; Strauss et al., 2000), indicating that the VSVT also affirmatively answers the second question as suggested by the new *Daubert* standard.

WHAT IS KNOWN ABOUT THE POTENTIAL ERROR RATE IN APPLYING THE PARTICULAR SCIENTIFIC THEORY OR TECHNIQUE?

With regard to the third question inherent in the new *Daubert* standard regarding the error rates, the VSVT is reported to have almost 100% specificity, which is paramount in any test assessing symptom validity (Slick et al., 1997). Such specificity helps to ensure that patients are not falsely identified as exhibiting response bias during an evaluation or worse, diagnosed as malingering, a diagnosis that carries with it some very negative consequences that may dramatically affect the quantity or quality of services that a patient is given access to in the future. Additionally, it should be noted that because the VSVT cut-off scores are based on binomial probability theory and are not norm-referenced, it is very unlikely that a patient who scores in the Invalid range on the VSVT will do so for any reason other than response bias or malingering. It should also be noted that Slick, Sherman, and Iverson (1999) suggested that common euphemisms such as insufficient effort or poor motivation not be used to characterize VSVT scores that fall in the Invalid range, as these scores are significantly below chance and therefore, require that the patient makes an effort to identify the correct answer and then to deliberately select the wrong answer. Therefore, these scores will be referred to as invalid responding, response bias, or malingering throughout the remainder of this article. Additionally, the VSVT includes a left-right preference score that could alert clinicians to one of the very few conditions that might cause spurious false positives on the VSVT (e.g., left neglect). However, a patient who only selected numbers on the right side would score in the Questionable range, as the target stimulus (i.e., the correct answer) is presented an equal number of times on the left and right side of the computer screen during the administration of the test to avoid this potential problem.

With regards to the known error rates of the VSVT, because the use of the VSVT is based on binomial probability theory, the probability or likelihood of any given score being obtained by chance is easily derived through binomial probability theory or by looking up previously derived probability values in Appendix C of the VSVT Professional Manual (Slick et al., 1997). Although it might be argued that the probability of an event occurring by chance is not the same value as error rate, such a value does provide a quantifiable measure that relates directly to the degree of certainty or confidence the clinician has in classifying the patient's VSVT scores. Correspondingly, the probability that any VSVT score is not the result of chance can be easily derived or obtained through using the Professional Manual (Slick et al., 1997). Therefore, if the clinician employs cutoffs to assess Valid, Invalid, or Questionable responding based on probability theory when using the VSVT, the exact probability of making a correct decision is known.

Recent studies have also shown the VSVT to have high diagnostic accuracy. Strauss et al. (2000) examined the ability of the VSVT to discriminate between a control group and a group of simulated malingerers and found that the VSVT exhibited excellent sensitivity and specificity as it correctly classified 88% of the controls and 89% of the simulated malingerers.

The use of the classification matrix, a matrix based on bayesian statistics found in Appendix B of the VSVT Professional Manual (Slick et al., 1997) allows the clinician to determine the likelihood that a given score is from a malingerer with respect to the estimated base rates of malingering in the population from which the patient who is being tested is assumed to be drawn. For example, if the clinician's practice is devoted extensively to forensic evaluations involving patients in litigation seeking compensation for alleged cognitive deficits, the base rate of malingering might be expected to be quite high, maybe as high as 50%. In the case of high base rates, the error rate of the VSVT would be low. In contrast, if the clinician sees primarily patients with dementia, the base rate might be quite low, perhaps 5%. In this case, the error rate for the VSVT would be significantly higher. For example, by using the Classification Confidence Matrix for Easy and Difficult Items Correct

Scores found in Appendix B on pages 64-65 of the Professional Manual (Slick et al., 1997), one can determine that a Difficult Items Correct Score of 13 corresponds to a 0.27 probability of feigning for an assumed base rate of 5% as compared to a probability of 0.88 for an assumed base rate of 50%.

Use of this classification matrix demonstrates how base rates can dramatically affect the positive and negative predictive power of tests such as the VSVT. Positive predictive power refers to the probability that a positive test result actually indicates the presence of a disorder. Positive predictive power is increased when there is a higher base rate (i.e., prevalence) of the disorder in a given population. Negative predictive power refers to the probability that a patient who obtains a negative test result does not have the disorder. Although there is considerable dispute about the base rate of malingering in compensation-seeking patients, one can see that, as the base rates increase, there are dramatic improvements in the ability of the VSVT to detect response bias or malingering. However, Slick et al. (1997) cautions the clinician about the limitations of using the above bayesian diagnostic probability values, citing that, like all actuarially based scores, these scores are limited by the representativeness of the sample size and test reliability, and therefore should not be used in isolation to make a diagnosis of malingering.

TO WHAT EXTENT HAS THE THEORY OR TECHNIQUE RECEIVED GENERAL ACCEPTANCE IN THE RELEVANT SCIENTIFIC COMMUNITY?

As previously mentioned, symptom validity tests such as the VSVT have enjoyed widespread acceptance in the scientific community as indicated by numerous publications of these tests in peer-reviewed journal articles. Symptom validity tests based on binomial probability theory are also published and sold by a variety of test publishers.

Implicitly stated in the *Daubert* standard is the need for tests used in scientific testimony to exhibit adequate reliability and validity. Studies of the VSVT's reliability described in the Professional Manual (Slick et al., 1997) using data pooled from Compensation- and Non-compensation-seeking groups revealed coefficient alpha values for the Easy, Difficult, and the combined set of 48 items of .82, .87, and .87, respectively. Test-retest reliability values obtained from administering the VSVT to 28 Compensation-seeking patients, with a median test-rest interval of

31 days was 0.84 for Total Items Correct score, 0.83 for Easy Items Correct score, and 0.78 for Difficult Items Correct score. Test-retest reliability values for the Easy Items Response Latency scores and the Difficult Items Response Latency scores were 0.56 and 0.84, respectively. It should be noted that because of the effects of range restriction in VSVT Total, Easy, and Difficult Items Correct scores, the test-retest reliability coefficients for the Control Group did not accurately reflect the stability of the VSVT, and therefore, they were not listed in the Professional Manual.

Another measure of reliability, the stability of patients' initial group classification as determined by their VSVT scores (i.e., Valid, Questionable, and Invalid) over a test-retest interval was examined. It was discovered that although the overall classification of patients based on their VSVT scores remained relatively stable (i.e., the contingency coefficient for these groups was $r = .75, p < .001$), further inspection of the data revealed the stability of patients' classifications (i.e., Valid, Invalid, Questionable) varied considerably with respect to their *initial* classification. That is, 100% of the Control group retained their initial classification, whereas only 86% of the Compensation-seeking patients retained their original classification. An examination of the Compensation-seeking patients whose classification differed upon retesting revealed that the majority of these patients (approximately 40%) were initially classified as belonging to the Questionable group. Overall, these findings suggest that the VSVT exhibits adequate reliability and suggests that changes in classification across test-retest intervals most likely reflect the VSVT's sensitivity to changes in the effort or performance exhibited by patients and not error variance. A published review of the VSVT drew a similar conclusion, reporting that, in regards to changes in the classification of VSVT scores, "The greater variability of compensation-seeking subjects likely says more about subjects than the reliability of this measure" (Denney, 1999, p. 91). Additionally, reliability studies suggest greater stability of scores over time for patients who obtained more extreme scores (i.e., Valid and Invalid groups). It should also be noted that because the VSVT is computer-administered, all test stimuli are presented to patients in a standardized and invariant manner, which enhances its reliability by minimizing any error variance which might be associated with minor variations in the manner in which different clinicians might otherwise administer this test.

Testimony based on scientific test data should also be valid in order to meet the question implicitly stated in the *Daubert* standard. Initial validity studies of the VSVT as reported in the Professional Manual (Slick et al., 1997) demonstrate convergent validity by showing its significant correlations with other tests used to ascertain the validity of a patient's responses. Significant correlations have been reported (*r*s = .77 and .69) between the Easy and Difficult Items Correct scores (Slick et al., 1997) and the raw scores on the Rey 15-item Test (Lezak, 1995), another measure believed to be fairly sensitive to malingering, but also sensitive to genuine memory impairment (Guilmette, Hart, Giuliano, & Leininger, 1994; Schretlen, Brandt, Kraft, & Van Gorp, 1991); however, sample sizes were rather limited ($n = 9$).

Although the Minnesota Multiphasic Personality Inventory-2 (MMPI-2; Butcher, Dahlstrom, Graham, Tellegen, & Kaemmer, 1989) validity scales are intended to assess the validity of a patient's endorsement of psychopathology and not to assess for response bias or the feigning of memory impairments, both the VSVT and the validity scales of the MMPI-2 attempt to assess whether the patient approached endorsement of test items in a valid manner. An examination of the relationship between the VSVT Easy and Difficult Items Correct scores and the MMPI-2 validity scales (e.g., F scale, F − K raw score, and Fake-Bad raw scores) revealed modest negative correlations (e.g., the correlation between Easy Items Correct scores and the MMPI-2 F scale T score was $r = -.29$; Slick et al., 1997). In other words, higher MMPI-2 F scale T scores were moderately associated with lower VSVT Easy Items Correct scores. In contrast, VSVT Easy and Difficult Item Response Latency scores were minimally correlated with MMPI-2 validity scales with the exception of moderate correlations with the Fake-Bad scale (Slick et al., 1997). Easy and Difficult Items correlations with the Fake-Bad scale were $r = .42$ and $r = 43$, respectively.

Demonstration of divergent validity of tests used for scientifically based courtroom testimony is of crucial importance, as a false positive result can be devastating. That is, if a test were to incorrectly classify patients as malingerers based on their poor test performance, when in fact their poor performance was attributed to actual cognitive impairments, this may dramatically reduce the likelihood that these patients would receive needed treatment or financial compensation for their impairments. Not surprisingly, protection against false positives is also built into our legal system for the very same reason, as courts fail to convict if reasonable doubt exists. Therefore, it would be problematic if a symptom validity test correlated even moderately with frequently used neuropsychological tests assessing attention, executive functioning, verbal and visual memory, and intelligence. Fortunately, correlations between the VSVT Easy and Difficult Items Correct scores and a variety of widely and frequently used neuropsychological measures including the Wechsler Intelligence Scale-Revised Full Scale IQ and Digit Span subtest (Wechsler, 1981), the Wechsler Memory Scale-Revised Logical Memory subtests (Wechsler, 1987), the Rey Complex Figure Test (Lezak, 1995; Meyers & Meyers, 1995), the Trail Making Test (Reitan & Wolfson, 1993), and the Wisconsin Card Sorting Test (Heaton, Chelune, Talley, Kay, & Curtiss, 1993) have been quite low (ranging from .00 to .23), demonstrating good discriminant validity (Slick et al., 1997). Although most neuropsychological measures showed little relationship to VSVT scores, a slightly higher correlation was noted between the VSVT Easy and Difficult Items Correct scores and the Word Trial ($r = -.28$ and $r = -.21$, respectively) of the Stroop Color Word Test, Victoria Revision (Regard, 1981). It should be noted that the Easy and Difficult Items Response Latency scores showed less divergent validity as they were moderately correlated with attentional and processing speed measures such as Digit Span (Wechsler, 1981) and the Trail Making Test. The latter findings also highlight the authors' recommendations that the VSVT response latencies not be used in isolation to classify a patient's scores; rather the response latencies should be used in an ancillary manner to support decisions based primarily on VSVT Total, Easy, and Difficult Items Correct scores (Slick et al., 1997).

Studies of the VSVT have also noted good predictive validity as significant group effects are found for the number of Easy and Difficult Items correct (Slick et al., 1997). Patients in the Feigning group earned on average Difficult Items Correct scores that were 9 points lower than their Easy Items Correct scores ($t = 11.3, p < .001$). Similarly, the Compensation-seeking group's mean Difficult Items Correct score was 3 points lower than their mean Easy Items Correct score ($t = 11.2$, $p < .001$). In contrast, patients in the Control and Non-compensation-seeking groups obtained mean Easy and Difficult Items Correct scores that were within 1 point of each other (Slick et al., 1997). Examination of distribution data in the form of percentiles also revealed that the score distributions for all groups, with the exception of the Compensation-seeking and Feigning groups were positively skewed suggesting that normal and even non-compensation-seeking head injured patients had little difficulty earning near perfect scores on the VSVT. This conclusion is readily seen by examining the Total Items Correct scores (out of a possible score of 48 items correct) for the four groups examined in the study, which were as follows: Controls, mean = 47.41; Non-compensation-seeking group, mean = 46.16; Compensation-seeking group, mean = 43.50, and the Feigning group, mean = 31.26. It is also interesting to note that an examination of the standard deviations for the Total Items Correct scores for the four groups revealed little variability in the scores for the Control group ($SD = 0.92$), while significant variation was noted in the Feigning group ($SD = 9.05$). Not surprisingly, more recent studies have demonstrated that increased variability in an individual's VSVT responses, which will be discussed later, has also been shown to be helpful in alerting clinicians to the possibility of response bias or malingering (Strauss et al., 2000).

RECENT STUDIES OF THE VSVT

A number of studies have demonstrated the VSVT's ability to identify response bias or malingering since its publication in 1997. In an attempt to cross-validate and to extend the findings of the original VSVT standardization study, a recent study by Grote et al. (2000) examined the ability of the VSVT to discriminate between compensation-seeking patients (CS) with mild traumatic brain injury ($n = 53$) and non-compensation-seeking patients (NCS) with intractable seizures ($n = 30$). These authors suggested that cut-off scores based on binomial probability theory that were frequently used in forced-choice symptom validity tests were not the most efficient in identifying response bias or malingering (i.e., did not produce the highest hit rates). Because most NCS patients with moderate to even severe traumatic brain injuries tend to perform at or significantly above chance on symptom validity tests, it was hypothesized that cut-off scores could be adjusted upward to reflect empirically derived cut-off scores to enhance the sensitivity of symptom validity tests while minimally affecting specificity. This idea has been previously supported by Guilmette et al. (1994) and Guilmette, Whelihan, Hart, Sparadeo, and Buongiorno (1996) who also cited the need for empirically based cut-off scores to enhance the sensitivity of the Abbreviated Hiscock Forced Choice Procedure (A-HFCP; Guilmette et al., 1996), a symptom validity test. A previous review of the VSVT by Denney (1999) was also somewhat critical of the sensitivity of the VSVT when using theoretically based cut-off scores. Denney noted that most of the Feigning group obtained Difficult Items Correct scores in the chance to below chance ranges. Although the VSVT was designed to be very conservative so as to minimize false positives, the authors of this test also suggested "additional samples of non-litigating mild to moderate head injury patients will likely facilitate the derivation of more robust norm-referenced scoring systems for the VSVT" (Slick et al., 1997, p. 58). In examining the utility of empirically based cut-scores, Grote et al. (2000) discovered that 100% of the NCS epilepsy patients in their study obtained Difficult Items Correct Scores of 18 or greater (out of a possible 24 Difficult Items). Furthermore, 93.3% of these patients obtained scores of at least 21. Grote et al. (2000) pointed out that Berry (cited in Slick et al., 1997) also reported that, in a study of 30 patients with moderate to severe traumatic brain injuries, 90% obtained Difficult Items Correct scores of 19 or greater. Similarly, the VSVT standardization study (Slick et al., 1997) noted that all patients in the NCS group obtained Difficult Items Correct scores of 20 or greater. Because 93% of NCS patients obtained Difficult Items Correct scores of 21 or greater, Grote et al. (2000) suggested that the range of Difficult Items Correct scores previously viewed as Valid, that is scores ranging from 16-24, be adjusted upward to reflect the fact that patients with even moderate to severe head injuries tend to obtain Difficult Item Corrects scores of 21 or greater. That is, they suggested that Difficult Items Correct scores that fall within the range of 16-20 should "not be thought of as valid, but instead as a level of performance that is rarely seen among NCS patients with documented brain disease" (Grote et al., 2000, p. 717). These findings suggest that, rather than relying upon theoretically derived cut-off scores to identify response bias or malingering, "a more appropriate strategy may be to refer to empirically-derived distributions of memory scores achieved by non-compensation-seeking samples in this and other studies" (Grote et al., 2000, p. 716).

Grote et al. (2000) also examined VSVT block data to determine if other empirically derived cut-off scores for within-block performance might enhance the sensitivity of the VSVT. (It should be pointed out that the VSVT Professional Manual indicates that there are 3 blocks of 16 items each that are comprised of 8 Easy Items and 8 Difficult Items. However, Grote et al. (2000) refer to 6 blocks containing 8 items each, apparently meaning that they are dividing each of the 3 blocks into 2 blocks for a total of 6 blocks, each containing 8 Easy and 8 Difficult items.) These authors found that in the 30 NCS patients examined, out of 180 blocks of scores (i.e., 30 patients × 6 blocks of scores), 179 of these blocks contained at least 5 or more correct Easy or Difficult items (not to be confused with 5 or more total items correct). Grote et al. (2000) suggested that because a score of 5 or less Easy or Difficult items correct in any block of 8 items was extremely uncommon in the NCS group, a cutoff of 5 or less Easy or Difficult Items correct within a block could be used to accurately identify patients exhibiting response bias or malingering.

One of the more interesting findings of Grote et al. (2000) was that only one-third of the compensation-seeking patients correctly answered at least 90% of the VSVT Difficult items, whereas two-thirds of the patients in this group scored below this level. These authors concluded that, although the representativeness of this sample of compensation-seeking patients was not known, this finding should alert clinicians to routinely give tests assessing response bias or symptom validity to patients who are seeking compensation for alleged cognitive deficits.

These authors also examined the use of the mean Easy and Difficult Items Response Latency scores and found them to be of little or no diagnostic utility, as they misclassified a significant percentage of NCS patients and because these scores were not independent of the memory items scores (i.e., the number of total VSVT items correct). In other words, response latencies were not independent of the number of items correct on the VSVT, because the CS patients who scored in the Questionable/Invalid range on the VSVT Difficult Items exhibited response latencies that were significantly longer than CS patients who obtained VSVT scores that fell within the Valid range. Similarly, Slick et al. (1997) suggested that despite the large group differences in *mean* response latency scores, the observed overlap between the 95% confidence intervals for response latencies in Valid, Questionable, and Invalid groups suggested that mean response latency scores should not be used to make clinical decisions regarding malingering. However, when Grote et al. (2000) examined *individual* response latency scores, they found that latencies in excess of 4 seconds were sufficiently rare among the NCS patients so that when latencies of this or greater magnitude are observed "an interpretation of response bias should be considered" (Grote et al., 2000, p. 717).

CASE EXAMPLE

The VSVT was administered in conjunction with several other measures to assess for possible response bias or malingering in a married, right-handed, middle-aged patient whose chief complaint was severe anterograde memory problems that were preventing a return to work. The patient reported that cognitive problems had developed approximately a year earlier following an episode of sudden diplopia and light-headedness. Diagnostic tests including a CT scan, an MRI, an MRA, and two spinal taps were negative. The patient also had two EEGs. Per patient report, the first EEG revealed some mild abnormality; however, the patient could not recall the nature of this abnormality. The second EEG was negative. After numerous evaluations and diagnostic tests, the patient was eventually diagnosed as having a connective tissue disease.

Since being diagnosed with this disease, the patient reported experiencing chronic fatigue, vertigo, constipation, difficulties concentrating, memory problems, severe headaches, a feeling of bruising in parts of the scalp, and intermittent tingling in the base of the head. In addition, the patient reported sleeping more than usual, having reduced energy levels, and consequently no longer pursued many previously enjoyed activities. However, there was no reported decrease in the patient's sexual activity or appetite. After the initial episode described above, the patient also reported discontinuing driving, as it had become overwhelming due to a feeling of sensory overload. That is, the patient felt unable to adequately process the multitude of visual images that were encountered while driving. The patient also reported difficulties following conversations when in group settings and was, in general, more sensitive to noise. Interestingly, despite these severe impairments, the patient was able to perform financial transactions on the computer without any assistance. The patient's spouse, who had stopped working in order to stay home and care for the patient, noticed personality changes in the patient who had become more emotional and who was described as exhibiting a more exaggerated range of positive and negative emotions. The spouse also reported that the patient was less gregarious and had difficulties coping with situations where there were many people due to a tendency to be easily overwhelmed.

Previous neuropsychological testing revealed evidence of cognitive impairments that included severe memory impairments, severe impairments on a task of visual search and attention, a mild decline in right hand fine motor speed, and a mild decline in verbal fluency. Interestingly, the patient performed normally on the VSVT at that time. However, an assessment of personality functioning with the MMPI-2 revealed elevations on clinical scales suggesting that the patient endorsed a number of physical symptoms and had indicated worries about physical health, depression, and possible suicidal ideation.

Before the onset of the purported cognitive problems, the patient was employed in a managerial position, which was reportedly enjoyable, but very stressful. With regard to education, the patient completed two years of college.

The patient reported being on disability and that a re-evaluation was needed in order to continue to receive disability payments. It was also noted that, during the initial interview the patient frequently looked to the spouse, who was present only during the interview, to answer specific questions about the patient's medical history and memory problems.

Prior to the evaluation, instructions were given to the patient to ask that instructions be repeated or further explained, if needed, and/or to request a break if fatigued, as it was important to obtain the patient's best performance.

As part of routine procedures for evaluating patients where potential financial incentives exist for convincingly feigning cognitive impairments or malingering, the patient was given the VSVT before the administration of any other tests. This is consistent with previous studies, which have recommended administering symptom validity tests at the beginning of the evaluation to optimize their sensitivity (Grote et al., 2000; Guilmette et al., 1994; Guilmette et al., 1996). Additionally, because the VSVT is computer scored, administering it first enabled the examiner to inspect the patient's scores and give additional measures to assess for response bias or malingering, since the patient's VSVT Difficult Items Correct score fell in the Questionable range. Alternatively, if the patient's response latencies exceeded the cut-off score or if the number of items correct fell below the cut-off score suggested by Grote et al. (2000), it could have also alerted the examiner to the need to administer additional measures of response bias or malingering.

The patient correctly answered 33 of the 48 VSVT items. This performance was significantly above chance (p = 0.9972) with a Total Items Correct score falling in the Valid range. Further inspection of the VSVT results revealed that all 24 of the 24 Easy Items were correctly answered ($p > .9999$, Valid range) indicating that the patient understood the task and had demonstrated a capacity to perform normally. In contrast, the patient only answered 9 of the 24 Difficult Items correctly, a performance that fell within the Questionable range ($p = 0.1537$). These findings, particularly when viewed in the context that all 24 Easy Items were answered correctly, suggested that the patient knew the correct answer and, for items perceived as being more difficult, the patient made an effort to choose the wrong answer in an attempt to feign cognitive impairment. Therefore, although a score in the Questionable range was not of sufficient magnitude to unequivocally indicate invalid responding, it raised strong suspicions of this possibility.

In addition, although the scores of the previously administered VSVT were unavailable, it was reported that the patient "performed normally" on this test, thus arousing further suspicion of invalid responding. This is because relatively small inconsistencies in VSVT performance across testing sessions or "intra-individual variability" have been shown to be clinically useful in detecting malingering across serial testing with the VSVT (Strauss et al., 2000). These authors suggested that increases or decreases of 2 or more points on VSVT Difficult Items Correct score or changes of 1 or more points on the Easy Items Correct score warrants suspicion.

The empirically derived cut-off scores proposed by Grote et al. (2000) were also retrospectively examined to determine whether they would have assisted in correctly identifying this patient as exhibiting response bias or malingering. Initial inspection of the protocol revealed that the patient's Difficult Items Correct score of 9 fell significantly below their empirically derived cut-off score of 21, which patients with even moderate to severe head injury equaled or exceeded, and therefore, the patient would have been correctly diagnosed using this empirically based decision rule. A cut-off score of 5 or less items correct within any of the "6" blocks of 8 items was also found by these authors to be extremely uncommon in non-compensation-seeking patients. Inspection of the patient's VSVT performance revealed the following scores: Block 1, Easy Items Correct score = 8, Difficult Items Correct score = 4; Block 2, Easy Items Correct score = 8, Difficult Items Correct score = 2, and Block 3, Easy Items Correct score = 8, Difficult Items Correct score = 3. It can be seen that by using the empirically validated cut-off score of 5 or less Difficult items correct on any of the three blocks would have led to classifying the patient's scores as Invalid. In contrast, using the more conservative theoretical binomial based cut-off scores to classify the above Difficult Item Correct scores resulted in a Questionable classification for the Difficult Items Correct scores of 4, 2, and 3 with probabilities of 0.6367, 0.1445, and 0.3633 respectively. These findings demonstrate how the use of these empirically validated cut-off scores for block data can be used to enhance the sensitivity of the VSVT.

The patient's response latencies across all 48 VSVT items were examined to determine if any exceeded the four-second cut-off score suggested by Grote et al. (2000). Inspection of these response latencies revealed that 18 of the 48 response latencies exceeded 4 seconds and of these, 8 exceeded 6 seconds and 1 was 10.93 seconds. Response latencies of this magnitude are extremely unlikely and are sufficiently rare to warrant a conclusion of response bias (Grote et al., 2000).

The patient was also administered selected subtests of the Wechsler Adult Intelligence Scale-Third Edition (WAIS-III; The Psychological

Corporation, 1997) that included Digit Span and Vocabulary. Mittenberg, Theroux, Zielinski, and Heilbronner (1995) had previously demonstrated the ability of the Vocabulary-Digit Span difference score as well as a discriminant function they developed to accurately identify malingered head injury on the Wechsler Adult Intelligence Scale-Revised (WAIS-R; Wechsler, 1981). Mittenberg et al. (in press) recently demonstrated that the Vocabulary-Digit Span difference and the discriminant function could be similarly used to accurately identify malingering on the WAIS-III. Although this formula has not yet been used to identify malingering in connective tissue disorders, it was retrospectively applied to the results of this evaluation to determine if the patient's pattern of performance was consistent with what is shown in malingered head injury. Using previously provided tables from their original study, it was determined that the observed 8-point difference between the patient's Vocabulary age corrected scaled score of 11 and a Digit Span age corrected scaled score of 3 corresponded to a 0.88346 probability of malingering.

Testing was conducted over two sessions and again, at the beginning of the second testing session, the importance of putting forth one's best effort was stressed. The patient was also encouraged to request that instructions be clarified or repeated, if needed, to best understand them. At the beginning of the second session the patient was administered the Test of Memory Malingering (TOMM; Tombaugh, 1996) and earned a score of 22 out of a possible 50 points on Trial 1, a score of 24 out of a possible 50 points on Trial 2, and a score of 25 out of 50 points on the Retention Trial. These findings provided additional evidence of symptom exaggeration or malingering.

The Wechsler Memory Scale-Third Edition (WMS-III; The Psychological Corporation, 1997) was also administered during the second half of the evaluation, and it was found that the patient was unable to recall several of the six items on the Delayed Recognition Logical Memory subtest that are answered correctly by persons who have never heard the Logical Memory stories. Applying this Rarely Missed Index (RMI), an index developed through discriminant function analysis by Killgore and DellaPietra (2000), to the patient's responses resulted in a score that fell below the cutoff score of 136, a score shown to identify malingering.

After completing approximately three-fourths of the evaluation, the patient was given the Rey 15 Item Test (Rey, 1941, 1964). The patient correctly recalled only 9 of the 15 items, which is just at the cutoff of 9 items that is frequently used to identify malingering (Lezak, 1995), although other authors have recommended a lower value to minimize false positives (Lee, Loring, & Martin, 1992).

The patient was also administered the MMPI-2. An inspection of the Validity scales revealed an elevated Lie scale (T = 71), suggesting that the patient's responses were of questionable validity. This finding suggested that the patient might have attempted to minimize psychological difficulties. Not surprisingly, none of the Clinical scales were significantly elevated. Although the reason for the patient's attempt to minimize psychological difficulties was not known, it may have been an attempt to suggest that the previously noted cognitive impairments were not functional in nature (i.e., not due to or exacerbated by the effects of anxiety or depression), but were neurologically based.

DISCUSSION

It is not unusual for this author to administer multiple measures to assess for response bias or malingering during a clinical evaluation where there is potential secondary gain for a patient who can convincingly feign cognitive impairments. However, it was unusual for one patient to exhibit poor performance on four different measures assessing response bias. Nevertheless, the patient's multiple extreme scores across a variety of theoretically and empirically validated (i.e., norm-referenced) tests assessing response bias or malingering provides compelling evidence that the patient's neuropsychological results were invalid. These findings indicate that using conservative cut-off scores derived from binomial probability theory to identify response bias with the VSVT can result in a Questionable classification. If a patient falls within this classification, the clinician should administer additional tests of response bias. Additionally, the clinician may wish to use empirically based cut-off scores that can enhance the sensitivity of the VSVT without compromising its specificity. In this regard, the "90% rule" appears promising. That is, using empirically based cut-off scores that represent the lowest score that 90% of moderate to severe head injured patients equal or exceed to identify response bias may help to increase the sensitivity of symptom validity tests while preserving their high specificity.

The findings of Grote et al. (2000) that two-thirds of their compensation-seeking patients correctly answered less than 90% of the VSVT Difficult Items demonstrates the need for tests assessing for response bias to be routinely given to patients who are seeking compensation for alleged cognitive deficits. This need is also indicated by Doss et al.

(1999) who noted that a high proportion of their compensation-seeking patients performed in the Questionable and Invalid ranges on the VSVT. In fact, because these authors found invalid responding in their non-compensation-seeking sample, they suggested that clinicians consider using such tests in all evaluations.

Several studies have also suggested that symptom validity tests such as the VSVT should be given at the very beginning of the evaluation in order to further enhance their sensitivity (Grote et al., 2000; Guilmette et al., 1994; Guilmette et al., 1996). The degree to which administering the VSVT first enhances its sensitivity is not certain. However, at the very least, administering this test first and then inspecting the scores can alert the clinician to the need to administer additional symptom validity tests and/or to include tests for which discriminant function derived malingering formulas have been developed (Mittenberg, Rotholc, Russell, Heilbronner, 1996; Mittenberg et al., in press).

The administration or application of multiple malingering measures during one evaluation may not as yet enjoy widespread use. However, considerable evidence suggests that the approach malingerers use to feign deficits on neuropsychological tests can vary considerably (Lezak, 1995; Pankratz & Binder, 1997) and that coaching or warning patients can reduce the sensitivity of tests designed to detect malingering (Johnson & Lesniak-Karpniak, 1997; Thompson et al., 1996). Thompson et al. (1996) found that limited coaching significantly reduced the sensitivity of the A-HFCP in the detection of simulated malingerers. They also noted that when simulated malingerers were provided with nine specific symptoms frequently associated with head trauma (from Gouvier, Cubic, Jones, Brantley, & Cutlip, 1992), this limited information resulted in further reductions in the test's sensitivity. Administering multiple and/or repeated measures to assess response bias or malingering would also likely make it increasingly more difficult for a patient to be coached to convincingly feign impairment across multiple measures. In addition, by giving more than one malingering test it is more likely that a particular malingering test will ". . . be relevant to a specific patient's functional or genuine complaints, or both. Thus the best use of a single test will be in combination with other tests–always within the context of a patient's history and clinical presentation–which together will reduce the likelihood of prediction error" (Lezak, 1995, p. 792). Additionally, the finding that a patient passes a single test of response bias or malingering does not exclude the possibility that the patient did not exaggerate cognitive impairments throughout the remainder of the evaluation, particularly when considering the lengthier testing typically performed in forensic settings where compensation for deficits can be considerable. A similar opinion was expressed by Spreen and Strauss (1998) who stated, "Given the current state of affairs, it is our view that multiple approaches must be used in the diagnostic process and that statements regarding incomplete effort should not be based on a single test score" (p. 668). This increasingly popular view is also shared by Bianchini et al. (2001) who not only see the need to administer multiple symptom validity measures to identify malingerers, but to help rule out malingering so that patients with valid cognitive impairments can obtain appropriate treatment and compensation.

In addition to the added clinical value of administering multiple tests to assess for response bias or malingering, one may recall that a negative finding on the VSVT or other symptom validity or malingering test does not exclude the possibility of malingering. Although there is some dispute as to whether a single test score should be used to make statements about incomplete effort or malingering, there is a clearly quantifiable degree of certainty or probability of performing significantly below chance on a binomial based symptom validity test, which is known (e.g., $p = 0.0500$). In contrast, the certainty or likelihood that a patient who obtained a score in the Valid range on one such symptom validity test exhibited valid effort throughout the entire evaluation or test battery is not known, particularly since symptom validity tests have been shown to be sensitive to coaching. Given this uncertainty, it seems prudent to administer several different measures of response bias at different points during an evaluation. Because of this uncertainty, it could be argued that testifying to a jury that a lack of malingering was found on one symptom validity test might be unduly prejudicial. Therefore, a court might rule that such testimony was inadmissible. By administering multiple tests assessing response bias or malingering, the clinician will likely help to ensure the admissibility of expert testimony related to the results of these tests.

A similar concern for potentially prejudicial evidence appears to be shared by others in the legal system, as the Federal Rules of Evidence requires the potential prejudicial effect of scientific testimony to be carefully balanced against its probative value (Saxe & Ben-Shakhar, 1999). Therefore, the use of multiple malingering measures might also help to provide this "balance" in a manner that is more consistent with the standards set for the admissibility of scientific evidence in the court. For example, expert testimony indicating that a plaintiff passed multiple measures assessing for response bias or malingering would likely provide the court with information it would need to decide with a high degree of confidence or certainty that the purported cognitive impairments were valid and that the plaintiff needed to be compensated appropriately. Additionally, the use of multiple tests assessing for response bias or malingering, particularly when extreme scores on these tests are noted, can provide clinicians with the evidence they need to make accurate diagnostic decisions while addressing the concerns about the effects of low base rates on positive predictive power that have been raised by researchers (Rosenfeld, Sands, & van Gorp, 2000).

CONCLUSION

The VSVT is likely to meet the *Daubert* standard for the admissibility of expert scientific testimony based on neuropsychological evaluations for numerous reasons. These include the features utilized in the VSVT to enhance its sensitivity, its strong psychometric characteristics, and its binomial-based three category classification system that allows it to be generally used to assess for response bias or malingering in a variety of different diagnostic groups (i.e., groups other than mild traumatic brain injury) without adversely affecting its very high specificity. The VSVT is also able to generate graphs and reports that can be used to accurately convey results derived from binomial probability theory to assist the courts in making accurate decisions regarding the validity of a plaintiff's symptoms, without the requirement that the jury or the court have an extensive understanding of the theoretical underpinnings of probability theory. Its ease of use, its short administration time, and other positive characteristics further suggest that clinicians might wish to include the VSVT as one of several tests routinely given at the beginning of a neuropsychological evaluation to assess for response bias or malingering, particularly in compensation-seeking patients where very strong financial incentives are involved.

REFERENCES

Allen, L. M., Conder, R. L., Green, P., & Cox, D. R. (1997). *CARB '97 Manual for the Computerized Assessment of Response Bias*. Durham, NC: CogniSyst, Inc.

American Psychology-Law Society. (2001, Winter). *American Psychology-Law Society News*, *21*(1), 1-26.

Beetar, J. T., & Williams, J. M. (1995). Malingering response styles on the Memory Assessment Scales and Symptom Validity Tests. *Archives of Clinical Neuropsychology*, *10*, 57-72.

Bianchini, K. J., Mathias, C. W., & Greve, K. W. (2001). Symptom validity testing: A critical review. *The Clinical Neuropsychologist 15*, 19-45.

Binder, L. M. (1993). Assessment of malingering after mild head trauma with the Portland Digit Recognition Test. *Journal of Clinical and Experimental Neuropsychology, 15*, 170-182.

Butcher, J., Dahlstrom, W. G., Graham, J., Tellegen, A., & Kaemmer, B. (1989). *Minnesota Multiphasic Personality Inventory (MMPI-2): Manual for administration and scoring*. Minneapolis, MN: University of Minnesota Press.

Denney, R. L. (1999). Test Review: *Victoria Symptom Validity Test Version 1.0., Journal of Forensic Neuropsychology, 1*(1), 89-94.

Doss, R. C., Chelune, G. J., & Naugle, R. I. (1999). *Victoria Symptom Validity Test:* Compensation-seeking vs. non-compensation seeking patients in a general clinical setting. *Journal of Forensic Neuropsychology, 1*(4), 5-20.

Gouvier, W. D., Cubic, B., Jones, G., Brantley, P., & Cutlip, Q. (1992). Postconcussion symptoms and daily stress in a normal college population. *Archives of Clinical Neuropsychology, 7*, 193-211.

Graham, J. R. (1990). *MMPI-2: Assessing personality and psychopathology*. New York: Oxford University Press.

Greiffenstein, M. F., Baker, W. J., & Gola, T. (1994). Validation of malingered amnesia measures with a large clinical sample. *Psychological Assessment, 6*, 218-224.

Grote, C. L., Kooker, E. K., Garon, D. C., Nyenhuis, D. L., Smith, C. A., & Mattingly, M. L. (2000). Performance of compensation seeking and non-compensation seeking samples on the Victoria Symptom Validity Test: Cross validation and extension of a standardization study. *Journal of Clinical and Experimental Neuropsychology, 22*, 709-719.

Guilmette, T., Hart, K., Giuliano, A. J., & Leininger, B. E. (1994). Detecting simulated memory impairment: The Rey Fifteen-Item Test and the Hiscock Forced-Choice procedure. *The Clinical Neuropsychologist, 3*, 283-294.

Guilmette, T., Whelihan, W., Hart, K., Sparadeo, F., & Buongiorno, G. (1996). Order effects in the administration of a forced-choice procedure for detection of malingering in disability claimants' evaluations. *Perceptual and Motor Skills, 83*, 1007-1016.

Heaton, R. K., Chelune, G. J., Talley, J. L., Kay, G., & Curtiss, G. (1993). *Wisconsin Card Sorting Test manual: Revised and expanded.* Odessa, FL: Psychological Assessment Resources.

Hiscock, M., & Hiscock, C. K. (1989). Refining the forced-choice method for the detection of malingering. *Journal of Clinical and Experimental Neuropsychology, 11*, 967-974.

Johnson, J. L. & Lesniak-Karpniak, K. (1997). The effect of warning on malingering on memory and motor tasks in college samples. *Archives of Clinical Neuropsychology, 9*, 437-450.

Killgore, W. D. S. & DellaPietra, L. (2000). Using the WMS-III to detect malingering: Empirical validation of the Rarely Missed Index (RMI). *Journal of Clinical and Experimental Neuropsychology, 22*, 761-771.

Lee, G. P., Loring, D. W., & Martin, R. C. (1992). Rey's 15-Item Visual Memory Test for the detection of malingering. Normative observations on patients with neurological disorders. *Psychological Assessment, 4*, 43-46.

Lezak, M. D. (1995). *Neuropsychological Assessment* (3rd ed.). New York: Oxford University Press.

Meyers J. E., & Meyers K. R. (1995). *Rey Complex Figure Test and Recognition Trial Professional Manual.* Odessa, FL: Psychological Assessment Resources.

Mittenberg, W., Rotholc, A., Russell, E. & Heilbronner, R. L. (1996). Identification of malingered head injury on the Halstead-Reitan Battery. *Archives of Clinical Neuropsychology, 11*, 271-281.

Mittenberg, W., Theroux, S., Aquila-Puentes, G., Bianchini, K., Greve, K., & Rayls, K. (in press). Identification of malingered head injury on the WAIS-3. *The Clinical Neuropsychologist.*

Mittenberg, W., Theroux, S., Zielinski, R. E., & Heilbronner, R. L. (1995). Identification of malingered head injury on the Wechsler Adult Intelligence Scale-Revised. *Professional Psychology: Research and Practice, 26*, 491-498.

Pankratz, L. (1979). Symptom validity testing and symptom retraining: Procedures for the assessment and treatment of functional sensory deficits. *Journal of Consulting and Clinical Psychology, 47*, 409-410.

Pankratz, L., & Binder L. M. (1997). Malingering on intellectual and neuropsychological measures. In R. Rogers (Ed.), *Clinical Assessment of Malingering and Deception* (2nd ed., pp. 223-236). New York: Guilford Press.

Psychological Corporation (1997). *WAIS-3/WMS-3 Technical Manual.* San Antonio, TX: Author.

Psychological Corporation (1997). *The Wechsler Memory Scale, 3rd Edition.* San Antonio: Harcourt Brace & Co.

Regard, M. (1981). *Cognitive rigidity and flexibility: A neuropsychological study.* Unpublished PhD dissertation, University of Victoria, British Columbia.

Reitan, R. M., & Wolfson, D. (1993). *The Halstead-Reitan Neuropsychological Test Battery: Theory and Clinical Interpretation.* Tucson, AZ: Neuropsychology Press.

Rey, A. (1941). L'examen psychologique dans les cas d'en-cephalopathie traumatigue [The psychological exam in cases of traumatic encephalopathy]. *Archives de Psychologie, 28*(112), 286-340.

Rey, A. (1964). *L'examen clinique en psychologie* [The clinical exam in psychology]. Paris: Press Universitaire de France.

Rosenfeld, B., Sands, S. A., & Van Gorp, W. G. (2000). Have we forgotten the base rate problem? Methodological issues in the detection of distortion. *Archives of Clinical Neuropsychology, 15*, 349-359.

Saxe, L., & Ben-Shakhar, G. (1999). Admissibility of polygraph tests: The application of scientific standards post-*Daubert. Psychology, Public Policy, and Law 5*(1), 203-223.

Schretlen, D., Brandt, J., Kraft, L., & Van Gorp (1991). Some caveats in using the Rey 15-Item Memory Test to detect malingered amnesia. *Psychological Assessment, 3*, 667-672.

Slick, D., Hopp G., Strauss E., & Thompson, G. B. (1997). *Victoria Symptom Validity Test version 1.0 Professional Manual.* Odessa, FL: Psychological Assessment Resources.

Slick, D. J., Sherman E. M., & Iverson, G. L. (1999). Diagnostic criteria for malingered cognitive dysfunction: Proposed standards for clinical practice and research. *The Clinical Neuropsychologist, 13*, 545-561.

Spreen, O., & Strauss, E. (1998). *A Compendium of Neuropsychological Tests: Administration, Norms and Commentary* (2nd Ed). New York: Oxford University Press.

Strauss, E., Hultsch, D. F., Hunter, M., Slick D. J., Patry, B., & Levy-Bencheton, J. (2000). Using intraindividual variability to detect malingering in cognitive performance. *The Clinical Neuropsychologist, 14*, 420-432.

Thompson, G. B., Arruda, J. E., Jarvorsky, D. J., Dahl, K., Somerville, J. A., Guilmette, T. J, & Stern, R. A. (1996). *The effects of coaching on detection of malingering using the Abbreviated Hiscock Forced-Choice Procedure*. Poster presented at the annual meeting of the National Association of Neuropsychology, New Orleans, LA.

Tombaugh, T. N. (1996). *Test of Memory Malingering (TOMM).* Toronto, Canada: Multi-Health Systems, Inc.

Wechsler, D. (1981). *Wechsler Adult Intelligence Scale-Revised.* San Antonio, TX: The Psychological Corporation.

Wechsler, D. (1987). *Wechsler Memory Scale-Revised.* San Antonio, TX: The Psychological Corporation.

The Test of Memory Malingering (TOMM) in Forensic Psychology

Tom N. Tombaugh

Carleton University

SUMMARY. The Test of Memory Malingering (TOMM) is described with particular emphasis directed towards the historical setting within which the TOMM was developed. This includes a review of the criteria for developing a memory malingering test, and the use of the empirically derived decision along with a discussion of the relative merits of empirically based vs. statistically based rules for detecting malingering. Data from a series of five experiments showing the sensitivity of the TOMM to feigned memory impairments, guidelines for interpretation of TOMM scores, and answers to frequently asked questions about the TOMM are provided. Finally, the ability of the TOMM to meet the *Daubert* guidelines is addressed. *[Article copies available for a fee from The Haworth Document Delivery Service: 1-800-HAWORTH. E-mail address: <getinfo@haworthpressinc.com> Website: <http://www.HaworthPress.com> © 2002 by The Haworth Press, Inc. All rights reserved.]*

KEYWORDS. Malingering, neuropsychological assessment, TOMM

Tom N. Tombaugh is affiliated with Carleton University, Ottawa, ON.

Address correspondence to: Tom N. Tombaugh, PhD, Psychology Department, Carleton University, Ottawa, ON, Canada K1S 5B6.

The Test of Memory Malingering (TOMM) is published by Multi-Health Systems, 3770 Victoria Park Avenue, Toronto, ON, Canada M2H 3M6.

[Haworth co-indexing entry note]: "The Test of Memory Malingering (TOMM) in Forensic Psychology." Tombaugh, Tom N. Co-published simultaneously in *Journal of Forensic Neuropsychology* (The Haworth Medical Press, an imprint of The Haworth Press, Inc.) Vol. 2, No. 3/4, 2002, pp. 69-96; and: *Detection of Response Bias in Forensic Neuropsychology* (ed: Jim Hom, and Robert L. Denney) The Haworth Medical Press, an imprint of The Haworth Press, Inc., 2002, pp. 69-96. Single or multiple copies of this article are available for a fee from The Haworth Document Delivery Service [1-800-HAWORTH, 9:00 a.m. - 5:00 p.m. (EST). E-mail address: getinfo@haworthpressinc.com].

© 2002 by The Haworth Press, Inc. All rights reserved.

The issue of malingering is becoming increasingly important in the field of forensic psychology as more and more psychologists and neuropsychologists are being called upon to serve as expert witnesses. This is particularly true in cases involving traumatic brain injury (TBI) where alleged memory impairment is used to seek personal compensation, forms the basis for disability petitions, or constitutes a defense against prosecution for various crimes. In cases such as these, the psychologist must determine whether or not the person's cognitive abilities were diminished by the index injury. Part of this determination involves evaluating if the person had put forth maximum effort on each of the tests administered. In fact, one of the basic assumptions underlying the interpretation of results from any psychometric test is that the person was performing to the best of his/her ability. The failure to do so seriously questions the validity of the results, and in the absence of factors such as fatigue and depression raises the question of malingering.

The TOMM was developed to provide an objective, criterion-based psychometric test that is capable of discriminating between individuals with a *bona fide* memory impairment and those who feign symptoms of an impaired memory. Research on the TOMM was prompted by several factors, all of which indicated (1) the need for a specific test to detect feigning of a memory impairment, and (2) the failure of methods available in the mid 1990s to meet this need. The initial impetus for the development of the TOMM was the highly cited, but tragically flawed, article entitled *Accident Neurosis* (Miller, 1961). The gist of this article is that physical injury has no bearing on the symptoms associated with a concussion and patients recover spontaneously from concussions after their legal case is settled. However, subsequent research has failed to substantiate either the premise or the conclusion of this article (see reviews by Alexander, 1995; Binder, 1986; King, 1997).

A second source of influence was a series of articles that centered around the ongoing debate in the late 1980s and early 1990s as to whether neuropsychologists were able to detect malingering on the basis of neuropsychological test scores (Arkes, Faust, & Guilmette, 1990; Barth, Ryan, & Hawk, 1992; Bigler, 1990; Faust, Guilmette et al., 1988; Faust, Hart, Guilmette, & Arkes, 1988; Matarazzo, 1991; Schmidt, 1989). Although the debate was never conclusively decided, most evidence suggested that detection of malingering solely on the basis of neuropsychological test scores was, at best, problematic. Within this context, consensus exists among neuropsychologists, forensic psychologists, and psychiatrists that psychometric inconsistency is the hallmark of malingering. This inconsistency can range from a grossly exaggerated difference between feigned and *bona fide* symptoms, to a pattern of scores that does not make "neurological sense." Table 1 provides a list of commonly used qualitative signs and symptoms of malingering (also see Brandt, 1988; Franzen, Iverson, & McCracken, 1990; Nies & Sweet, 1994; Pankratz, 1988; Rogers, 1988; Ruff, Wylie, Tennant, 1993; Trueblood, 1994; Trueblood & Schmidt, 1993, Wasyliw & Cavanaugh, 1989; Zielinski, 1994). Although the idea of using these various indicators and patterns of inconsistency to identify malingering is conceptually appealing, its practical application is limited (Franzen, Iverson, & McCracken, 1990; Mittenberg, Azrin, Millsaps, & Heilbronner, 1993; Trueblood, 1994; Trueblood & Schmidt, 1993). This is primarily because the invalidity signs appear relatively infrequently. Moreover, even when invalidity signs are present, considerable overlap existed between them and valid symptoms (Mittenberg et al., 1993; Trueblood & Schmidt, 1993).

The failure to find diagnostically useful patterns of qualitative features prompted some neuropsychologists to determine if quantitative patterns of malingering could be established through the application of statistical procedures, such as discriminant function analyses. This approach was pioneered by Heaton et al. (1978), who reported that multivariate procedures were superior to clinical judgment in identifying malingerers. Although other authors have reported moderate success us-

TABLE 1. Qualitative Signs of Malingering on Tests of Cognitive Abilities

1. Memory impairment is disproportionate with the severity of the injury.
2. Discrepancies occur between scores on tests measuring similar abilities.
3. Inconsistencies are observed between memory complaints and observed behavior.
4. Failing easy items on a test while passing more difficult ones.
5. High frequency of "I don't know" answers.
6. High frequency of near misses or approximate answers.
7. Pronounced decline in performance on delayed retention test.
8. Scores on recognition tests are relatively lower than scores on recall tests.
9. Profile of test scores does not make "neurological sense."

ing multivariate procedures, several drawbacks have been identified. Most studies employing these techniques have compared the performance of malingerers with that of non-clinical participants. Very little evidence exists showing how well malingerers can be differentiated from other diagnostic groups. The evidence that does exist suggests that a separate set of empirically derived discriminant functions would be needed each time a different set of tests was used or when a different diagnostic category was involved (Bernard, Houston, & Natoli, 1993).

The general dissatisfaction with the previously discussed detection strategies led the present author to search the literature for some type of quantitative, criterion-based test that was capable of detecting feigned memory impairment. A review of the existing tests failed to reveal any single test that was judged to be adequate. In spite of this, there did seem to be an overall trend that the most sensitive malingering tests utilized some type of a recognition paradigm. The most prominent of these were the "symptom validity tests" (SVT) patterned after the research of Pankratz and associates (Pankratz, 1979; Pankratz, 1983; Pankratz, Fausti, & Peed, 1975). In this procedure, a stimulus is shown to the patient. Then, following a short delay, two stimuli are presented, and the patient is required to select the one seen previously. In this two-choice procedure the person can obtain a score of 50 percent by chance. Consequently, malingering is indicated by lower-than-chance performance. Several SVT procedures have been developed. All of these used numbers as stimuli (Binder, 1990, 1993; Bolter & Niccolls, 1993; Greiffenstein, Baker, & Gola, 1994; Guilmette, Hart, Giuliano, & Leininger, 1994; Hiscock & Hiscock, 1989; Rose, Hall, & Szalda-Petree, 1995; Slick, Hopp, Strauss, Hunter, & Pinch, 1994). For example, Hiscock and Hiscock (1989) used a 5-digit number as the stimulus to be remembered across short retention intervals. The basic procedure consists of presenting a card containing a 5-digit number for a brief study period. Then after a short delay (5s, 10s and 15s), a second card containing the original number and a new number is presented, and the person is required to identify the original number. Non-malingering participants typically identify the correct number on all of the trials, while malingering subjects make increasingly more errors as the length of the retention interval increases. An individual is assumed to be malingering when the number of errors falls below that expected by chance. However, research using the below-chance performance as the criterion for malingering has reported unacceptably low rates of identifying individuals who were asked to simulate the performance of brain-injured patients. Most participants who were simulating TBI symptoms performed at above-chance levels of accuracy and were misclassified as not malingering (Binder & Willis, 1991; Guilmette, Hart, & Giuliano, 1993; Martin, Gouvier, Todd, Bolter, & Niccolls, 1992; Prigatano & Amin, 1993). Particularly noteworthy is the fact that even though performance was greater-than-chance, it was still substantially below the performance of brain-injured or cognitively-intact individuals. This suggests that a decision rule based on the performance of a comparison group rather than on statistical probabilities might more adequately detect malingering.

Based on this observation, detection of malingering has relied increasingly on different types of norm-based criteria such as scores occurring below the lowest score obtained from a TBI group (Binder & Willis, 1991), scores lower than 90% correct (Guilmette, Hart, & Giuliano, 1993), or scores falling 1.3 standard deviations below the average TBI score (Greiffenstein, Baker, & Gola, 1994). Although these approaches have met with differing degrees of success, they have several disadvantages including the lack of a universally accepted criterion score, their sensitivity to various types of neurological impairments, the duration of time required for their administration, and their low degree of face validity as a memory test.

Despite these shortcomings, a substantial body of literature suggested that some type of a recognition procedure was the best candidate for developing a specific test to detect memory malingering. In light of this evidence, the TOMM was conceived and developed. The original idea for the TOMM stemmed from research in two related but independent fields–neuropsychology and cognitive psychology.

Prior to beginning research on the TOMM, a set of criteria was developed that contained the essential features that any test designed to detect malingering of a memory disorder should fulfill. These are enumerated below.

1. A malingering test should be *sensitive* to the feigning of memory deficits.
2. A malingering test should not be sensitive to any other factors that typically produce a memory deficit. That is, the malingering test should be *insensitive* to the effects of demographic variables (e.g., age, education, IQ, and gender), TBI and other neuropsychological disorders, and affective disorders such as depression.
3. The perceived difficulty of the malingering test should be greater than the actual difficulty of the malingering test.

4. The malingering test should have high face validity as a test of memory.
5. The malingering test should have universal application.

The reasoning underlying the first two criteria is obvious–a malingering test should only be sensitive to malingering. The clinical utility of a malingering test is decreased if it is affected by age, education, or various neurological/psychological variables. For example, if a malingering test is designed to differentiate between TBI patients who have a *bona fide* memory deficit and those who are feigning a memory deficit, the scores from these two groups should not be similar. Ideally, the two sets of scores should be distinct and separate, so that individuals in the two groups can be clearly discriminated by the test score. Although it is possible to compensate for the effects of some variables by providing norms stratified across different levels of the variable (e.g., age), this is much more difficult to achieve when the *bona fide* effects of the neurological insult overlap with the simulated effects of the same injury. Thus, in the case of TBI, it was considered essential to develop a memory malingering test that was not sensitive to the cognitive effects typically associated with TBI.

The third criterion was included because research has shown that individuals feigning memory impairments will be more readily detected when they believe that a test is difficult and they adjust their performance accordingly (Bickart, Meyer, & Connell, 1991; Slick et al., 1994). Keeping this in mind, the stimulus materials used in any malingering test should create the impression that the test is relatively difficult, while in reality the test should be relatively easy. Consequently, malingerers who think the test would be difficult for people with memory impairments should perform poorly, while individuals with impaired memory ability should have little difficulty with the task. Construction of a test along these lines also helps fulfill the first two criteria by producing a test that is sensitive to malingering but is insensitive to neurological impairments.

The fourth criterion addresses the issue of transparency. A memory malingering test will not be effective if it is readily perceived to be a malingering test. Recognition that it is a malingering test will greatly reduce, if not eliminate, the likelihood that the malingerer will malinger. Thus, it is essential that any memory malingering test should be perceived to be a legitimate measure of memory.

The final criterion was included to eliminate the need for translating the test to meet the needs of different language groups. Every attempt should be made to create a test that has the broadest possible range of application.

Research in the field of cognitive psychology suggested that all of these criteria could be achieved by using a recognition procedure that utilized pictures or line drawings of ordinary objects. Several studies have shown that cognitively-intact individuals have a remarkably high capacity for storing and retrieving pictorial information of objects commonly seen in everyday life (Nickerson, 1965, 1968; Shepard, 1967; Standing, Conezio, & Haber, 1970). In view of these findings, a recognition procedure using pictures of common objects served as the basis for developing the TOMM. The initial development and validation of the TOMM occurred over a 4-year period. Continued validation is ongoing.

TEST DEVELOPMENT AND VALIDATION

Test development and initial validation with non-clinical participants is fully described elsewhere (Tombaugh, 1996, 1997) and will only be summarized here.

Test Construction

The TOMM consists of two learning trials and a retention trial. The learning trials involve a study and a test phase. The study portion of each learning trial contains 50 line-drawn pictures (targets), each presented for 3 seconds with a 1-second interval between pictures. The same 50 pictures are used on each learning trial. However, they are presented in a different order on the second trial. During the test phase, each target is paired with a new line drawing (distractor). The person is required to select the correct picture (i.e., target) from each panel. For each answer, the examiner provides feedback about the correctness of the response. A delayed retention trial, consisting only of the test phase, is administered approximately 15-20 minutes after completion of the two learning trials.

The line drawings used as stimuli were selected from a pool of approximately 550 line drawings created specifically for the TOMM. Line drawings, rather than photographs, were used to ensure a greater homogeneity of stimulus material. A large pool of drawings was needed because each distractor is used only once. Only the target pictures are presented more than once.

Validation with a Non-Clinical Sample

Following development of the stimulus booklets, the TOMM was administered to 475 community-dwelling adults ranging in age from 17-84 years (Leger & Tombaugh, 1995; McIntyre, 1996). In order to obtain an estimate of the perceived difficulty of the TOMM, participants were asked at the beginning of each test phase to estimate how many of the pictures they thought they would be able to recognize.

Figure 1 shows the number of correct responses (obtained scores) and the number of estimated correct responses (estimated scores) for each trial. Two major findings are evident in this figure. First, participants were highly accurate in their ability to recognize previously seen pictures. On the first trial, approximately 95% of the targets were correctly identified. On the remaining two trials, the average number of correctly identified targets exceeded 99%. Multiple regression analyses performed on these data showed that age and education accounted for less than 8% of the variance. Second, the highly accurate performance of participants stands in marked contrast to how well they anticipated they would perform. This contrast is most evident on Trial 1, where esti-

FIGURE 1. Mean obtained and estimated scores on the TOMM for 475 cognitively-intact adults ranging in age from 17-84 years.

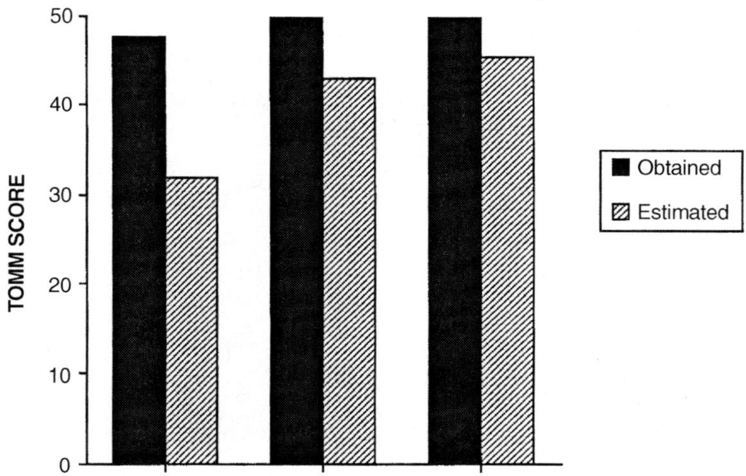

mated scores were significantly lower than obtained scores. The substantially higher estimates that occurred on the other two trials suggest that experience with the test permitted participants to upgrade their estimates. Nevertheless, under-estimations of performance were the rule rather than the exception.

The overall results from this study show that neurologically-intact individuals achieve exceptionally accurate performance. Moreover, comparisons of estimated and obtained performance indicate that the perceived difficulty exceeded the actual difficulty. This finding suggests that the TOMM should have high face validity as a memory test when administered as part of a battery of neuropsychological tests.

Validation with a Clinical Sample

The next stage in the development of the TOMM was to obtain scores from a clinical sample (1) to determine if performance on the TOMM was affected by various types of neurological impairments, and (2) to provide a set of clinically-based norms that would allow direct comparison between TOMM scores obtained from a person suspected of malingering and TOMM scores obtained from patients with similar levels of neurological insult but not suspected of malingering. That is, the clinically-based norms would provide a baseline whereby the performance of TBI patients suspected of malingering could be compared to the performance of non-malingering TBI patients.

The clinical sample consisted of 138 consecutive neuropsychological assessments from the Veterans Administration Medical Center, Boston, Massachusetts, and 23 TBI patients from an ongoing Ph.D. thesis (Rees, 1996). These patients were divided into five major groups based on their primary diagnosis: no cognitive impairment (n = 13), cognitive impairment (n = 42), aphasia (n = 21), TBI (n = 45), and dementia (n = 40). None of the TBI patients were engaged in compensation hearings or litigation. Estimated performance was not requested because preliminary testing revealed that asking for performance estimates substantially increased a patient's anxiety. Figure 2 shows the performance of each group. Comparison of the results with those in Figure 1 shows a remarkable similarity. With the exception of the dementia group, performance was exceptionally high on Trial 2 and on the Retention trial. In addition to scores from the TOMM, 81% of the patients also had scores from a visual learning task and a verbal learning task. Although these scores varied across the groups, they generally fell within the impaired range. Correlational analyses between these scores and

FIGURE 2. Mean obtained scores on the TOMM for five different groups of clinical patients: No Cognitive Impairment (NCI); Cognitive Impairment (CI); Aphasia, Traumatic Brain Injury (TBI), and Dementia.

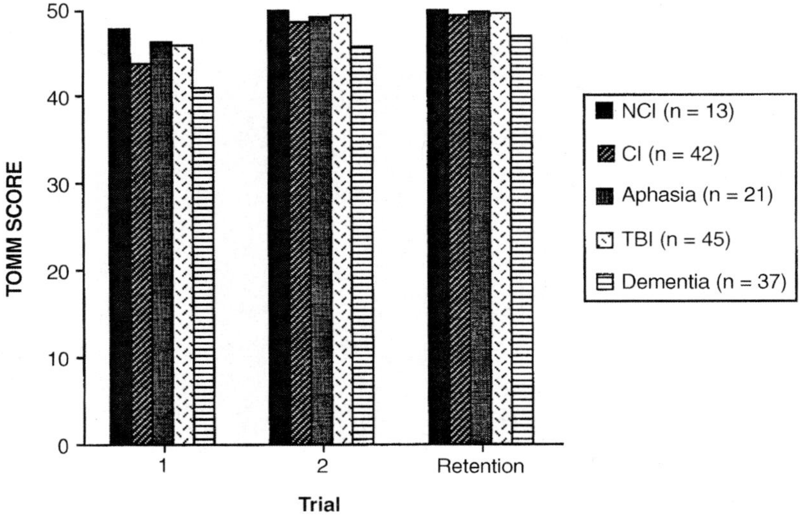

those obtained on the TOMM ranged from .20 to .35. This lack of substantial correlation is important, because it demonstrates that the TOMM is relatively insensitive to learning and memory dysfunctions associated with various neurological impairments. This fact, of course, should increase the TOMM's sensitivity to malingering in patients with impaired memory abilities.

Conspicuously absent from this clinical sample were patients with a primary diagnosis of depression. One of the defining features of depressive disorders is decreased motivation that often manifests itself as a pervasive lack of interest or decreased effort to perform to the best of one's ability. Moreover, depressive symptoms often accompany TBI and may contribute to impaired performance on psychometric tests. Thus, it is important to systematically evaluate what effect, if any, different levels of depression have on the TOMM. Consequently, after the initial publication of the TOMM, Rees, Tombaugh, and Boulay (2001) administered the TOMM to 26 inpatients whose primary diagnosis was a major depressive disorder. Scores on the Beck Depression Inventory (BDI) classified 6 patients as mildly depressed (BDI = 3-14), 8 patients as moderately depressed (BDI = 17-29), and 12 patients as severely depressed (BDI = 30-51). The scores from the depressed group were compared to TBI and community controls. The results showed that all three groups performed at comparable levels. In fact, no depressed patient scored lower than 49 on Trial 2 or on the Retention Trial. This includes 4 patients who were undergoing ECT.

ESTABLISHING AN EMPIRICALLY BASED CRITERION SCORE

The next step in the development of the TOMM was to establish a criterion score or decision rule that could be used to detect malingering. Based on the results previously described, performance on Trial 2 and on the Retention Trial was used as the point of reference. Inspection of the distribution of correct responses for all of the cognitively-intact participants and the clinical patients showed that most non-demented individuals achieved a perfect score on these trials. Moreover, rarely did a non-demented patient obtain a score lower than 45. In view of these results, the criterion score of 45 on Trial 2 or on the Retention Trial was selected. That is, any score lower than 45 should raise concern that an individual is not putting forth maximum effort and is likely malingering.

Since it was reasonable to assume that none of the community-dwelling participants or members of the clinical groups were feigning a memory impairment, the criterion score could be used to determine the degree to which it was able to correctly classify these participants as not malingering (i.e., specificity of the TOMM). The criterion score of 45 correctly classified 100% of the community-dwelling participants and 95% of the non-demented clinical patients (cognitively impaired = 90%, aphasia = 95%, TBI = 98%, depressed = 100%, and dementia = 73%).

It should be noted that below-chance performance also can be used as a statistical decision rule. This rule is based on the fact that a person can correctly identify 50% of the pictures by guessing. Thus, a score of 25 represents chance level of performance on the TOMM. Moreover, application of the binomial distribution (Siegel, 1956) shows that at the 95% confidence interval chance performance ranges from 18 to 32. Consequently, scores below 18 are unlikely to occur by chance. These low scores imply that the person knew some of the pictures were correct, but intentionally picked the incorrect picture.

VALIDATION OF CRITERION SCORE WITH "MALINGERING" SAMPLES

The evidence presented above shows that the TOMM met all of the previously discussed criteria except one–the ability to detect malingered memory performance. The greatest validity for a malingering test would be obtained from patients who have admitted to malingering–either before or after taking the test. However, malingering patients rarely make such an admission. A second approach is to use another test to classify participants into a malingering and a non-malingering group and then determine the accuracy of the TOMM in correctly identifying members of the two groups. Unfortunately, at the time the TOMM was being developed, no "gold standard" test was available to provide an a priori classification. Consequently, determination of the sensitivity of the TOMM to malingering relied on two general types of research designs. The first approach employed neurologically-intact individuals who simulated the performance of TBI patients. The second approach used individuals who had sustained some type of neurological insult and who were "at-risk" for malingering, such as occurs with compensation-seeking patients.

Simulation Studies

Overview: Four simulation studies were undertaken. All studies used the same basic procedure. A simulation group and a control group were used. Participants in the simulation group met with the experimenter 1 week before testing. At that time, the nature of the experiment was described, and participants were given a brief scenario describing an individual who was seeking compensation for a head injury caused by a motor vehicle accident. Participants were told they would be given a series of neuropsychological tests and were asked to *realistically* simulate the test performance of an individual who was still suffering from brain damage in order to be awarded compensation (for further details on scenario see Rees, Tombaugh, Gansler & Moczynski, 1998; Tombaugh, 1996, 1997). They were given 1 week to prepare and told that they could use any resource available to them. They returned approximately 1 week later to be tested. At that time, they were asked to reread the scenario. The procedure was the same for members of the control group except they did not receive the scenario and were asked to perform to the best of their ability.

Experiment 1: Forty-one volunteers from an introductory psychology class were randomly assigned to one of the two groups. During testing, the TOMM was administered. Table 2-Experiment 1 shows the mean obtained scores. On each trial, controls scored significantly ($p <$ .001) higher than simulators. On Trial 2, all of the controls scored higher than 48. In comparison, none of the simulators scored higher than 42. Using the cut-off score of 45, all of the controls and all of the simulators were correctly identified (i.e., 100% specificity and 100% sensitivity). Application of the same criterion score on the Retention Trial produced identical results. The distribution of scores on Trial 2 for the simulation group also was examined to determine what percentage of scores fell below chance performance. If chance is viewed as less than 25, then only 40% of simulators would have been correctly identified. Based on a 95% confidence interval (score of 19), none of the simulators would have been identified. Thus, it is evident that the empirically based criterion score of 45 is superior to the statistically based chance level of performance.

Experiment 2: One possible shortcoming of Experiment 1 is that the participants lacked any experience with the TOMM. This naivete about the TOMM may have restricted their ability to produce a credible simulated performance. That is, in the absence of knowledge about the relative difficulty of the TOMM, the simulators may have over-reacted to

TABLE 2. Means (SD) for Three Simulation Studies Using the TOMM

	Group	
Measure	Simulator	Control
Experiment 1		
Trial 1	27.2 (6.8)	47.8 (2.5)
Trial 2	27.9 (7.2)	49.9 (0.8)
Retention	26.4 (7.5)	49.7 (1.1)
Experiment 2		
Trial 1	30.3 (5.8)	49.3 (1.0)
Trial 2	31.9 (7.7)	50.0 (0.0)
Retention	27.5 (9.4)	50.0 (0.0)
Experiment 3		
Trial 1	32.6 (7.8)	48.8 (1.7)
Trial 2	35.7 (8.9)	49.9 (0.2)
Retention	34.3 (8.2)	50.0 (0.0)

its perceived difficulty and unrealistically lowered their performance. In order to evaluate the effects of test sophistication on the ability of the TOMM to discriminate between simulating and control participants, the present experiment used a within-subject design in which 20 students from an introductory psychology class were administered the TOMM under two counterbalanced instructional sets–to simulate and to "try your best" (Rees et al., 1998). The results from this study are shown in Table 2-Experiment 2. Inspection of this table shows essentially the same results as previously reported–simulators performed significantly lower than controls. Statistical analysis appropriate to a two-way mixed design showed only the effects of instruction to be significant ($p < .001$). Application of the < 45 criterion score to Trial 2 or to the Retention Trial correctly identified 95% of the simulators (simulate first = 91% vs. simulate second = 100%) and 100% of the controls. Application of the < 25 chance level criterion correctly identified only 10% of the simulators on Trial 2 (5% at the 95% level of confidence), and 30% of the simulators on the Retention Trial (20% at the 95% level of confidence).

Experiment 3: The consistent finding in the first two experiments that the TOMM accurately discriminated between simulators and controls used a different procedure from that used in clinical situations. That is, only a single neuropsychological test was administered. Typically a malingering test is embedded within a battery of neuropsychological tests. Because the individual has the opportunity to compare the malingering test with other tests measuring the same cognitive ability, the clinical situation presents a distinctively different environment to detect malingering than occurred in the first two experiments. It is possible that when the TOMM was presented in isolation, its true purpose is less obvious than when administered in conjunction with other neuropsychological tests. Experiment 3 tested this hypothesis by embedding the TOMM within a series of other tests: California Verbal Learning Test (Delis, Kramer, Kaplan, & Ober, 1987), Mental Control, Digit Span, and Visual Reproduction subtests of the Wechsler Memory Scale-Revised (Wechsler, 1987); Trail Making Test–Parts A and B (Reitan & Wolfson, 1985); Ruff Figural Fluency Test (Ruff, 1988); Controlled Oral Word Association (FAS & Animals; Lezak, 1995); Information subtest from the Wechsler Adult Intelligence Scale-Revised (Wechsler, 1987), and Finger Tapping Test (Reitan & Wolfson, 1985). The TOMM was administered between the WMS-R Visual Reproduction Test and WAIS-R Information subtest, approximately 30 minutes after the beginning of the test session.

Forty-four students from an introductory class were randomly assigned to the simulation or control group (Rees, 1996). Mean scores for the TOMM are shown in Table 2-Experiment 3. Essentially the same relationship occurred in Experiment 3 that was described in the first two experiments. The TOMM accurately discriminated between the two groups on each trial ($p < .001$) When the cut-off score of 45 was applied to Trial 2 and to the Retention Trial, 100% of the control participants were identified, and 84% and 88% of the simulators were identified, respectively. Application of the < 25 chance criterion correctly identified only 12% of the simulators on Trial 2 (4% at the 95% level of confidence) and 12% of the simulators on the Retention Trial (8% at the 95% level of confidence).

Experiment 4: In spite of the convergent evidence presented above, it is possible that the sensitivity of the TOMM to detect feigned memory impairment may have reflected, at least in part, the participants' lack of knowledge about the cognitive effects of TBI. Even though the participants were encouraged to learn about head injuries in the week immediately preceding their participation, it is very possible that they did not use this time to increase their knowledge about TBI. Even if they had "researched" the topic, knowledge gained from secondary sources may not have been sufficient to ensure an adequate presentation of memory deficits compared with knowledge acquired through the actual experience of the trauma.

In order to ensure that participants were truly knowledgeable about the types of cognitive impairments caused by TBI, 18 individuals were recruited for Experiment 4 who had actually suffered a TBI. Approximately half of them were randomly assigned to a TBI simulation group and half to a TBI control group. For reasons of comparison, the scores from these two groups were compared to a cognitively-intact control group (Rees, Tombaugh, Gansler, & Moczynski, 1998). Inspection of Figure 3 reveals that virtually the same relationship occurred in this experiment as occurred in the first three experiments. That is, TBI simulators scored significantly lower than both the TBI control group and the cognitively-intact control group on each trial ($p < .001$). Application of the cut-off score of 45 on Trial 2 and on the Retention trial yielded 100% correct classification for the TBI simulators and greater than 98% for the two control groups. Chance level performance correctly classified only 6% of the TBI malingerers on Trial 2 and 38% on the Retention Trial (0% at the 95% level of confidence on both trials). Overall, the results from Experiment 4 show that when individuals with preexisting knowledge of the effects of TBI on cognitive abilities are asked to

FIGURE 3. Mean obtained scores on the TOMM for TBI simulators, TBI controls, and cognitively-intact controls.

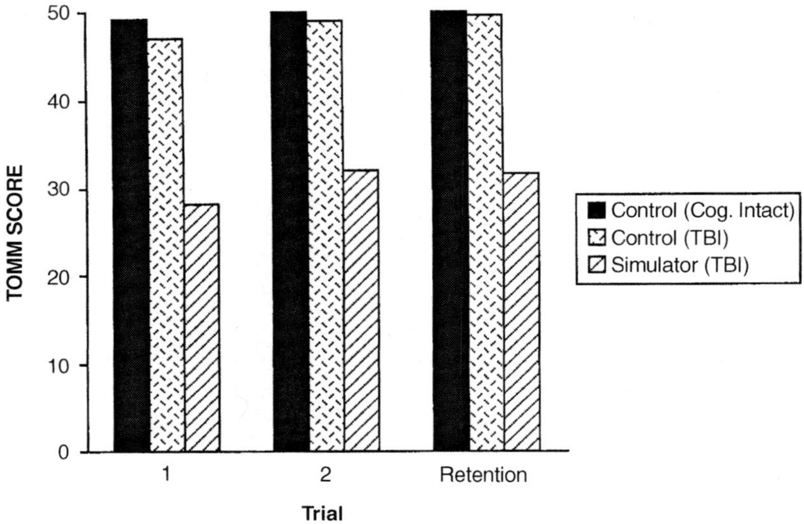

simulate malingering, they performed substantially lower than TBI controls. This finding is similar to the performance of university students asked to malinger, and indicates that the results from the first three experiments can not be attributed to the participants' lack of first-hand knowledge about the effects of TBI.

Litigating vs. Not Litigating Comparison

The research strategy employed in the present experiment (Gansler, Tombaugh, Mocyznski, & Rees, 1995) was to evaluate individuals in situations where the likelihood of malingering is great. A prime example is when the opportunity for financial compensation exists, such as occurs in personal liability suits or disability petitions. Traditionally, this strategy has been implemented by comparing the performance of people who are litigating with those who have a similar neurological insult but who are not litigating. This strategy is employed in the present study as another way of providing converging evidence that the TOMM is a clinically useful measure of malingering.

Three groups of participants were used: TBI litigating (n = 13); TBI non-litigating (n = 13) and hospital controls (n = 13). The TOMM was administered as part of a complete neuropsychological assessment. The results, presented in Figure 4, demonstrate that the scores for the TBI litigating group are significantly lower on each trial ($p < .001$) than those for the other two groups. On Trial 2 and on the Retention Trial, the TOMM correctly identified 77% of the TBI litigating group, and 100% of the two control groups. Although the 77% detection rate is somewhat lower than reported in the previous studies, it must be noted that this detection rate does not refer to the detection of patients who were asked to malinger but merely identifies individuals who were in the "high-risk" condition. In this context, these results suggest that 77% of the patients in the TBI litigating group were probably feigning some type of memory disorder for personal gain. Using chance performance as a decision rule identified only 23% of the litigating group on Trial 2 (15% at the 95% level of confidence) and 15% of the litigants on the Retention Trial (0% at the 95% level of confidence).

CONCLUSION

The results from the five experiments provide convergent evidence that the TOMM readily differentiated between malingering and non-

FIGURE 4. Mean obtained scores on the TOMM for TBI litigating patients, TBI not litigating patients, patient controls, and cognitively-intact controls.

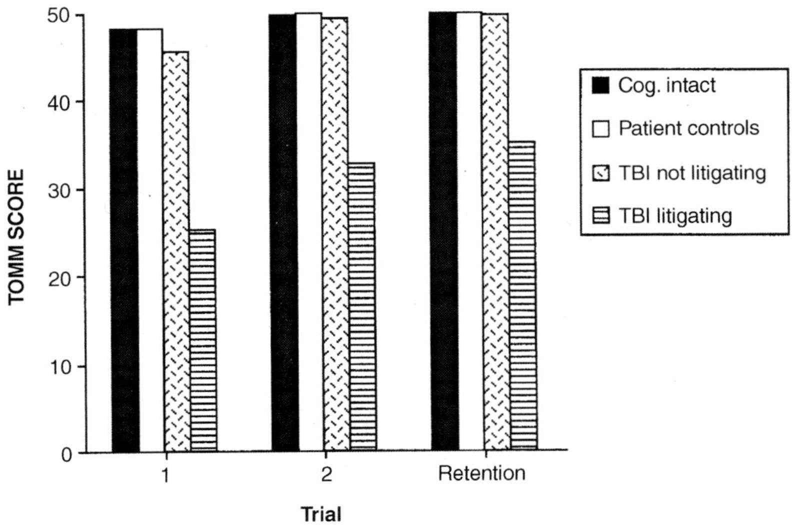

malingering individuals, and suggest that the TOMM is a useful psychometric test for detecting exaggerated or deliberately faked memory impairment. High levels of accuracy were obtained with different types of participants and different types of experimental designs. Moreover, this high degree of accuracy occurred when the comparison was between groups as well as when each participant served as his/her own control. Similar results were obtained when the TOMM was administered alone or within the context of a full neuropsychological battery.

The clinical utility of the TOMM was further indicated by the fact that the TOMM was not sensitive to the effects of age or years of education. Moreover, performance on the TOMM was not affected in a clinical sample of cognitively impaired, depressed, aphasic, and TBI patients. In fact, the only clinical sample that produced lower TOMM scores was a dementia group. Even here, these individuals still obtained an average score of greater than 92% on Trial 2. However, this finding is not a particularly negative finding for using the TOMM to detect malingering in a general clinical sample. That is, it is unlikely that feigning memory impairment is a major issue when dementia patients undergo neuropsychological assessment.

The results obtained from these experiments also illustrate how detection of malingering depends on the type of decision rule employed. In each experiment, care was taken to contrast the detection rates using two types of decision rules: below-chance performance and an empirically derived criterion. Classification based on the statistically based decision produced unacceptably low rates of detection. This finding is consistent with previous research showing that individuals suspected of feigning memory impairment or asked to simulate the performance of brain-injured patients perform at above-chance-levels of accuracy (Beeter & Williams, 1995; Binder & Willis, 1991; Guilmette et al., 1993; Martin, Gouvier, Todd, Bolter, & Niccolls, 1992; Prigatano & Amin, 1993; Slick et al., 1994). In contrast, the use of an empirically based criterion score yielded high levels of detection accuracy. This finding illustrates the value of validating a malingering test with an appropriate clinical reference group. In the present instance, the reference group selected was one that contained TBI patients. (The issue of criterion groups will be addressed more fully later in the paper.)

Before turning to other issues, it should be noted that the failure of the below-chance decision rule to correctly identify most members of a simulation group does not necessarily mean that it is not a useful criterion, but only that it should not be used as the sole basis for detecting feigned memory impairment. That is, instances where below-chance performance does occur provide powerful evidence that a person is malingering. In fact, performance on a forced-choice recognition test that is significantly below chance has the same interpretive thrust as does performance that is significantly above chance–the individual has a good memory!

INTERPRETING THE TOMM

The conclusion that a person is malingering should *never* be made *solely* on the basis of the score that a patient obtains on the TOMM. Any statement concerning whether a person is malingering or feigning a memory impairment depends on many factors starting with the basic conceptual issue of how "malingering" is defined. It should be quite obvious from its title that the Test of Memory Malingering was developed with a definite, preconceived notion that malingering was situation specific. That is, contrary to the impression of many individuals who have contacted the present author with specific questions about how to interpret the TOMM, the TOMM is *not* a malingering test, *per se*. It is a test to determine whether or not an individual is feigning or malingering a *memory* impairment. Consequently, the TOMM does not measure a general trait called "malingering." In forensic assessments, the TOMM is not an appropriate test to evaluate whether or not a person is faking a psychiatric disorder any more than it would be appropriate to use it to determine if a person is faking a back injury. Moreover, the interpretation of the TOMM should not be used to identify a "malingerer," but rather to indicate that a person is malingering. Although individuals "malinger," malingering should not be viewed as a personality trait. That is, malingering in one instance does not necessarily mean that the person will always malinger or that the person will ever malinger again. In many instances, individuals with TBI who malinger are "good" people caught in "bad" situations. It must also be remembered that malingering is not an all-or-none phenomenon, but that it exists in different degrees ranging from minor exaggeration of existing symptoms to flagrant faking of non-existent symptoms. The fact that malingering is motivated by external incentives suggests that it varies across situations. In addition, it is expected the individuals will be selective in the symptoms they distort.

Thus, it is apparent that the interpretation of the TOMM is based on how malingering is defined. The definition of malingering has been postponed until this time because it has as much impact on the interpreting of a test score as it exerts on the development of a test. In essence, malingering is a specific type of motivational disorder which DSM-IV (American Psychiatric Association, 1994) defines as the "intentional production of false or grossly exaggerated physical or psychological symptoms, motivated by external incentives such as avoiding military duty, avoiding work, obtaining financial compensation, evading criminal prosecution or obtaining drugs" (p. 683). This definition has three critical components. First, there is a conscious intent or motivation. Second, symptoms are either invented or exaggerated. Third, there is an external incentive. A low score on the TOMM only addresses the second issue. Evidence about intentionality and the motivational basis of the behavior must come from other sources. In most cases, it is difficult, if not impossible, to demonstrate conclusively that falsification of symptoms represents an intentional behavior motivated solely by external gains. Even when conscious deception occurs, it may not be possible to rule out that the fabrication served, at least in part, to preserve the person's psychological integrity by unconsciously serving other psychological needs. One potential solution to this problem in forensic assessments is to circumvent the entire issue of intentionality by viewing a low score as an indication that the person failed to put forth his/her best effort without attributing this motivational bias to any particular source. While this approach may be criticized for its atheoretical bias, it does emphasize that a low score on the TOMM has serious implications for the validity of scores obtained from other neuropsychological or intellectual tests. At the very least, a low TOMM score raises serious questions about the person's motivation to perform well on other tests and should raise concerns regarding the validity of scores from these tests.

The validity of neuropsychological test scores requires that individuals put forth maximum effort. If this effort is lacking, the motivation underlying suboptimal performance may stem from non-neurological sources that do not involve the conscious desire to seek external gain through deception. That is, an individual's failure to put forth maximum effort does not necessarily mean the person is a "malingerer." It often represents a "cry for help," or it may reflect other motivational factors such as a psychiatric disorder, anxiety, fulfillment of emotional needs, a desire to obtain retribution, or fulfillment of unconscious needs. The variety of reasons that may lead to suboptimal effort may be referred to collectively as "motivational disorders." Viewed in this context, the acronym "TOMM" could mean "Test of Memory Motivation."

Given the above, it is obvious that the most forthright answer to the frequently asked question "Does a below-criterion score on the TOMM mean the person is malingering?" is "No, a low score is only suggestive of malingering." The criterion score should be viewed as a guideline, with the likelihood of malingering increasing as the person's score deviates further from the normative baseline for the specific diagnostic group. The TOMM score should be viewed as the starting point for a diagnosis of malingering, not as the end point.

Any diagnosis of malingering requires considerable clinical judgement. Making the diagnosis of malingering is no different from any other diagnosis, and the process should follow the existing guidelines and conceptual principles governing all diagnostic processes. It should reflect the same inferential processes and careful examination of all relevant information that occurs in any other neuropsychological diagnosis. The conclusion that a person is noncompliant or feigning symptoms should be based on convergent evidence gathered from a variety of other sources, including scores from other malingering tests and "invalidity signs" (see Table 1). Information about the onset, duration, and severity of the impairment is particularly critical in determining if the symptoms make "neurological sense." Level of pre-injury functioning, as well as the context in which the examination occurred, must be considered. Thus, to paraphrase Larrabee (1990), a score on a test does not diagnose malingering; rather the diagnosis is made by a skilled psychologist.

Finally, it should be mentioned that the existence of malingering does not exclude the possibility that *bona fide* symptoms might exist. For example, a person may be exaggerating existing symptoms. Ironically, a person's attempt to obtain compensation by exaggerating symptoms often makes it difficult, if not impossible, to determine if genuine impairments actually exist. In a forensic setting, establishing that a person is feigning a memory impairment may be of assistance to the legal process, but it has little clinical utility for the individual. The "diagnosis" of malingering merely establishes that a person did not put forth optimal effort; it does not attempt to provide any answers as to the reasons underlying the suboptimal effort other than the tacit assumption that the person is trying to avoid prosecution or obtain compensation.

INQUIRIES FROM USERS OF THE TOMM

Since the publication of the TOMM, there have been several inquiries about the administration and interpretation of the TOMM. Most of these center around the question as to whether it is appropriate to administer the TOMM to individuals when appropriate norms are not available. Most often this question arises in forensic cases that involve developmentally handicapped individuals whose IQ falls in the low average to borderline range (i.e., 70-89 on the WAIS) and who have been charged with some type of a criminal offense. Frequently, attorneys will attempt to defend the behavior of these individuals on the basis of their lowed cognitive abilities, focusing particularly on their diminished ability to remember certain events and facts. The specific question that arises concerns the availability of norms for the intellectually challenged. Unfortunately, no published norms are currently available. However, this is certainly a topic that needs further research and one for which the present author would be more than happy to supply the materials to any investigator interested in pursuing this topic.

Although this answers the specific question pertaining to the availability of norms for the developmentally handicapped, it does not address the more general question as to whether it is appropriate to administer the TOMM to an individual for whom norms are not available. The simplest and most psychometrically sound answer to this question is that the TOMM should be administered only when appropriate norms are available and there is an issue about diminished memory. Certainly, the interpretation of below-criterion scores for an individual lacking the appropriate normative base is clearly unwarranted and ill advised. However, a recent discussion with W. Mittenberg (personal communication) indicated that there may be at least two instances where the TOMM might provide useful information in the absence of norms. This first is when the score falls below chance levels, thereby indicating that the person may be feigning a memory disorder. The second is where the score is greater than the criterion score of 45. A score in this range provides evidence that the individual is putting forth maximum effort on at least one test and may serve as a source of converging evidence for determining the person's motivational set. Keeping the above in mind, it seems that the issue is not whether it is appropriate to administer the TOMM in the absence of appropriate norms, but rather what types of scores are legitimately interpretable in the absence of norms.

One unique inquiry deserves special attention. This inquiry concerned a challenge to the reliability of the TOMM that was based on the fact that when the TOMM was administered (and videotaped in the office of the defendant's lawyer), the interval between the pictures was different than the 3 seconds cited in the manual as the correct inter-stimulus interval (ISI). The challenge presented evidence that the ISI averaged 2.7 seconds rather than 3.0 seconds. Although this seems like a trivial challenge and one that can be easily rebutted, it illustrates how important it is, particularly in forensic cases, to adhere strictly to the prescribed administrative procedures. In order to avoid challenges based on imprecise administrative procedure, a computerized version of the TOMM is available.

DAUBERT GUIDELINES

The degree to which any psychometric instrument meets scientific criteria has always been a concern for test developers and publishers. In addition to those generally accepted standards contained in any standard text on psychometrics, the *Daubert* guidelines provide the generally accepted standards to assist judges in determining the scientific admissibility of evidence, particularly when presented by expert witnesses. Since results from the TOMM often are used to support the contention that an individual is feigning a memory impairment, it is essential that the TOMM is able to meet each of the *Daubert* guidelines. Each of the four guidelines is listed below in the form of a question, followed by an answer.

Question 1. "Has the technique (i.e., TOMM) been tested or is subject to being tested?"

Answer: Most certainly! All of the research described previously demonstrates that the TOMM has been fully tested using a variety of different types of procedures and samples.

Question 2. "Has the TOMM been subjected to peer review and publication?"

Answer: Most certainly! Three major articles have been published in peer reviewed journals (Tombaugh, 1996; Rees, Tombaugh, Gansler, & Moczynski, 1998; Rees, Tombaugh, & Boulay, 2001). The TOMM has been reviewed and published by Multi-Health Systems, a major publisher of psychological tests. Numerous workshops on the TOMM have been presented in Canada, United States, Australia, and New Zealand.

Question 3. "What is the known or potential rate of error in applying the TOMM?"

Answer: The review of the TOMM cited evidence from cognitively-intact individuals varying in age, education and gender. Error rate for misclassification of these individuals was 0% (i.e., specificity = 100%). Research with TBI patients had an error rate of 2%. This extremely low error rate is particularly critical because the TOMM is typically used with this type of injury. Low error rates were also found with depressed patients (0% error) and aphasia patients (5%). Research performed with cognitively-impaired individuals with varying degree of impairment (excluding TBI patients) misclassified only 10% of the participants–all of these patients were severely impaired (Korsakoff, pontine infarct, right frontal craniotomy, and right thalamic infarct). Thus, overall, it is very unlikely to misclassify a non-malingering individual as malingering. A review of the research studies using simulated groups and groups at-risk for malingering also revealed a very low misclassification rate. That is, the rate of detecting malingering was very high. For example, the detection rate for all of the simulation studies performed was greater than 90%.

Question 4. "To what extent has the TOMM been accepted in the relevant scientific community?"

Answer: The acceptance of the TOMM can be judged by the number of articles that have been published in peer reviewed journals that support its scientific basis (see above), the number of favorable reviews that have been published (Gierok & Dickson, 2000; Hubley & Zumbo, 1996; Smith & Haley, 1998; Spreen & Strauss, 1998; Vallabhajosula & van Gorp, 2001), and prevalence of use. All of these indicators clearly demonstrate that the TOMM has been highly accepted by the scientific community.

REFERENCES

Alexander, M.P. (1995). Mild traumatic brain injury: Pathophysiology, natural history, and clinical management. *Neurology*, *45*, 1253-1260.

American Psychiatric Associataion. (1994). *Diagnostic and Statistical Manual of Mental Disorders* (4th edition). Washington, DC: American Psychiatric Association.

Arkes, H.R., Faust, D., & Guilmette, T.J. (1990). Response to Schmidt's (1988) comments on Faust, Hart, Guilmette, and Arkes (1998). *Professional Psychology; Research and Practice*, *21*, 3-4.

Barth, J.T., Ryan, T.V., & Hawk, G.L. (1992). Forensic neuropsychology: A reply to the method skeptics. *Neuropsychology Review*, *2*, 251-266.

Beetar, J.T., & Williams, J.M. (1995). Malingering response styles on the Memory Assessment Scales and symptom validity tests. *Archives of Clinical Neuropsychology, 10*, 57-72.

Bernard, L.C., McGrath, M.J., & Houston, W. (1993). Discriminating between simulated malingering and closed head injury on the Wechsler Memory Scale-Revised. *Archives of Clinical Neuropsychology, 8*, 539-551.

Bickart, W.T., Meyer, R.G., & Connell, D. (1991). The symptom validity technique as a measure of feigned short-term memory deficit. *American Journal of Forensic Psychology, 9*, 3-11.

Bigler, E.D. (1990). Neuropsychology and malingering: Comment on Faust, Hart, and Guilmette (1988). *Journal of Consulting and Clinical Psychology, 58*, 244-247.

Binder, L.M. (1986). Persisting symptoms after mild head injury: A review of the postconcusive syndrome. *Journal of Clinical and Experimental Neuropsychology. 8*, 323-346.

Binder, L.M. (1990). Malingering following minor head trauma. *The Clinical Neuropsychologist, 4*, 25-36.

Binder, L.M. (1993). An abbreviated form of the Portland digit recognition test. *The Clinical Neuropsychologist, 7*, 104-107.

Binder, L.M., & Willis, S.C. (1991). Assessment of motivation after financially compensable minor head trauma. *Psychological Assessment: A Journal of Consulting and Clinical Psychology, 3*, 175-181.

Bolter, J.F., & Niccolls, R. (1993). *Multi-Digit Memory Test*. San Luis Obisbo, CA: Wang Neuropsychological Laboratories.

Brandt, J. (1988). Malingered amnesia. In R. Rogers (Ed.). *Clinical Assessment of Malingering and Deception* (pp. 65-83). New York: Guilford Press.

Delis, D.C., Kramer, J.H., Kaplan, E., Ober, B.A. (1987). *The California Verbal Learning Test (CVLT)*. New York: The Psychological Corporation.

Faust, D., Guilmette, T.J., Hart, K., Arkes, H.R., Fishburne, F.J., & Davey, L. (1988). Neuropsychologists' training, experience, and judgement accuracy. *Archives of Clinical Neuropsychology, 3*, 145-163.

Faust, D., Hart, K., Guilmette, T.J., & Arkes, H.R. (1988). Neuropsychologist's capacity to detect adolescent malingers. *Professional Psychology: Research and Practice, 19*, 508-515.

Franzen, M.D., Iverson, G.L., & McCracken, L.M. (1990). The detection of malingering in neuropsychological assessment. *Neuropsychology Review, 1*, 247-279.

Gansler, D., Tombaugh, T.N., Moczynski, N.P., & Rees, L.M. (1995). Test of Memory Malingering (TOMM): Initial validation in a traumatic brain injury cohort. Poster presented at the Annual Meeting of the National Academy of Neuropsychology, San Francisco, CA.

Gierok, S.D., & Dickson, A.L. (2000). Test of Memory Malingering. *Archives of Clinical Neuropsychology, 15*, 649-651.

Greiffenstein, M.F., Baker, W.J., & Gola, T. (1994). Validation of malingered amnesia measures with a large clinical sample. *Psychological Assessment, 6*, 218-224.

Guilmette, T.J., Hart, K.L., & Giuliano, A.J. (1993). Malingering detection: The use of a forced-choice method in identifying organic versus simulated memory impairment. *The Clinical Neuropsychologist, 7*, 59-69.

Guilmette, T.J., Hart, K.J., Giuliano, A.J., & Leninger, B.E. (1994). Detecting simulated memory impairment: Comparison of the Rey Fifteen-Item Test and the Hiscock Forced-Choice presentation. *The Clinical Neuropsychologist, 8*, 283-294.

Heaton, R.K., Smith, H.H., Lehman, R.A.W., & Vogt, A.T. (1978). Prospects for faking believable deficits on neuropsychological testing. *Journal of Consulting and Clinical Psychology, 46*, 892-900.

Hiscock, M., & Hiscock, C.K. (1989). Refining the forced-choice method for the detection of malingering. *Journal of Clinical and Experimental Neuropsychology, 11*, 967-974.

Hubley, A. M., & Zumbo, B. D. (1996). A report on the Test of MemoryMalingering (TOMM). *International Test Commission Newsletter, 6*(2), 24-25.

King, N. (1997). Mild head injury: Neuropathology, sequelae, measurement and recovery. *British Journal of Clinical Psychology, 36*, 161-184.

Larrabee, G.J. (1990). Cautions in the use of neuropsychological evaluations in legal settings. *Neuropsychology, 4*, 239-247.

Leger, H.M., & Tombaugh, T.N. (1995). Normative data for the two-choice TOMM. Unpublished data, Carleton University, Ottawa, Ontario.

Martin, R.C., Gouvier, D., Todd, M.E., Bolter, J.F., & Niccolls, R. (1992). Effects of task instruction on malingered memory performance, *Forensic Reports, 5*, 393-397.

Matarazzo, J. (1991). Psychological assessment is reliable and valid: Reply to Ziskin and Faust. *American Psychologist, 46*, 882-884.

McIntyre, N. (1996). *The Recognition Memory Battery: Normative data from age 16 to age 85*. Unpublished Ph.D. dissertation, Carleton University, Ottawa, Ontario.

Miller, H. (1961). Accident neurosis. *British Medical Journal, 1*, 919-925 and 992-998.

Mittenberg, W., Azrin, R., Millsaps, C., & Heilbronner, R. (1993). Identification of malingered head injury on the Wechsler Memory Scale-Revised. *Psychological Assessment, 5*, 34-40.

Nickerson,.R.S. (1965). Short-term memory for complex meaningful visual configurations: A demonstration of capacity. *Canadian Journal of Psychology, 19*, 155-160.

Nickerson, R.S. (1968). A note on long-term recognition memory for pictorial material. *Psychonomic Science, 11*, 58.

Nies, K.J., & Sweet, J.J. (1994). Neuropsychological assessment and malingering: A critical review of past and present strategies. *Archives of Clinical Neuropsychology. 9*, 501-552.

Pankratz, L. (1979). Symptom Validity Testing and symptom retraining: Procedures for the assessment and treatment of functional sensory deficits. *Journal of Consulting and Clinical Psychology, 47*, 409-410.

Pankratz, L. (1983). A new technique for the assessment and modification of feigned memory deficit. *Perceptual and Motor Skills, 57*, 367-372.

Pankratz, L. (1988). Malingering on intellectual and neuropsychological measures. In R. Rogers (Ed.), *Clinical Assessment of Malingering and Deception* (pp. 169-192). New York: Guilford Press.

Pankratz, L., Fausti, A., & Peed, S. (1975). A forced-choice technique to evaluate deafness in the hysterical or malingering patient. *Journal of Consulting and Clinical Psychology, 43*, 421-422.

Prigatano, G.P., & Amin, K. (1993). Digit memory test: Unequivocal cerebral dysfunction and suspected malingering. *Journal of Clinical and Experimental Neuropsychology, 15*, 537-546.

Rees, L.M. (1996). *A Test of Memory Malingering: A simulation study and clinical validation*. Unpublished Ph.D. dissertation, Carleton University, Ottawa, Ontario.

Rees, L.M., Tombaugh, T.N., & Boulay, L. (2001). Depression and the Test of Memory Malingering. *Archives of Clinical Neuropsychology, 16*, 501-506.

Rees, L.M., Tombaugh, T.N., Gansler, D., & Moczynski, N. (1998). Five validation experiments of the Test of Memory Malingering (TOMM). *Psychological Assessment, 10*, 10-20.

Reitan, R.M., & Wolfson, D. (1985). *The Halstead-Reitan Neuropsychological Test Battery*. Tucson, AZ: Neuropsychology Press.

Rogers, R. (1988). *Clinical Assessment of Malingering and Deception*. New York: Guilford Press.

Rose, F.E., Hall, S., & Szalda-Petree, A.D. (1995). Portland Digit Recognition Test-Computerized: Measuring response latency improves the detection of malingering. *The Clinical Neuropsychologist, 9*, 124-134.

Ruff, R.M. (1988). *The Ruff Figural Fluency Test*. San Diego, CA: Neuropsychological Resources.

Ruff, R.M., Wylie, T., & Tennant, W. (1993). Malingering and malingering-like aspects of mild closed head injury. *Journal of Head Trauma Rehabilitation. 8*, 60-73.

Schmidt, J.P. (1989). Why recent researchers have not assessed the capacity of neuropsychologists to detect malingering. *Professional Psychology: Research and Practice, 209*, 140-141.

Siegel, S. (1956). *Nonparametric Statistics for the Behavioral Sciences*. New York: McGraw-Hill.

Shepard, R. (1967). Recognition memory for words, sentences and pictures. *Journal of Verbal Learning and Verbal Behavior, 6*, 156-163.

Slick, D., Hopp, G., Strauss, E., Hunter, M., & Pinch, D. (1994). Detecting dissimulation: Profiles of simulated malingerers, traumatic brain-injury patients, and normal controls on a revised version of Hiscock and Hiscock's forced-choice memory test. *Journal of Clinical and Experimental Neuropsychology, 16*, 472-481.

Smith, G., & Haley, J.A. (1998). Test Review: Test of Memory Malingering. *American Psychology-Law Society News*, Spring, 16-18 & 29-30.

Spreen, O., & Strauss, E. (1998). *A Compendium of Neuropsychological Tests: Administration, Norms, and Commentary* (2nd edition). New York: Oxford University Press.

Standing, L., Conezio, J., & Haber, N. (1970). Perception and memory for pictures: Single-trial learning of 2500 visual stimuli. *Psychonomic Science, 19*, 73-74.

Tombaugh, T.N. (1997). The Test of Memory Malingering (TOMM): Normative data from cognitively intact and cognitively impaired individuals. *Psychological Assessment, 9*, 260-268.

Tombaugh, T.N. (1996). *The Test of Memory Malingering (TOMM)*. Toronto, Canada: Multi-Health Systems.

Trueblood, W. (1994). Qualitative and quantitative characteristics of malingered and other invalid WAIS-R and clinical memory data. *Journal of Clinical and Experimental Neuropsychology, 16*, 597-607.

Trueblood, W., & Binder, L.M. (1997). Psychologists' accuracy in identifying neuropsychological test protocols of clinical malingerers. *Archives of Clinical Neuropsychology, 12*, 13-27.

Trueblood, W., & Schmidt, M. (1993). Malingering and other validity considerations in the neuropsychological evaluation of mild head injury. *Journal of Clinical and Experimental Neuropsychology, 15*, 578-590.

Vallabhajosula, B., & van Grop, W.G. (2001). Post-*Daubert* admissibility of scientific evidence on malingering of cognitive deficits. *Journal of the American Academy of Psychiatry and the Law, 29*, 302-215.

Wasyliw, O.E., & Cavanaugh, J.L. (1989). Simulation of brain damage: Assessment and decision rules. *Bulletin of the American Academy of Psychiatry and Law, 17*, 373-386.

Wechsler, D. (1987). *The Wechsler Adult Intelligence Scale-Revised*. San Antonio, TX: The Psychological Corporation.

Zielinski, J.J. (1994). Malingering and defensiveness in the neuropsychological assessment of mild traumatic brain injury. *Clinical Psychology: Science and Practice, 1*, 169-183.

The Word Memory Test and the Validity of Neuropsychological Test Scores

Paul Green

Neurobehavioural Associates

Paul R. Lees-Haley

Independent Practice

Lyle M. Allen III

CogniSyst, Inc.

SUMMARY. The Word Memory Test (WMT; Green, Allen, & Astner, 1996) contains measures that are very sensitive to exaggeration or poor effort but insensitive to all but the most extreme forms of cognitive impairment. The WMT is unique among symptom validity tests because of its extensive validation in clinical forensic settings, rather than relying on simulation research with healthy volunteers. Effort measured by the WMT predicted 50% of the variance in a total of 30,736 neuropsychological test results from 904 consecutive patients involved in com-

---

Paul Green is affiliated with Neurobehavioural Associates, Edmonton, AB.

Paul R. Lees-Haley is in independent practice, Huntsville, AL.

Lyle M. Allen III is affiliated with CogniSyst, Inc., Durham, NC.

Address correspondence to: Paul Green, PhD, Suite 201, 17107-107 Avenue, Edmonton, AB, Canada, T5S 1G3 (E-mail: paulgreen@shaw.ca).

[Haworth co-indexing entry note]: "The Word Memory Test and the Validity of Neuropsychological Test Scores." Green, Paul, Paul R. Lees-Haley, and Lyle M. Allen III. Co-published simultaneously in *Journal of Forensic Neuropsychology* (The Haworth Medical Press, an imprint of The Haworth Press, Inc.) Vol. 2, No. 3/4, 2002, pp. 97-124; and: *Detection of Response Bias in Forensic Neuropsychology* (ed: Jim Hom, and Robert L. Denney) The Haworth Medical Press, an imprint of The Haworth Press, Inc., 2002, pp. 97-124. Single or multiple copies of this article are available for a fee from The Haworth Document Delivery Service [1-800-HAWORTH, 9:00 a.m. - 5:00 p.m. (EST). E-mail address: getinfo@haworthpressinc.com].

© 2002 by The Haworth Press, Inc. All rights reserved.

pensation claims. In group data, WMT-measured effort was sufficient to eliminate or reverse major effects, such as the presence of greater impairment in people with severe versus mild head injuries. The removal of invalid data from people failing the WMT was found to make a major difference to the conclusions of several studies. Properly interpreted, the WMT will meet *Daubert* challenges. *[Article copies available for a fee from The Haworth Document Delivery Service: 1-800-HAWORTH. E-mail address: <getinfo@haworthpressinc.com> Website: <http://www.HaworthPress.com> © 2002 by The Haworth Press, Inc. All rights reserved.]*

KEYWORDS. Effort, malingering, brain injury, symptom validity

INTRODUCTION

When the Word Memory Test (WMT; Green, Allen, & Astner, 1996) was invented, it was already clear from a growing literature that there was a risk of concluding that a person had impairment of a certain ability, such as verbal memory, when the real reason for the low test score was deliberate exaggeration or insufficient effort to produce valid data. There was no *a priori* reason for assuming that misleading test results would only be found in people with a particular diagnosis, and so the WMT was given to every outpatient referred to the first author for neuropsychological assessment. Over several years, the WMT has been given to over 1,000 consecutive adults in this series, all involved in compensation or disability claims. This has become the central data set from which much of the WMT research has evolved. Each patient was given two days of assessment, including neuropsychological tests, along with various other measures of symptom validity for cross-validation. These included the Computerized Assessment of Response Bias (CARB; Allen, Conder, Green, & Cox; 1997), the Recognition Hits and Logit Formula derived from the California Verbal Learning Test (CVLT; Delis, Kramar, Kaplan, & Ober, 1987; Millis, 1999) and Warrington's Recognition Memory Test for Words and Faces (WRMT; Warrington, 1984). A number of patients were also given the English version of the Amsterdam Short Term Memory Test (ASTMT; Schmand, Lindeboom, Schagen, Heijt, Koene, & Hamburger, 1998) or the 21 item test (Iverson, 1998).

The main sample included 535 patients with head injuries and 89 neurological patients with strokes, aneurysms, multiple sclerosis, tumor, epilepsy or other miscellaneous conditions. Also included were patients referred with major depression (n = 85) anxiety disorders (n =

18), orthopedic injuries (n = 77), chronic fatigue syndrome (n = 34), chronic pain syndrome or fibromyalgia (n = 61) and various other conditions (n = 101). Various other groups are described below, including patients who were asked to simulate memory impairment. With data from the series of 1,000 consecutive cases, we can study not only effort itself but, more importantly, we can determine the influence of varying degrees of effort on many neuropsychological test scores and symptom rating scales. These data have revealed unexpectedly large and widespread effects of effort on test scores. It will be shown that, in the samples studied, poor effort, as measured by the WMT, had a much larger effect on neuropsychological test scores than did severe brain injury or neurological diseases.

STRUCTURE OF THE WMT

The WMT is a test of verbal learning and memory, designed to allow the evaluation of a person's effort to do well in the course of taking the test, so that a determination can be made about whether or not the person's test scores are valid estimates of ability. The WMT measures the ability to learn a list of 20 word pairs (e.g., pig-bacon, fish-fin, dog-cat) presented orally or on a computer screen. The effort components of the WMT were designed to avoid confusing actual impairment with deliberate exaggeration. They are virtually insensitive to all but the most extreme forms of impairment of learning and memory, and the range of genuine scores is very narrow, as shown below.

After being shown 20 word pairs on the computer screen, the person is required to choose the word from the original list in each of 40 new word pairs (e.g., "dog" from "dog-rabbit"). This is the immediate recognition trial (IR), the first measure of effort. Feedback regarding correctness is given to assist motivated patients in learning for later subtests. After a half-hour delay, the delayed recognition trial (DR) is presented, which is very similar to IR, but it includes different foil words (e.g., "dog-rat"). Several measures of response consistency are computed, including the consistency of responses between the 40 paired IR and DR trials, which correlates very highly with results from the IR and DR subtests.

Following the main effort measures, the patient is given four separate measures of *memory* ability: the Multiple Choice subtest (MC), in which the person is shown the first word from each pair and is asked to choose the matching word from eight options; Paired Associates (PA), in which the person is given the first word from each pair by the tester and is asked to tell the tester the second word; Delayed Free Recall (DFR), in which the person is asked to recall as many words as possible from the list in any order. The Long Delayed Free Recall subtest (LDFR) may also be given after a further 20-minute delay. The computer printout shows the patient's results in two graphs and lists the person's raw scores on all measures of the WMT. A table shows the patient's scores compared with the mean scores obtained from each of a number of reference groups, including patients with moderate to severe brain injury, neurological patients, patients with normal verbal memory, patients with impaired verbal memory and bright normal controls.

A cardinal feature of the WMT is that it consists of multiple subtests that vary widely in their objective difficulty level. Only one other test that measures symptom validity shares this primary characteristic, the Validity Indicator Profile (VIP; Frederick, 1997). However, unlike the VIP, the WMT was designed with the dual purpose of measuring both effort and actual ability, and the WMT measures the most common form of exaggeration, which is exaggeration of memory difficulties. Given the structure of the WMT, it is very difficult for a person who is not making a full effort to produce a plausible profile. Users of the WMT will recognize that there are many other WMT results and statistics listed in the computer printout that may be useful in the detection of exaggeration and in quantifying memory ability. The WMT can be administered orally or partially unattended on a PC-compatible computer. The two forms of the WMT appear to be equivalent, but the majority of WMT research to be discussed below has employed the computerized form.

WMT SCORES IN PATIENTS WITH BRAIN INJURIES AND NEUROLOGICAL DISEASES

Table 1 shows the mean scores on the WMT effort subtests from 40 healthy volunteers (Iverson, Green, & Gervais, 1999), compared with 57 patients with moderate to severe brain injuries whose mean Glasgow Coma Scale score was 9. These patients were described in detail by Allen and Green (1999) in a supplement to the WMT manual. The mean scores from the brain-injured patients on both IR and DR were above 95% correct (i.e., above 38 out of 40 correct). The mean score on the three WMT effort measures in the healthy volunteers was 97.8% correct, compared with 95.1% correct in the patients with brain injuries.

TABLE 1. Performance on WMT Subtests from 40 Healthy Community Volunteers versus 57 Patients with Moderate to Severe Brain Injuries (Mean Glasgow Coma Scale Score = 9.6; *SD* = 4.1)

	Brain-injured patients (n = 57)		Healthy volunteers (n = 40)	
	Mean	SD	Mean	SD
Effort measures				
WMT-IR	95.5%	5.1	98.0%	2.8
WMT-DR	96.1%	3.9	98.6%	2.4
IR/DR Consistency	92.8%	6.4	96.8%	3.8
CARB Total Test	98.3%	2.6	-	
WMT Memory subtests				
Multiple Choice (MC)	85.4%	16.1	95.4%	6.7
Paired Associates (PA)	78.3%	19.8	92.6%	9.6
Delayed Free Recall (DFR)	45.4%	15.2	63.7%	12.5

Allen and Green (1999) also showed that, within the brain-injured patients, the WMT effort measures (IR, DR and Consistency) were unrelated to major measures of head injury severity, including Glasgow Coma Scale scores, duration of post-traumatic amnesia and duration of loss of consciousness.

Further evidence that the WMT effort scores are relatively insensitive to brain disease is listed in Table 2, showing the mean scores from 40 patients with neurological diseases, including brain tumors, strokes, multiple sclerosis and ruptured cerebral aneurysms. These patients are described both individually and as a group by Green and Allen (1999). The neurological patients were divided into two groups of equal size, based on scoring above or below the groups' median on the learning trials of the CVLT. Despite a significant difference on the CVLT in these two subgroups, there were no significant differences in their scores on the WMT effort measures nor on an independent effort measure, the CARB (Table 2). These data show that the WMT effort scores are relatively insensitive to actual cognitive impairment and, in particular, are unaffected both by neurological diseases and by memory impairment in this sample. On the other hand, the scores on the WMT subtests designed to measure memory (MC, PA, DFR and LDFR) were all significantly lower in the neurological patients with impaired CVLT scores

TABLE 2. No Difference in Mean Scores on CARB and the WMT Effort Measures Between Neurological Patients with "Normal Range" versus "Impaired" Memory Scores on the CVLT

	Impaired memory (n = 20)		Normal range memory (n = 20)		
Effort Tests	Mean	SD	Mean	SD	P value
WMT-IR	96.1%	3.3	96.2%	3.6	0.92 ns
WMT-DR	94.9%	5.5	96.2%	4.9	0.44 ns
WMT-CONS	93.0%	5.9	93.8%	5.5	0.57 ns
CARB total	96.8%	5.6	97.4%	3.3	0.58 ns
Memory Tests					
CVLT 1 to 5	40.9	7.2	54.4	7.8	0.0001
CVLT-SD	6.5	3.1	10.7	2.8	0.0001
CVLT-LD	7.3	2.9	11.4	2.6	0.0001
Recog.hits	13.5	2.2	14.3	1.3	0.17 ns
WMT-MC	81.0%	12.4	90.0%	10.4	0.014
WMT-PA	70.8%	18.3	84.0%	13.8	0.014
WMT-DFR	36.7%	10.9	50.2%	14.8	0.002
WMT-LDFR	35.8%	14.9	50.6%	17.3	0.01
VIQ	93.4	12.4	101.2	15.4	0.08
Educ (yrs)	13.4	3.1	13.2	3.0	0.8

than in those with normal range CVLT scores. These data show that what the latter subtests are measuring (memory) is not the same as what the effort subtests measure (effort).

There is a strong ceiling effect on the WMT effort measures. For example, on WMT IR, even neurological patients with impaired verbal memory scored a mean of almost 100% correct (96.1%, *SD* = 3.3), which is almost identical to the mean score from those with normal verbal memory. In marked contrast, the neurological patients with impaired memory, as defined by their CVLT results (Table 2), scored only 36.7% correct (*SD* = 10.9) on the WMT free recall subtest (WMT-DFR). WMT effort scores are not normally distributed, but the WMT memory scores are normal.

SEVERITY OF HEAD INJURY

We might expect WMT effort scores to decline as the severity of brain injury increases. Paradoxically, the opposite pattern was found in a large sample of head injury patients of mixed severity (Green, Iverson, & Allen, 1999). On average, those with the most mild head injuries obtained significantly *lower* WMT effort scores than the patients with the most severe brain injuries. Such a result is the exact opposite of what would be expected if we were using a test sensitive to brain injury and if all test results were valid. It was argued that, as a group, the patients with mild head injuries were more inclined to exaggerate their impairment. This was supported by significantly lower scores in the mild head injury group on an independent test of effort, the CARB. When cases failing CARB were excluded, there were no longer any significant differences between the mild and the severe brain injury patients on any of the WMT effort scores. This provided more evidence that the WMT effort scores are sensitive to effort but insensitive to brain injury in the vast majority of outpatients studied.

ABNORMAL BRAIN SCAN RESULTS AND EFFORT SCORES

In the current series of 1,000 patients, there were 187 patients referred for assessment after a head injury who had abnormal results on CT or MRI scans of the brain and 149 who had normal brain scan results. The mean Glasgow Coma Scale scores in these two groups were, respectively, 10.3 ($SD = 4.2$) and 14.7 ($SD = 1.2$). Also, the median duration of post traumatic amnesia was 48 hours in those with abnormal scans, but it was zero in the group with normal brain scans. The mean WMT-DR score in those with abnormal brain scans (90.7% correct, $SD = 13$) was found to be paradoxically significantly *higher* than the mean WMT-DR score in those with normal brain scans (82.5% correct, $SD = 18.4$; Mann-Whitney U test, $z = 4.3$, $p < .0005$). This difference cannot be explained as a result of more severe cognitive impairment in one group than the other, because the results are directly contrary to this hypothesis. Instead, it is more likely that, on average, symptom exaggeration was greater in those with normal brain scans than those with abnormal brain scans in this sample of patients assessed in the course of compensation claims. Indeed, on the Memory Complaints Inventory (MCI; Green & Allen, 1997), it was found that those with normal brain scans complained of significantly *more* memory problems than those with abnormal brain scans (mean MCI scores of 36.3%, *SD* = 17 versus 25.0%, *SD* = 17, F [2,300] = 9.9, p < .0005). In further support of the effort hypothesis, the mean score on an independent effort test, the CARB, was significantly higher in those with abnormal brain scans (mean 96.1% correct, *SD* = 9.4) than in those with normal scans (mean 91.1%, *SD* = 15.3; z = 3.3, p = .001). Higher WMT and CARB scores in those with the most severe brain injuries are most reasonably explained by the more severely injured patients making a greater effort to do well on these tests. The difference in scores obviously does not reflect differences in brain functioning between these two groups.

SCORES OF VOLUNTEER SIMULATORS, PATIENTS AND PATIENT SIMULATORS ON WMT

Table 3 shows the scores from 25 highly educated volunteers, mainly psychologists and physicians, who were asked to take the WMT and to act as if they had impaired memory. These simulators were told that the WMT was designed to detect exaggeration of impairment, and they were asked to try to circumvent the WMT effort measures and respond as if they had genuine memory impairment. Whereas 40 healthy volunteers obtained a mean score of 97.8% correct on the three WMT effort measures, the sophisticated simulators obtained a mean score of only 67.2% correct (Iverson, Green, & Gervais, 1999). On the delayed recognition subtest (DR), the simulators obtained a mean score which was *13 standard deviations lower* than the mean from the healthy volunteers who made an effort to score as well as they could (Table 3). Even though these data are not normally distributed, such figures give a clear indication of the magnitude of the difference between full effort versus incomplete effort in group data. The mean WMT-DR score of the sophisticated simulators was more than five standard deviations lower than the mean score from neurological patients known to have impaired verbal memory (Table 2) and more than seven standard deviations lower than the mean score from 57 patients with a mean Glasgow Coma Score of 9 (Table 1). Thus, volunteers who were trying to act as if they had impairment and who said that they tried hard to be subtle to avoid being detected actually scored many standard deviations below people with brain damage or brain disease. Clearly, they were not very successful in their goal.

Similar results were obtained from 20 consecutive patients tested

TABLE 3. Mean Scores (Percent Correct) and Standard Deviations on Each of the WMT Effort and Memory Scores from All Groups

Group	N	WMT-IR	WMT-DR	Consistency	Multiple Choice	Paired Associates	Delayed Free Recall
1) Community volunteers	40	98.0 (2.8)	98.6 (2.4)	96.8 (3.8)	95.4 (6.7)	92.6 (9.6)	63.7 (12.4)
2) Sophisticated simulators	25	70.9 (12.6)	67.2 (16.5)	63.5 (12.4)	46.8 (17.9)	48.2 (19.9)	35.0 (19.2)
3A)* Clinical cases making genuine effort	20	98.1 (3.1)	98.2 (3.0)	96.6 (3.8)	94.0 (8.0)	92.7 (10.1)	54.1 (13.7)
3B) Clinical cases asked to simulate	20	63.2 (12.6)	62.0 (12.0)	62.7 (8.9)	39.5 (14.3)	40.7 (17.1)	21.6 (9.6)
4)** Clinical cases exaggerating	20	63.5 (18.0)	62.8 (22.1)	62.4 (12.4)	46.3 (20.6)	38.0 (15.3)	26.2 (10.0)

* Group 3A scored significantly higher than groups 3B and 4 on all WMT measures.
** Group 4 was not significantly different from group 3B on any WMT measure.

clinically who passed the WMT effort measures during their regular disability examination. Their mean WMT-DR score was 98.2% correct (*SD* = 3), and so it was obviously very easy for them. They were asked to take the WMT again, but this time to fake memory impairment and make every effort to avoid being detected as exaggerating (Table 3). On retesting, their mean WMT effort score dropped from 98.2% to 62.6% correct. Their mean WMT-DR score of 62% was (a) *more than 12 standard deviations* lower than they were actually capable of achieving, as shown by their scores when they took the test the first time, and (b) 8.7 standard deviations lower than the mean score from patients with moderate to severe brain injuries. In using standard deviations with such data, there is no assumption of normality, and WMT effort test data are definitely not normally distributed. Whether data are normal or not, Tchebycheff's theorem (Hays, 1963) states that the *maximum* probability of a score in a given distribution that is k standard deviations from the mean is 1/k squared. Hence, in the patients with moderate to severe brain injuries in Table 1, a WMT-DR score of 62% is highly improbable (one in 76 or p = 0.013), and yet this was the mean score from patients trying to simulate impaired memory. Their WMT-DR scores were so low that it was highly unlikely that they were drawn from the same group as patients with brain injury.

It is very likely that the exaggeration shown by the patients who volunteered to simulate impairment on the WMT is similar to what would be exhibited by other patients who spontaneously exaggerate impairment. To examine this suggestion, a group of 20 patients who spontaneously failed the WMT effort measures on clinical testing was selected from a database with results from 1160 patients tested independently by Dr. Roger Gervais for disability. These 20 patients were selected to match the patients from group 3A in Table 3 in terms of diagnosis, age, gender and years of education. Their mean score on the WMT effort measures was 62.9% correct (Table 3), which is almost identical to the mean score from the patients who were asked to fake impairment without being detected (62.6% correct). This experiment demonstrates that, on average, patients who try to present themselves as having impaired memory on the WMT, when they are not really impaired, score in the region of 5 to 10 standard deviations below people known to have actual brain injury or disease. The experimental simulating patients, the matched patients who failed the WMT spontaneously, and the sophisticated simulators all produced mean WMT effort scores more than ten standard deviations below what they were actually capable of achieving.

In 949 consecutive patients of mixed diagnoses who took the computerized WMT, the 660 cases who passed the effort measures scored a mean of 96.7% correct (*SD* = 3.7) on IR, 96.8% correct (*SD* = 3.6) on DR and 94.7% (*SD* = 4.8) on Consistency. In contrast, for the 289 patients who failed any one of the computerized WMT effort measures, the mean scores on the same measures were 73.3% correct (*SD* = 15.8) on IR, 70.4% correct (*SD* = 16.5) on DR and 68.4% (*SD* = 11.5) on Consistency. On DR, for example, those who failed the WMT scored more than seven standard deviations lower than those who passed. Such enormous differences between the mean test scores of large patient groups are very unusual indeed in psychology. It may also be noted from the standard deviations that the variation in scores in those making inadequate effort greatly exceeds the variation in those making a good effort. Almost anyone making an effort to do so can score close to 100% correct on WMT effort measures, but the range of scores in exaggerators is wide.

EFFORT HAS A LARGER EFFECT ON NEUROPSYCHOLOGICAL TEST SCORES THAN SEVERE BRAIN INJURY

It is essential in validating effort tests to prove that, when the test is failed, the person's other test results are probably invalid. This step has not been taken in the validation of most effort tests, but much of the research with the WMT has been directed towards this fundamental goal. The results provide some of the strongest evidence that failure on the WMT implies invalid results on other tests. A hint of the likely effect of exaggeration of cognitive deficits on neuropsychological test results in general may be found in the mean memory test scores shown in Tables 1, 2 and 3. We know that the clinical cases discussed earlier, who were asked to simulate impairment, did not have impaired memory because they took the WMT and scored a mean of 54.1% correct (*SD* = 13.7) on delayed free recall of the word list. However, when they were later asked to exaggerate and simulate memory difficulties under experimental instructions, their mean score was 21.6% (*SD* = 9.6), which was more than thirty points (or 2.4 standard deviations) lower than their actual ability, as previously measured. This score was lower than the mean score from neurological patients with impaired memory (36.7%, Table 2), and it was less than half of the mean score of 45.4% correct, obtained from patients with head injuries sufficient to produce a mean Glasgow Coma Scale score of 9 (Table 1). In the 1,000 case series, the 289 patients who failed the computerized WMT effort measures obtained a mean free recall score (DFR) of 28.9% (*SD* = 12.6), which is also lower than the mean scores from patients with brain injuries or neurological diseases shown in Tables 1 and 2. These data provide one illustration of an important general finding in these groups of patients, which is that *poor effort or exaggeration of cognitive difficulties has a larger effect on memory test scores than brain injury or neurological disease.*

It is necessary to ask whether effort, as measured by the WMT, also has a pronounced effect on scores from other tests, which are in widespread use, such as the CVLT. One way of answering such a question is to examine the mean scores on an isolated CVLT measure, such as long delayed free recall, in people who score in all ranges on the WMT effort measures. In the 1,000 patients tested consecutively, 949 cases took both the CVLT and the computerized or oral WMT, and the correlation between WMT-DR and CVLT long delayed free recall was 0.56. It is very clear in Table 4 that effort, as measured by the WMT and as reflected in the mean WMT-DR score, is a continuum. The lower their WMT effort score, the lower the patients scored on CVLT long delayed free recall. In the group scoring 67% on WMT-DR (which is fairly typical of those making incomplete effort, irrespective of diagnosis) the long delayed free recall score was an average of 1.2 standard deviations lower than in those with a mean WMT-DR score of 97%, which is typical of good effort. Such large effects are not only found with the CVLT but with almost any test so far examined.

TABLE 4. Mean CVLT Long Delayed Free Recall Scores for People Scoring at Each Level on WMT Effort Measures

Number of cases	Mean WMT-DR % correct (SD)	Mean CVLT LD FREE score out of 16 (SD)	LD FREE SD units below top scoring group
624	97.6% (2.5)	11.0 (3.1)	0.0
136	87.5% (2.7)	8.9 (3.2)	−0.68 SD
76	77.1% (2.8)	8.0 (3.5)	−0.97 SD
49	67.6% (2.7)	7.2 (3.3)	−1.2 SD
38	56.7% (2.6)	5.1 (2.7)	−1.9 SD
46	42.0% (8.4)	3.9 (2.9)	−2.3 SD

Note: WMT-DR = Word Memory Test Delayed Recognition subtest; LDFREE = Long Delayed Free Recall score on the California Verbal Learning Test.

To examine the effects of effort on neuropsychological test scores in general, the scores from the widely used tests listed in Table 5 were studied, using data from 904 clinical patients from the present series (Green, Rohling, Lees-Haley, & Allen, 2001; Rohling, Green, Allen, & Lees-Haley, 2000). All of the measures were converted to z-scores relative to external normative groups and then averaged for each case. Using this technique, the mean score from normal controls would be a z-score of zero, and non-zero scores would represent standard deviations above and below the normal mean. A composite mean score, the overall test battery mean (OTBM), was calculated from the scores from up to 43 separate measures of ability, with a mean of 34 measures for each of 904 cases, yielding 30,736 ability test scores (Table 5). In these data, the mean score from the WMT effort measures was found to explain 49% of the variance in the OTBM (r = 0.7). In contrast, age and education, which are widely regarded as significant determinants of test scores, explained only 4% and 11% of the variance, respectively, indicating relatively small effects of age and education on the same OTBM data, when compared with the effects of effort.

EFFORT AS A CONFOUNDING VARIABLE IN GROUP STUDIES

Patients with mild head injuries who passed the WMT-DR effort measure produced a slightly below average OTBM mean z-score of

TABLE 5. Forty-Three Ability Measures Contributing to the Overall Test Battery Mean (OTBM-43), Grouped by Domain

Executive Functioning, EF (n = 6) Wisconsin Card Sorting Test–Categories achieved & Perseverative errors; Category Test–Errors; Thurstone Word Fluency; Ruff Figural Fluency–Total score and perseverations; Gorham's Proverbs

Memory and Learning, ML (n = 15) CVLT–Total, Trial 5, SDFR, LDFR, Recognition hits; Cognisyst Story Recall Test–Immediate & Delayed Recall; Word Memory Test–Paired Associates, Multiple Choice, Delayed recall, Long delayed recall; Rey CFT–Delayed Recall & Recognition; Warrington Recognition Memory Test–Words & Faces

Verbal Comprehension, VC (n = 4) WAIS-R VIQ or MAB VIQ; WRAT-3–Reading, Spelling & Arithmetic

Attention and Working Memory, AW (n = 8) Trail-Making Test–Parts A & B; Digit Span–Forward & Backward; Visual Memory Span–Forward & Backward; CVLT–Trial 1 & List B

Perceptual Organization, PO (n = 4) Rey Complex Figure Test–Copy & Recall; Benton's Judgment of Line Orientation; WAIS-R PIQ

Psychomotor Skills, PS (n = 6) Finger Tapping–Dom. & N'dom; Grip Strength–Dom. & N'dom; Grooved Pegboard–Dom & N'dom.

−0.12 (Green, Rohling, Lees-Haley, & Allen, 2001). That is, on average, they scored only 0.12 standard deviations below the normal mean on a wide range of neuropsychological tests, which was not significantly different from the mean score from people with orthopedic injuries and no head injury. In contrast, those with mild head injuries who failed WMT-DR produced a mean score of −1.36 on the OTBM. Thus, exaggeration, as shown by low WMT effort scores, caused the mean OTBM from the exaggerators to be *more than 10 times further below the normal mean* than scores from patients with similar mild head injuries but who were making a genuine effort. Also, patients with severe brain injuries who passed the WMT effort tests scored only 0.39 standard deviations below the normal mean on the OTBM. Hence, the effect of exaggeration in people with mild head injuries was to suppress their overall mean performance on an average of 34 tests to a degree which was more than three times greater than the effects of a severe brain injury (−1.36 versus −0.39).

If effort has such large effects, it could easily obscure real differences between groups. In fact, there was no significant difference between the mean OTBM score in patients with mild head injuries versus those with severe brain injuries or neurological diseases (Green, Rohling, Lees-Haley, & Allen, 2001; Rohling et al., 2000). If taken out of context, such results would suggest that many of the neuropsychological tests in common use are insensitive to the effects of brain injury or disease. However, when the data from patients failing the WMT were excluded because they were assumed to be invalid, it was found that the patients with severe brain injuries and neurological diseases scored significantly lower on the OTBM than patients with mild head injuries, as we would expect. In this study, we could only see that severe brain injury had more of an effect on test scores than mild head injury once we removed the invalid data created by people failing the WMT effort tests.

RANGES OF EFFORT AND OTBM SCORES

Failure on WMT-IR and DR means that a person has scored about three standard deviations or more below the mean score obtained by patients with moderate to severe brain injuries shown in Table 1. We can see in Table 6 that 374 people who scored at or above the mean WMT score from these patients with brain injuries obtained a mean OTBM score of exactly zero, meaning that they performed at the same level as normal controls on the mean of 34 test scores. However, the mean OTBM was −0.44 in the 271 cases who scored between 0 and 2 standard deviations below the severe brain injury mean on WMT effort measures. Scores in this range would not fall below the usual (conservative) cut-offs for incomplete effort. Those who scored more than six standard deviations below the mean from people with brain injuries on the WMT effort measures (n = 104) obtained a mean OTBM of −1.8 (Table 6). Thus, their mean score across an average of 34 measures was 1.8 standard deviations below the normal mean, which represents an extremely low level of performance, when we consider that the effect of a severe brain injury was only to produce a mean OTBM of −0.39. In this instance, poor effort led to a mean OTBM that was 4.6 times further below the normal mean on the OTBM than the mean score of patients with severe brain injuries. Again, incomplete effort had a far greater effect on the overall test battery mean than severe brain injury. This is all the more significant because more than half of all patients in the group with a mean OTBM of −1.8 were cases of mild head injury, and only 14 were cases of severe brain injury or neurological disease. Therefore, it is not plausible that the mean OTBM score of −1.8 is a valid reflection of the patients' abilities. These data show in another way how powerfully effort, as measured by the WMT, influences neuropsychological test scores.

TABLE 6. Means and Standard Deviations for up to 43 Neuropsychological Test Scores Expressed as z-Scores Relative to the Normal Mean (OTBM*)

WMT range relative to TBI group	Number of cases	Mean OTBM score	SD
Above TBI mean	374	0.0	0.6
Mean to −2 SD	271	−0.44	0.6
−2 SD to −4 SD	87	−0.97	0.6
−4 SD to −6 SD	60	−1.34	1.1
Less than −6 SD	104	−1.8	0.9

*OTBM = overall test battery mean derived from the mean of 43 test z-scores.
Note: Patients are grouped according to how they scored on the WMT compared with patients with moderate to severe traumatic brain injury (TBI). Ranges of WMT scores are in standard deviations from the mean from the latter patients.

EFFECTS OF EFFORT ON SPECIFIC COGNITIVE DOMAINS

In principle, effort might affect some ability tests more than others. In the study discussed above, each of the 43 test measures was assigned *a priori* to one of six domains of cognitive ability (see Table 5). For example, the Category Test was placed into the "executive function" domain, and others, such as CVLT scores, went into the "memory and learning" domain. Other tests were classified as measures of psychomotor skills, verbal comprehension, attention and working memory, or perceptual-organizational abilities. Within each domain, all available z-scores were averaged, yielding six domain scores per patient.

In Figure 1, the mean OTBM and domain scores are shown for five groups, broken down into the ranges within which people scored on the mean of the three main WMT effort measures. In the group on the far left, the patients' mean WMT effort z-scores were at or above the mean for brain-injured patients. The next group consists of people whose WMT z-scores were up to two standard deviations lower than the mean from brain injured patients. Similarly, scores which were three standard deviations below the brain-injured mean would be in the third range from the left in Figure 1, and those scoring more than six standard deviations lower than people with brain injuries would fall into the last range (far right), representing very poor effort indeed. The numbers of patients scoring in each range on the WMT measures shown in the fig-

FIGURE 1. Mean OTBM by level of WMT.

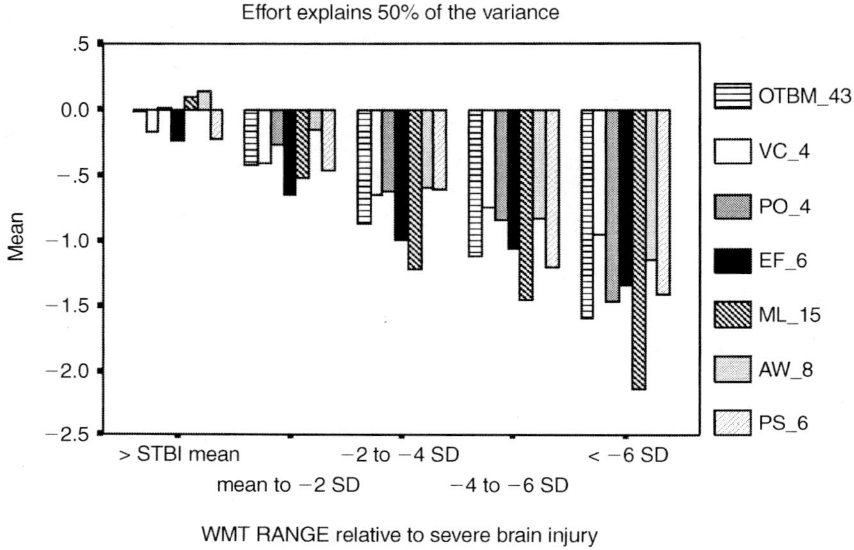

ure, from the highest to the lowest ranges of WMT scores, were 374, 271, 87, 60 and 104.

Figure 1 shows that effort, as measured by the WMT, has a powerful effect on test scores in all domains, but especially on the mean from 15 test scores in the domain of memory and learning (ML-15). Although the memory and learning results included the WMT ability measures, separate analyses excluding these subtests produced very similar results to those shown in Figure 1. In the current study, when people chose to exaggerate cognitive difficulties, they were most likely to exaggerate on memory tests. In 694 patients who passed WMT-DR, the mean z-score on the memory and learning domain was −0.23, compared with −1.88 in 188 cases who failed the DR effort measure. Figure 1 also shows that effort, as measured by the WMT, is a continuum, and that the lower that people score on the WMT effort measures, the lower they score across all domains. Hence, effort cannot be fully represented as two categories, which are "good effort" or "bad effort," because it is a continuum. It is a matter of degree.

A question might be raised about the representativeness of the main 1,000 patient sample used in the WMT research. The rates of exaggeration in forensic cases estimated by Larrabee (2000) suggest that the

28.9% failure rate on the WMT in the current series of 1,000 cases is no higher than and probably lower than average for neuropsychologists in private practice. Secondly, in a very large independent series of patients with brain injury, Rohling (personal communication) has found that, using effort measures other than WMT, it was possible to explain 50% of the variance in a battery of neuropsychological test results, strongly supporting the findings with the WMT.

OLFACTORY TEST SCORES, DEPRESSION, FIBROMYALGIA, CHRONIC PAIN AND EFFORT

In the above examples, the effects on neuropsychological test scores of exaggeration, measured by the WMT, were so large that they literally inverted or obscured known effects. A similar phenomenon was found in studies of olfactory discrimination. Green and Iverson (1997, 2001) and Green, Rohling, and Iverson (in press) showed that impaired smell test scores were far more common in patients with the most severe brain injuries than in those with the least severe head injuries. However, exaggeration of cognitive difficulties, as shown by failing the WMT, was strongly associated with exaggeration of impairment on the smell test. The excess of impaired olfaction in those with more severe brain injuries was found *only after removing* patients who failed the WMT effort measures and whose data were, therefore, of questionable reliability. Hence, in studies of olfaction in groups of patients, it is important to measure effort and to isolate and remove test scores whose validity is questionable because of invalid effort. Otherwise, false conclusions may be drawn from group data.

In a meta-analysis of many studies of depressed patients, Veiel (1997) showed that test scores, such as those on Trail Making, were significantly lower than normal in all depressed patient groups. In contrast, Rohling, Green, Allen, and Iverson (in press) showed that, after removing cases failing effort tests (either the WMT or CARB), leaving 420 patients in the sample, there was no association between self-reported symptoms of depression and any of numerous neuropsychological test scores, including finger tapping speed, grip strength, or Grooved Pegboard scores. While those with very high and very low Beck Depression Inventory scores differed on other self rating scales measuring depression, none of the 43 separate t-tests showed significant differences on the neuropsychological tests employed ($p > 0.05$ for all tests, uncorrected). If depression did not affect scores on relatively difficult neuropsychological tests, it was reasoned that depression could not explain failure on effort tests. This argument was recently given added weight by a study of depression and the Test of Memory Malingering ([TOMM; Tombaugh, 1996]; Rees, Tombaugh, & Boulay, 2001).

Other studies have shown that incomplete effort is a factor in many different diagnostic conditions, including whiplash (Schmand et al., 1998), chronic fatigue syndrome (Van der Werf, Prins, Jongen, van der Meer, & Bleijenbet, 2000) and fibromyalgia (Gervais, Russell, Green, Allen, Ferrari, & Pieschl, 2001). The latter authors found only a 4% rate of failure on the WMT or CARB in 50 fibromyalgia patients who were not making a disability claim. However, there was a 35% failure rate in fibromyalgia patients claiming disability or already receiving compensation. The vast majority (82%) of the fibromyalgia patients made a valid effort on both CARB and the WMT, and so the results do not suggest that symptom exaggeration on cognitive tests is strongly associated with fibromyalgia, in particular. Instead, the study suggests that symptom exaggeration is associated with the availability of financial incentives for disability. However, even in children with no financial incentive, it has been found that effort is often insufficient to produce valid test results (Flaro, Green, & Allen, 2000). It would not come as a surprise to most teachers that, when taking tests, some children "could do better." In another study, Gervais, Green, Allen, and Iverson (2001) showed that there was approximately a 42% failure rate on CARB and the WMT effort tests in a subgroup of patients with pain disorder. However, when the next series of patients was warned that CARB failure is not caused by pain or emotional distress, the failure rate on CARB dropped to 6%, whereas on the WMT, about which they were not warned, the failure rate remained unchanged. It was concluded that neither pain nor emotional distress could explain the patients' failure on the effort tests.

SENSITIVITY OF WMT

For clinical purposes, it is critical to assess both the sensitivity and specificity of the WMT in the identification of suboptimal performance. In the clinical patients asked to simulate impairment (Table 3), the sensitivity of the WMT to exaggeration was 100%, because all patients failed one or more of the effort measures. In the highly educated simulators, the sensitivity of the WMT was 96%, because all cases failed one or more of the effort measures but one person passed all the WMT effort measures. This subject also scored within the normal range on all memory subtests of the WMT, and so she did not present an impaired memory profile. However, her scores were probably lower than she could have obtained if trying her best. Combining these two groups of simulators, the sensitivity of the WMT to exaggeration would be 97.7%. None of the healthy volunteer controls failed any of the WMT effort measures, giving a specificity of 100% in this series. These are probably overestimates of the sensitivity of the test under realistic clinical conditions. Studies of healthy subjects making an effort or people simulating impairment experimentally are limited in terms of their generalizability to clinical cases, which is one reason that most of the WMT research has been carried out in a clinical setting with actual patients evaluated for compensation-related disability claims. In order to fail the main WMT effort measures (IR and DR), a person has to score about three standard deviations or more below people with severe brain injuries or neurological diseases. For this reason, we would expect the false positive rate to be very low.

One feature of people who exaggerate their cognitive difficulties is that they tend to make a poor effort on some tests but not on others. They will often pass one effort test but fail another one of objectively equal difficulty. They perform inconsistently, which is one reason why the WMT contains measures of consistency of performance. For example, out of 889 patients in the current series who were given both the WMT and CARB, 140 cases failed CARB, from which we may conclude that they were not producing reliable results. Of these patients, 110 cases failed the WMT, such that, *if CARB were used to define exaggeration*, the sensitivity of the WMT would be 78%. The specificity of the WMT as a predictor of CARB failure would be 83%, because 130 patients passed CARB but failed the WMT. Similarly, 44 patients from the 1,000 case series were given both the WMT and the ASTMT. There was agreement between these two tests about whether effort was adequate or inadequate in 86.4% of cases, but this means that more than 15% of the sample passed one of these effort tests but failed the other. Of those 10 cases who failed the ASTMT, 8 also failed the WMT. Of those 12 cases who failed the WMT, 8 also failed the ASTMT. It may be argued that, because tests like the WMT, TOMM, ASTMT and CARB are equally easy, inconsistent scores across these tests provide additional evidence of suboptimal effort and unreliable data.

The third author compiled a total of 694 patients from three different practices who were given the TOMM as well as the WMT. Seventy patients (10.1%) failed the TOMM and, of these, 67 cases failed the WMT, such that the sensitivity of the WMT to poor effort as defined by

TOMM failure was 96%. However, there were 111 cases who passed the TOMM but failed the WMT, or an *additional* 15.5% of the sample. The total WMT failure rate was over 2.5 times the failure rate for the TOMM. Hence, if the WMT were used to define incomplete effort, the TOMM would have a sensitivity of only 38.7% relative to the WMT. Green, Berendt, Mandell, and Allen (2000) studied 144 patients given the TOMM and the WMT. Even though none of them carried diagnoses associated with cerebral dysfunction, the patients who failed the WMT but who passed the TOMM scored significantly lower on the verbal memory subtests of the WMT than patients with severe brain injury. It was argued that these test results were implausible and a result of suboptimal performance. Why else should they score significantly worse than people known to have severe brain injuries, when they had no cerebral dysfunction? It is often stated that there is no gold standard for exaggeration. The nearest we have to a gold standard is that people with mild head injuries or diseases implying no cerebral dysfunction are not expected to score worse than people with severe brain injuries, and, if they do, their results are of doubtful validity. Such is the case with people who pass the TOMM and fail the WMT. Gervais et al. (1999) argued that more people in their study failed the WMT than the TOMM because the WMT is a verbal memory task, whereas the TOMM is based on recognition memory for pictures. Consistent with this reasoning, patients were far more likely to complain of verbal than visual spatial memory difficulties on a structured self-report measure of memory complaints (Green & Allen, 1996, 2000). These findings were consistent across all seven diagnostic groups in the sample, and were true of all groups whether they passed or failed any of the symptom validity measures used.

Green (2001) discusses many reasons why clinicians are prone to disagreement about the validity of test results. One reason is that effort tests using different types of stimuli (e.g., verbal versus visual-spatial) are unlikely to be equivalent to each other. The WMT produced very different results than the "Tenhula-Sweet" malingering formula based on how a person performs on the Category Test (Williamson, Green, Allen, & Rohling, 2000). More studies are needed to compare different methods for measuring effort with each other and to study their relationship with symptom reporting in different clinical populations. In comparing different effort measures, it will be helpful to ask how much variance in test scores, especially memory test scores, is explained by each effort measure. It may be hypothesized that the more sensitive a test is to variations in effort, the greater will be the variance in neuropsychological test scores explained by scores on the effort test.

FALSE POSITIVES IN CLINICAL INTERPRETATION

It is important to point out that failure on the WMT effort measures does not mean that a person will automatically be labeled as a malingerer. This is such a pejorative and emotionally laden term that most medical practitioners are extremely reluctant to use it. It may be most prudent to report WMT findings operationally and to keep any discussion of motivation separate from WMT results and the validity of other results. If a person fails the WMT effort measures, they fall into one of two categories. In most cases, the other ability test results obtained from that person at about the same time as the WMT testing will be invalid, because the person probably did not make sufficient effort to produce valid test results. It is likely that the person's test results will overestimate any impairment actually present. Alternatively, as with other effort measures, in relatively few cases, it may be concluded that the person was actually unable to pass the WMT effort measures because of very severe and widespread cognitive impairment.

The latter cases are quite rare and should be obvious to the clinician. In the 1,000 case series described above, it is thought that there were only about five cases of this type, and they can be used as a benchmark with which to compare possible "false positive" results. The diagnoses included multi-infarct dementia, present for at least the previous 7 years, in an 84 year-old diabetic woman. This woman believed that she was still living with her brother, who died years earlier. She was unable to take steps of more than two or three inches, even when supported under both shoulders, and was totally dependent on her daughter for feeding, transport, insulin injections and general daily care. She scored below the cut-offs on the CARB, the WMT and the TOMM but above the chance range of performance. Another was a woman with Korsakoff's syndrome who needed guardianship and trusteeship. A third was a man with a brain tumor the size of an orange, which had just been resected, who had recently received 20 whole-brain radiation treatments and who also had a left temporal lobe hemorrhage. None of these probable false positive cases would be able to drive safely, all were under 24 hour a day care from relatives or institutional staff, all had a clear-cut diagnosis implying extremely severe impairment, and all had clear abnormalities on CT or MRI brain scans, consistent with their diagnosis. If a person resembles the latter cases in these respects (e.g., needs constant care, has a definite brain disease, has an abnormal brain scan, and is not allowed to drive), the possibility of false positives on the WMT should be considered. When judging whether a certain patient (e.g., one with a mild head injury and no loss of consciousness) failed WMT despite making an effort, such cases should be borne in mind.

It is equally important to consider some of the cases who are severely impaired but who pass the WMT. For example, Dr. Arthur Shores of Australia (personal communication) reported on a woman with an extremely severe brain injury, whose intelligence score was 56 and whose daily behavior was very degenerated, including smearing feces. This woman easily passed both the WMT and the CARB. Similarly, Dr. Lloyd Flaro (personal communication) reported a boy aged nine years with an IQ of 65, who easily passed CARB and the WMT effort measures. Numerous cases with known severe brain disease who had no difficulty passing the WMT effort measures are described in the manual supplement by Green and Allen (1999). It may be argued that, just as there are now formal studies of many patients showing that failing the WMT indicates incomplete effort, we would also need formal studies to support any claim that people in a given category are unable to pass the WMT despite good effort.

DAUBERT AND THE WMT IN FORENSIC NEUROPSYCHOLOGY

Is the WMT admissible under *Daubert*? Clearly, the answer is yes. The WMT is a powerful component in the armamentarium of neuropsychologists seeking to provide scientific evidence for use by the Courts. There are several potential questions listed below, which we can anticipate in *Daubert* challenges to the admissibility of opinions based on the WMT:

Is the WMT grounded in scientific method? The critical element of grounding in scientific methodology is empirical verification. From the outset, the WMT has been developed from an empirical scientific perspective. No presuppositions were made that any group would put forth less effort than others. In a lengthy series of studies of differing diagnostic groups, the data have demonstrated the remarkable relationship between WMT effort and neuropsychological test scores.

Is the procedure reliable and valid? The WMT has been subjected to intensive scientific validation and cross validation with large samples drawn from different locations and multiple diagnostic categories. Unlike most research on tests used to address questions of malingering and test validity in forensic settings, the validation of the WMT has been based primarily on actual claimants in forensic settings rather than students and other simulators pretending various conditions.

- Patients with mild head injuries scored lower on the WMT effort tests than patients with severe brain injuries, a finding that can only be explained by lower effort on the part of those with mild head injuries. This is the closest we have to a gold standard in effort testing.
- The cut-offs described in the WMT manual identified with a high level of sensitivity people known to be exaggerating (simulators), but normal controls and patients with moderate to severe brain injuries or neurological diseases easily passed the WMT, demonstrating high specificity for assessing effort.
- Scores on the WMT effort measures were no different in neurological patients with and without verbal memory impairment.
- In 969 patients tested with the computerized WMT, correlations between the three main effort measures (IR, DR and Consistency), ranged from 0.86 to 0.89, showing high internal reliability. The correlations between the WMT memory measures (MC, PA, DFR and LDFR) ranged from 0.71 to 0.90.
- The power of the WMT to predict performance on neuropsychological testing has been demonstrated for a wide variety of tests evaluating different cognitive domains (Table 5). The WMT effort measures explained nearly 50% of the variance in 30,736 test scores (a mean of 34 neuropsychological test scores from each of 904 patients), whereas education explained only 11% of the variance in the same data.
- Alternative explanations have been considered and ruled out in more depth than has been the case with other measures. For example, neither depression, fibromyalgia, chronic pain, neurological diseases nor brain injury were able to explain WMT failure. Failure of the WMT in fibromyalgia patients was associated strongly with financial incentives to exaggerate as part of medical disability claims (35% failure rate), and it was almost non-existent in those with no financial incentive (4% failures).
- The validity of the WMT has been established through comparisons with other symptom validity measures as well as group comparisons and evaluation of individual results. The WMT attained

> 96% sensitivity relative to the TOMM in a combined sample of 694 patients drawn from three independent sites. The verbal memory format of the WMT and its high face validity may explain why the WMT failure rate in this sample was 2.5 times greater than the TOMM, which utilizes a visual-spatial task.

What is the error rate? The WMT enjoys the distinct advantage that it measures a pervasive construct relevant to all neuropsychological tests–effort. The sensitivity, specificity and overall hit rate of the WMT have been demonstrated at impressive levels in several ways. The WMT has been cross validated against other tests associated with malingering or exaggeration. It has been studied by examining and comparing groups with and without incentives to put forth poor effort. It has been applied to patients with objectively demonstrated brain injuries and other neurological conditions in order to verify empirically the ease with which truly impaired individuals can perform the task. As described above, there is abundant evidence of the accuracy of the WMT in detecting poor effort.

Has the procedure been subjected to peer review? Because the WMT is a relatively new test, some of the validation studies are still under review, but some studies have already been published (e.g., Gervais, Green, Allen, & Iverson, 2001; Gervais, Russell, Green, Allen, Ferrari, & Pieschl, 2001; Green, 2001; Green & Iverson, 2001; Green, Iverson, & Allen, 1999; Green, Rohling, Lees-Haley, & Allen, 2001; Iverson, Green, & Gervais, 1999), and a number of other papers have recently passed the journal peer review process and are currently in press. Dozens of studies have been submitted as poster presentations and abstracted in *Archives of Clinical Neuropsychology*.

Is the procedure generally accepted in the scientific community? The claim that assessment of effort is relevant and helpful to the trier of fact in forensic neuropsychological cases is beyond impeachment. The proposition that examinees must do their best on tests has been well recognized and generally accepted in the psychological testing community for the entire history of psychological testing (e.g., see Anastasi, 1954; Cronbach, 1949; Terman & Merrill, 1937). The overwhelming majority of psychological and neuropsychological assessment reports comment on the level of effort exerted by the examinee. The special value of the WMT is to add an empirical test of effort to the examiner's clinical impressions. The basic principles incorporated into the WMT have enjoyed wide acceptance in the neuropsychological community for years (e.g., Binder, 1993; Pankratz, Fausti, & Peed, 1975). The use of the

WMT itself is growing rapidly in many countries, both in English and in translations.

Falsification: Can the expert's opinion, conclusion, or theory be tested? The thesis that the WMT measures effort can be and has been tested repeatedly. For example, this assertion has been studied through comparison of levels of performance of WMT pass/fail groups on other measures of neuropsychological functioning. It has been assessed by comparison with other measures associated with test validity. It has been studied by examining the plausibility of scores, e.g., the finding that severe brain injury patients and other objectively impaired individuals can pass the WMT whereas financially motivated mild injury claimants often perform poorly.

The above arguments apply mainly to the validity of the WMT effort subtests as measures of effort. The use of the WMT to measure memory and the validity of the memory subtests is a separate and very large topic. It may be seen from Tables 1 and 2 that the WMT memory subtests are sensitive to the effects of brain injury and to neurological diseases, which cause impaired verbal memory. However, this paper is not meant to address the reliability and validity of the WMT memory subtests (MC, PA, DFR and LDFR), which will be the subject of another article.

CONCLUSIONS

Hartman (in press) states in a review of the WMT, "Based on current and upcoming publications, it appears that the *Word Memory Test* and its cousin, the CARB, published by the same company, will soon be the most researched effort tests available. Considering the preliminary findings of such research, it seems likely that future investigations of litigating populations, (e.g., fibromyalgia, multiple chemical sensitivity, mild traumatic brain injury) which omit such tests may come to be considered unpublishable and uninterpretable." Unlike other effort test scores, WMT scores have been shown to be major predictors of scores on many neuropsychological tests in large clinical samples. It is this aspect of the WMT research that is its major strength. Because of the WMT research, we now know that effort has a much larger effect on test scores in general than severe brain injury, at least in cases involved in compensation claims. Effort explains so much of the variance in other test results that the validity of neuropsychological results might be questioned in any case presented in a court of law, if measures of effort are not used to rule out invalid test data. Effort tests at present may be thought of as analogous to quality control instruments–a sort of *Daubert* challenge to the plaintiff that throws up a red flag saying, "Data from this plaintiff cannot be trusted." If a plaintiff produces invalid results on one or a few tests, it renders the other data doubtful as evidence of the patient's true abilities. Similarly, studies of various patient groups show that any group differences in test scores obtained without controlling for effort may be questioned, especially if some of the patients are engaged in a financial compensation claim.

REFERENCES

Allen, L., Conder, R.L., Green, P., & Cox, D.R. (1997). *CARB '97 Manual for the Computerized Assessment of Response Bias*. Durham, NC: CogniSyst.

Allen, L., & Green, P. (1999). *Severe TBI Sample Performance on CARB and the WMT*. (Supplement to the CARB '97 and Word Memory Test Manuals). Durham, NC: CogniSyst.

Allen, L., & Green, P. (1999). CARB and WMT effort test scores in 57 patients with severe traumatic brain injury. *Archives of Clinical Neuropsychology, 14*, 789.

Anastasi, A. (1954). *Psychological testing*. New York: Macmillan Co.

Binder, L.M. (1993). Assessment of malingering after mild head trauma with the Portland Digit Recognition Test. *Journal of Clinical & Experimental Neuropsychology, 15*, 170-182.

Cronbach, L.J. (1949). *Essentials of psychological testing*. New York: Harper.

Delis, D.C., Kramer, J.H., Kaplan, E., & Ober, B. (1987). *The California Verbal Learning Test: Research Edition*. New York: The Psychological Corporation.

Flaro, L., Green, P., & Allen, L.M. (2000). Symptom validity test results with children: CARB and WMT. *Archives of Clinical Neuropsychology, 15*, 840.

Frederick, R.I. (1997). *Validity Indicator Profile Manual*, Minnetonka, ST: NCS Assessments, Inc.

Gervais, R., Green, P., & Allen, L. (1999). Differential sensitivity to symptom exaggeration of verbal, visual and numerical symptom validity tests. *Archives of Clinical Neuropsychology, 14*, 746-747.

Gervais, R., Green, P., Allen, L.M., & Iverson, G.L. (2001). Effects of coaching on symptom validity testing in chronic pain patients presenting for disability assessments. *Journal of Forensic Neuropsychology, 2*, (2), 1-19.

Gervais, R.O., Russell, A.S., Green, P., Allen, L.M., Ferrari, R., & Pieschl, S. (2001). Effort testing in patients with fibromyalgia and disability incentives. *Journal of Rheumatology, 28*, 1892-1899.

Green, P. (2001). Why clinicians often disagree about the validity of test results. *Neurorehabilitation, 16*, 231-236.

Green, P., & Allen, L.M. (1997). *Memory Complaints Inventory, a computerised test of memory complaints*. Durham, NC: CogniSyst.

Green, P., & Allen, L.M. (1999). Performance of neurological patients on the Word Memory Test (WMT) and Computerised Assessment of Response Bias (CARB): *Supplement to the Word Memory Test and CARB '97 Manuals*. Durham, NC: CogniSyst.

Green, P., & Allen, L.M. (2000). Patterns of memory complaints in 577 consecutive patients passing or failing symptom validity tests. *Archives of Clinical Neuropsychology, 15*, 844-845.

Green, P., Allen, L., & Astner, K. (1996). *Manual for Computerised Word Memory Test*. Durham, NC: CogniSyst.

Green, P., Berendt, J., Mandel, A., & Allen, L.M. (2000). Relative sensitivity of the Word Memory Test and Test of Memory Malingering in 144 disability claimants. *Archives of Clinical Neuropsychology, 15*, 841.

Green, P., & Iverson, G. (1997). Exaggeration of anosmia in 80 litigating head injury cases. Paper presented at *National Academy of Neuropsychology* annual conference, Las Vegas, NV.

Green, P., & Iverson, G.L. (2001). Effects of head injury severity and cognitive exaggeration on anosmia in head injury compensation claims. *Neurorehabilitation, 16*, 237-243.

Green, P., Iverson, G.L., & Allen, L.M. (1999). Detecting malingering in head injury litigation with the Word Memory Test. *Brain Injury, 13*, 813-819.

Green, P., Rohling, M.L., & Iverson, G.L. (in press). Relationships between olfactory discrimination and head injury severity. *Brain Injury*.

Green, P., Rohling, M.L., Lees-Haley, P.R., & Allen, L.M. (2001). Effort has a greater effect on test scores than severe brain injury in compensation claimants. *Brain Injury, 15* (12), 1045-1060.

Hartman, D.E. (in press). The unexamined lie is a lie worth fibbing: Neuropsychological malingering and the Word Memory Test, *Archives of Clinical Neuropsychology*.

Hays, W.L. (1963). *Statistics for Psychologists*. Toronto: Holt, Rinehart & Winston.

Iverson, G. (1998). *21 Item Test Research Manual*, unpublished.

Iverson, G., Green, P., & Gervais, R. (1999). Using the Word Memory Test to detect biased responding in head injury litigation. *The Journal of Cognitive Rehabilitation*, March/April, 2-6.

Larrabee, G.J. (2000). Neuropsychology in personal injury litigation. *Journal of Clinical and Experimental Neuropsychology, 22*, 702-707.

Millis, S. (1999). CVLT Logit function (unpublished). Presented at the National Academy of Neuropsychology conference, San Antonio, TX.

Pankratz, L., Fausti, S.A., & Peed, S. (1975). A forced-choice technique to evaluate deafness in the hysterical or malingering patient. *Journal of Consulting & Clinical Psychology, 43*, 421-422.

Rees, L.M., Tombaugh, T.N., & Boulay, L. (2001). Depression and the Test of Memory Malingering. *Archives of Clinical Neuropsychology, 16*, 501-506.

Rohling, M.L., Green, P., Allen, L., & Iverson, G.L. (in press). Depressive symptoms and neurocognitive test scores in patients passing symptom validity tests. *Archives of Clinical Neuropsychology*.

Rohling, M.L., Green, P., Allen, L.M., & Lees-Haley, P.R. (2000). Effect sizes of impairment that are associated with symptom exaggeration versus severe TBI: An analysis of a sample of 657 patients and counting. *Archives of Clinical Neuropsychology, 15*, 843.

Schmand, B., Lindeboom, J., Schagen, S., Heijt, R., Koene, T., & Hamburger, H.L. (1998). Cognitive complaints in patients after whiplash injury: The impact of malingering. *Journal of Neurology, Neurosurgery and Psychiatry, 64*, 339-343.

Terman, L.M., & Merrill, M.A. (1937). *Measuring intelligence: A guide to the administration of the new revised Stanford-Binet tests of intelligence*. Boston: Houghton Mifflin.

Tombaugh, T.N. (1996). *Test of Memory Malingering*. Toronto: Multi-Health Systems.

Van der Werf, S.P., Prins, J.B., Jongen, P.J., van der Meer, J.W., & Bleijenberg, G. (2000). Abnormal neuropsychological findings are not necessarily a sign of cerebral impairment: A matched comparison between chronic fatigue syndrome and multiple sclerosis. *Neuropsychiatry, Neuropsychology and Behavioural Neurology, 13*, 199-203.

Veiel, H.O.F. (1997). A preliminary profile of neuropsychological deficits associated with major depression. *Journal of Clinical and Experimental Neuropsychology, 19*, 587-606.

Warrington, E.K. (1984). *Recognition Memory Test Manual*, Windsor, England: NFER-Nelson Publishing Company.

Williamson, D., Green, P., Allen, L.M., & Rohling, M. (2000). Who's exaggerating? The Category Test and Word Memory Test give different answers. *Archives of Clinical Neuropsychology, 15*, 845.

Review of the Validity Indicator Profile

Richard I. Frederick

U.S. Medical Center for Federal Prisoners

SUMMARY. The Validity Indicator Profile (VIP™; Frederick, 1997) is a two-alternative forced-choice test procedure intended to identify when the results of cognitive and neuropsychological testing may be invalid because of malingering or other problematic response styles. The test consists of 100 problems that assess nonverbal abstraction capacity and 78 word-definition problems. The VIP attempts to establish whether an individual's performance in an assessment battery should be considered representative of his or her true overall capacities (valid or invalid). This paper reviews the development and cross-validation of the VIP, and the paper discusses how demonstrations of the construct validity of the VIP support a conclusion that its use as described above fulfills *Daubert* evidentiary standards. The author discusses the benefits of using the VIP and identifies some potential challenges for using the VIP in making decisions about the response styles of individuals who are having their cognitive abilities assessed. *[Article copies available for a fee from The Haworth Document Delivery Service: 1-800-HAWORTH. E-mail address: <getinfo@haworthpressinc.com> Website: <http://www.HaworthPress.com> © 2002 by The Haworth Press, Inc. All rights reserved.]*

Richard I. Frederick is affiliated with the U.S. Medical Center for Federal Prisoners, Springfield, MO.

Address correspondence to: Richard I. Frederick, PhD, Department of Psychology, U.S. Medical Center for Federal Prisoners, Springfield, MO 65807 (E-mail: richardfrederick@yahoo.com).

The conclusions and opinions reported in this paper do not necessarily represent the views of the Federal Bureau of Prisons or the U.S. Department of Justice.

"VIP" is a trademark of NCS Pearson, Inc.

[Haworth co-indexing entry note]: "Review of the Validity Indicator Profile." Frederick, Richard I. Co-published simultaneously in *Journal of Forensic Neuropsychology* (The Haworth Medical Press, an imprint of The Haworth Press, Inc.) Vol. 2, No. 3/4, 2002, pp. 125-145; and: *Detection of Response Bias in Forensic Neuropsychology* (ed: Jim Hom, and Robert L. Denney) The Haworth Medical Press, an imprint of The Haworth Press, Inc., 2002, pp. 125-145. Single or multiple copies of this article are available for a fee from The Haworth Document Delivery Service [1-800-HAWORTH, 9:00 a.m. - 5:00 p.m. (EST). E-mail address: getinfo@haworthpressinc.com].

© 2002 by The Haworth Press, Inc. All rights reserved.

KEYWORDS. Malingering, neuropsychological assessment, psychological evidence, effort

OVERVIEW

The Validity Indicator Profile (VIP™; Frederick, 1997) is a measure of response validity which is intended to be administered concurrently within a battery of cognitive tests. The VIP consists of two subtests; each can be administered and scored separately. The VIP nonverbal subtest (VIP-NV) presents 100 picture-matrix problems that require simple matching, complex matching, analogous decision making, progression, addition, subtraction, and abstraction. The VIP verbal subtest (VIP-V) consists of 78 word definition problems. Test-takers are presented with a stimulus word (e.g., *carpet*) and are asked to choose one of two possible answers that is more similar in meaning to the stimulus (e.g., *rug* or *shoe*). For both subtests, the items have a hierarchy of difficulty but are presented randomly with respect to item difficulty. Once administered, the items are scored and then re-ordered by difficulty.

As its fundamental analysis of response validity, the items are re-ordered by difficulty, scored (0 = incorrect, 1 = correct), and plotted to generate a performance curve demonstrating the average performance of the test taker across an increasingly difficult range of test items. The plotted points of the performance curve are *running means*, computed by averaging a set of 10 consecutive scored item responses. Responses to items 1 through 10 are averaged to yield the first plotted running mean, representing the individual's average performance on the 10 easiest items. Responses 2 through 11 are averaged to compute the second plotted running mean. This process continues until the last (most difficult) item has been included in the plot of the last running mean. The performance curve is then a plot of the running mean on the vertical axis against the plot of its serial position (i.e., 1, 2, 3, and so on) on the horizontal axis.

Performance Curves Representing Compliance

For the two-alternative forced-choice format, individuals who exert full effort to respond correctly should generate perfect (i.e., running mean values = 1.0) or near-perfect (e.g., running mean = 0.9 or 0.8) performance within the range of their capacity to answer items correctly, transitioning to random responding (i.e., running mean values approximate 0.5) once the test taker has reached his/her ceiling of ability (see Figure 1). This means that performance curves for compliant test takers should be fairly similar in shape regardless of differences in ability.

Performance Curves Which Are Unexpected for Compliant Responding

Significant deviations from this expected curve have meaning and allow for some reasonable conclusions about the response style of the individual. For example, an individual who performs at 80% throughout most of the test (see Figure 2, Line A) may intend to respond correctly but may also be expending insufficient effort (*careless responding*). Such an inconsistent performance suggests the test taker could have performed perfectly on much easier items, given that he/she correctly solved 80% of the moderately difficult items. Another deviation from the expected curve might be for an individual who performs at about 50% throughout the entire test (Figure 2, Line B). Such an individual is probably marking answers without regard to item content (*irrelevant responding*). As a final example, consider an individual who demonstrates a consistent increase in correct responding as the test items be-

FIGURE 1. Expected shape of performance curve for compliant performance on the VIP. For the easiest items, perfect performance is expected for most individuals. As test item difficulty increases and the test-taker reaches a ceiling, accuracy drops off, but will remain at about 50%, because guessing on two-alternative items will result in about 50% correct responses.

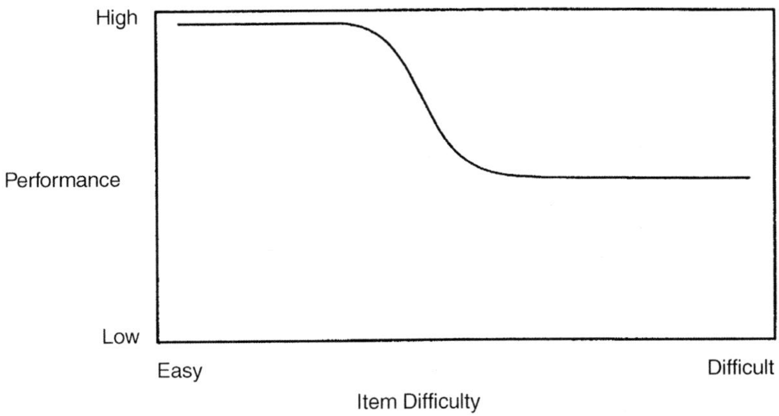

FIGURE 2. Unexpected performances for compliant performance on the VIP. Line A represents carelessness or inconsistent responding. The individual's imperfect responding for the easiest items is inconsistent with a similar level of performance accuracy for items of significantly greater difficulty. Line B represents irrelevant or random responding. Consistent performance accuracy at 50% indicates that responses were irrelevant to item content. Line C represents malingering. The improved performance as items become more difficult is best explained by intentional incorrect responding within the range of capacity to answer correctly and *improved* performance to 50% accuracy when the ceiling of ability is reached.

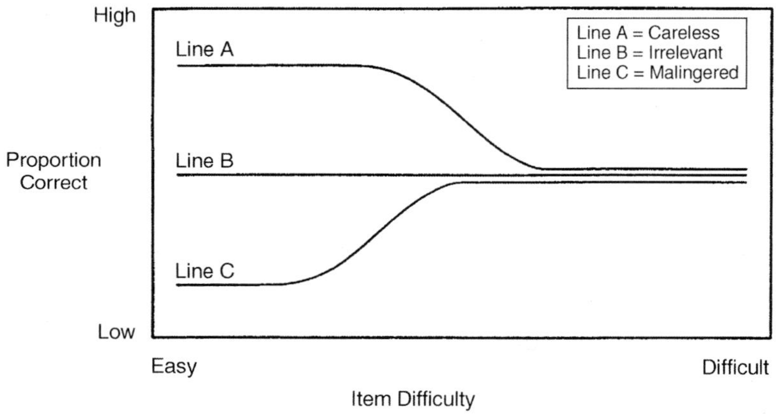

come more difficult (Figure 2, Line C). Such an individual is most likely intentionally choosing the wrong answer despite knowing the correct solution (*malingering*) and responding randomly only when the correct answer is not known.

In consideration of these four types of observed *performance curves*, Frederick (1997) postulated that the potential validity of performance on cognitive testing is a function of two test-taking characteristics: *motivation* and *effort*. Motivation refers to the intention of the test taker to perform well or poorly. Effort refers to the intensity of application of true ability to perform well or poorly (e.g., low effort or high effort). In this scheme, effort and motivation are independent constructs. Invalid assessments result from motivation to perform poorly or from poor effort when motivated to perform well.

This cross-classification of motivation and effort results in four *response styles*: compliant, careless, malingered, and irrelevant (see Figure 1). *Compliant* responding is characterized by *high effort* and *mo-*

tivation to perform well (alternatively, an *intention to respond correctly*). Compliant test-takers are cooperative with testing procedures, and their performance accurately represents their ability. *Careless,* or inconsistent, test-taking is also characterized by the *motivation to perform well*. However, it differs from compliant responding in that there is *incomplete effort* to respond correctly. Careless test-taking may result from inattention, distraction, or fatigue. *Malingering* is characterized by *high effort when motivated to perform poorly*, in which the test-taker strives to feign cognitive deficits in a convincing manner. Finally, *irrelevant*, or random, responding is characterized by *token effort when motivated to perform poorly* (alternatively, *no intention to respond correctly*). Irrelevant test-takers may be disengaged from the task of responding correctly, perhaps not caring about the outcome of the assessment.

Only Compliant performance curves are considered to represent Valid performances, providing strong evidence of the best effort of the test-taker to respond correctly. Careless, Irrelevant, and Malingering performance curves are considered to represent Invalid performances, each type of curve providing strong evidence of insufficient effort or motivation to perform poorly. The VIP was designed to generate Compliant, Careless, Irrelevant, and Malingering curves to represent, respectively, compliant responding, carelessness, irrelevant responding, and malingering.

DEVELOPMENT PHASE

Participants

The development sample included clinical and nonclinical groups. Participants in the nonclinical group (n = 944) were college students and employees of National Computer Systems, Inc. (NCS). Clinical participants (n = 104) were adults undergoing neuropsychological evaluation. Some were involved in litigation; others were being evaluated as part of ongoing clinical care. Compliant and Noncompliant groups were established based on random assignments for college students and NCS employees. Clinical participants were assigned to Compliant and Noncompliant groups based on a priori clinical judgments about the likelihood they would fake cognitive impairment or based on their performance on collaterally administered malingering tests. Methods of group assignments and participant instruction are reported in Frederick and Foster (1991), Frederick, Sarfaty, Johnston, and Powel (1994), Frederick (1997), and Frederick and Crosby (2000).

Classifying Valid and Invalid Performances

Performance on the VIP is first classified as Valid or Invalid by decision rules related to the consistency of responding correctly to test items across the test. Consistency is determined in several ways, each way examining in a different manner whether items of equivalent difficulty are answered correctly. Other decision rules evaluate whether the performance curve has a characteristic shape for compliant responding, or whether features of the curve deviate substantially from the shape shown in Figure 1. Frederick (1997) and Frederick and Crosby (2000) explain how these rules work. Decision rules for assignment to Valid or Invalid categories (Primary Validity Indicators [PVI]; Frederick, 1997) were established in the development sample and evaluated with the cross-validation sample. PVI decision rules were defined in the development phase so that the false-positive rate (equal to 1.0 minus specificity) would be approximately 10%. Test statistics were derived from an observation of the rate at which Compliant and Noncompliant participants were assigned to the VIP performance categorizations of Valid and Invalid, respectively. We attempted to maximize the sensitivity of the test while keeping a reasonably high bound on specificity.

CROSS-VALIDATION PHASE

Participants

The cross-validation sample consisted of normal adults, patients with traumatic brain injury, computer-generated cases of random responding, and patients at risk for malingering cognitive deficits. Normal adults were assigned to Compliant or Noncompliant criterion groups on an a priori basis. Compliant participants were instructed to complete the test, giving their best effort. Noncompliant normal participants were asked to feign believable brain impairment in completing tests. They watched a videotaped presentation of the nature of the research and a description of how brain injuries might affect individuals. Noncompliant normal participants were also provided with printed literature designed to help individuals understand the potential impact of mild brain injuries on behavior, mood, and thinking. They were offered meaningful financial incentives for successful feigning. All participants completed the Portland Digit Recognition Test (Binder, 1993) and the Rey malingering tests[1] (Frederick, 1997).

Diagnostic Efficiencies

Classification rates for the VIP-NV and VIP-V are reported in Table 1. The VIP-NV demonstrated an overall classification rate of 79.8%, with 73.5% sensitivity and 85.7% specificity. The VIP-V demonstrated an overall classification rate of 75.5%, with 67.3% sensitivity and 83.1% specificity. Table 2 reports the rate of agreement between the VIP-NV and VIP-V ($n = 310$, kappa = .70, $p < .001$). Breakdowns of Invalid performances subclassified as Careless, Irrelevant, or Malingering are given for the VIP-NV and VIP-V in Table 3.

Most members of the Compliant criterion groups (98.1% or 98.8%) were classified as "motivated to respond correctly" (Compliant or Careless) on the VIP-NV and VIP-V, respectively. About half of the Noncompliant criterion group members (42.0% or 47.7%) were classified as "motivated to respond incorrectly" (Irrelevant or Malingering) on the VIP-V and VIP-NV, respectively. These values are very close to the specificity (99.5%) and sensitivity (48.5%) reported for the Structured Interview of Reported Symptoms (SIRS; Rogers, Bagby, & Dickens, 1992, p. 24).

Table 4 compares the classification rates of the VIP subtests with the Rey malingering tests and the PDRT. As reported in Frederick and Crosby (2000), two hierarchical logistic regression analyses were performed to compare the incremental validity of the PDRT with the VIP. For both analyses, the Rey tests were entered on the first step (model chi-square = 22.7, df = 3, $p < .0001$) and correctly classified 66.7% of the cases. On the second step, either the PDRT or VIP (VIP-NV and VIP-V) classifications were entered. On the third step, the remaining test was entered. When the VIP classifications were entered as the third step, added to the PDRT, correct classifications improved from 69.8% to 77.3% (improvement chi-square = 41.0, df = 2, $p < .0001$). In contrast, when the PDRT classifications were entered as the third step, added to the VIP, correct classifications improved only from 76.5% to 77.3% (improvement chi-square = 7.7, df = 1, $p < .01$). Hierarchical logistic regression analyses in which the Rey tests were entered as the third step were nonsignificant and demonstrated no improvement over the PDRT and VIP classifications, which together correctly classified 77.3% of the cases.

TABLE 1. Analysis of Test Classification for the Nonverbal and Verbal Subtests of the Validity Indicator Profile Cross-Validation Sample

	Test Classification			
	Nonverbal Subtest			
	Valid		Invalid	
Criterion Group	*n*	%	*n*	%
Compliant Group				
Honest Normals	93	93	7	7
Brain Injured	45	74	16	26
Noncompliant Group				
Coached Normals	13	25	39	75
Suspected Malingerers	27	55	22	45
Random Responding	0	0	50	100
	Verbal Subtest			
	Valid		Invalid	
Criterion Group	*n*	%	*n*	%
Compliant Group				
Honest Normals	95	95	5	5
Brain Injured	38	63	22	37
Noncompliant Group				
Coached Normals	14	27	38	73
Suspected Malingerers	35	73	13	27
Random Responding	0	0	50	100

© 1997 NCS Pearson, Inc. All rights reserved. Reproduced with permission.

CONSTRUCT VALIDATION OF THE VIP

Evidence of the construct validity of these subclassifications was reported in Frederick, Crosby, and Wynkoop (2000). They examined data for a large sample of criminal defendants who were completing court-ordered examinations of competency and criminal responsibility. Classifications of response style by VIP performance curve characteristics were supported by an analysis of concurrently administered Rey malingering tests when matched on essential VIP measures of test perfor-

TABLE 2. Cross-Tabulation of Validity Indicator Profile Verbal and Nonverbal Subtest Classification Rates

	Verbal Subtest	
Nonverbal Subtest	Invalid	Valid
Invalid	157	21
Valid	25	107

Note. $n = 310$. Kappa = .70, $p < .001$.
© 1997 NCS Pearson, Inc. All rights reserved. Reproduced with permission.

mance to control for potential effects from cognitive capacity. Large to very large effect sizes on malingering test performance were seen for individuals classified as "motivated to perform well" (Compliant and Careless classifications) when compared to individuals classified as "motivated to perform poorly" (Irrelevant and Malingering). Moderate to large effect sizes on malingering test performance were seen for differences in motivation even when the effort of subjects was presumed to be low (Irrelevant vs. Careless performance curves). There were zero-order effects on malingering test performance when Compliant test takers were compared with those classified as Careless (i.e., both classes presumed motivated to perform well, but different in effort expended), but defendants classified as Careless had significantly higher scores on MMPI-2 carelessness indicators when compared to defendants classified as Compliant.

Furthermore, Frederick, Crosby, and Wynkoop (2000) hypothesized a mechanism of careless responding and simulated that process by computer for 4000 Compliant curves. The simulation of careless responding resulted in the predicted changes to the performance curve features which are used to describe responding as Careless.

DISCUSSION

Considerations in Light of Daubert

As noted above, reports on the VIP development and cross-validation (including the potential rate for error) and assessment of construct validity have been published in peer-reviewed journals which enjoy general acceptance in the field of neuropsychology and psychological

TABLE 3. Analysis of Response Style Classification of Invalid Performances on the Validity Indicator Profile Cross-Validation Sample

	Response Style Classification					
	Nonverbal Subtest					
Criterion Group	Careless		Irrelevant		Malingered	
	n	%	*n*	%	*n*	%
Compliant Group						
Honest Normals	7	7	0	0	0	0
Brain Injured	14	23	2	3	0	0
Noncompliant Group						
Coached Normal	20	38	16	31	3	6
Suspected Malingerers	18	37	4	8	0	0
Random Responding	1	2	48	96	1	2
	Verbal Subtest					
Criterion Group	Careless		Irrelevant		Malingered	
	n	%	*n*	%	*n*	%
Compliant Group						
Honest Normals	5	5	0	0	0	0
Brain Injured	19	32	3	5	0	0
Noncompliant Group						
Coached Normal	26	50	8	15	4	8
Suspected Malingerers	11	23	2	4	0	0
Random Responding	1	2	48	96	1	2

© 1997 NCS Pearson, Inc. All rights reserved. Reproduced with permission.

assessment. The test has received generally favorable reviews (Gamache, 1998; Ivens, 2001; Ross & Adams, 1999) and comments (Vallabhajosula & van Gorp, 2001), with some accompanying criticisms, concerns, and cautions (Gamache, 1998; Gebart-Eaglemont, 2001; Ross & Adams, 1999). Using performance curve characteristics as a means of examining the potential for response invalidity has received endorsement for cognitive tests other than the VIP (Gudjonsson & Shackleton, 1986; McKinzey, Podd, Krehbeil, & Raven, 1999; Rogers, Harrell, & Liff,

TABLE 4. Comparison of Classification Rates Among Malingering Tests Within Cross-Validation Sample

Test	Sensitivity	Specificity	Overall Classification Rate
VIP Nonverbal Subtest	73.5	85.7	79.8
VIP Verbal Subtest	67.3	83.1	75.5
Portland Digit Recognition Test	17.0	99.4	67.7
Rey 15-Item Memory Test	4.9	97.5	61.4
Rey Word Recognition Test	8.8	100.0	64.6
Rey Dot Counting Test	11.8	97.5	64.1

© 1997 NCS Pearson, Inc. All rights reserved. Reproduced with permission.

1993). Tatsuoka and Tatsuoka (1982, 1983) demonstrated the use of consistency measures used in the PVI decision rules to examine consistency of performance in cognitive tests. The VIP also compares proportion of total correct responses to that expected for no ability as an indicator of test-taking intention. This technique has received wide general acceptance as an indication of response validity for some time (e.g., Brady & Lind, 1961; Pankratz, 1979; Rogers et al., 1993; Theodor & Mandelcorn, 1973). These factors suggest the VIP should easily surpass scrutiny in a *Daubert* hearing concerning its use as a measure of response validity for cognitive assessment.

Criticism of the VIP

Lees-Haley, Dunn, and Betz (1999) criticized the VIP process of subclassification, stating: "This further classification confuses the issues by appearing to exclude irrelevant and careless performances from the definition of malingering, when, in fact, sub-optimal performances are specifically associated with malingering" (p. 12). Actually, the subclassifications of the VIP were never intended to speak definitively about the *ultimate goal* of the test-taker in the examination process. For example, the VIP manual (Frederick, 1997) includes this statement: "It is important to remember that the VIP classification of test performance and response style is made in the absence of any other information about the test taker (p. 37)." Similar statements appear routinely in the interpretive report, for example:

> The descriptions, inferences, and recommendations in this report should be evaluated in the context of other information that is available about the client. Such information may include clinician observations, the client's presenting complaint, scores from other assessment instruments, and an evaluation of situational factors that may influence test performance.

Subclassifications are intended to accurately identify the *intention* of the test taker in completing concurrently administered cognitive tests (i.e., "to respond correctly" or "to respond incorrectly") and to accurately categorize the *level of effort* produced by the examinee to fulfill the intention (i.e., "high effort" or "low effort"). A decision to use the term "Malingering" for only those *performance curves* obviously resulting from a strong effort to answer incorrectly certainly does not exclude suboptimal performance from the definition of a malingering *response style*. The criticism by Lees-Haley and his colleagues does not comport with statements about the process of interpretation in the VIP manual, for example, "An individual who intends to perform poorly and who make a conscious effort at deception might produce results that appear to be careless or irrelevant rather than malingered. This can occur, for example, if a malingerer answers the easiest items correctly" (p. 38). Even Compliant performance curves routinely contain this language in the interpretive report:

> Performances classified as valid are assumed to represent compliance. Individuals classified as compliant demonstrate a predictable decrement in performance as the items increased in difficulty. However, performance that follows such a pattern does not necessarily ensure that the test-taker made his or her best effort. The clinician should make that determination based on all available information.

Again, the use of Malingering as a classificatory label for pronounced positively-sloped performance curves does not indicate at all that malingerers must not instead produce Irrelevant, Careless, or even Compliant curves. For example, the interpretive report for Careless curves routinely contain this statement:

> Careless responding can result from many factors, the most probable of which is an insufficient effort to do well. Occasionally, however, Performance Curves that are classified as careless can result

> from an individual's deliberate attempt to do poorly but not poorly enough to be classified as a malingerer or as an irrelevant responder.

Ostensibly, Lees-Haley and his colleagues were concerned that conclusions that examinees had feigned aspects of their presentation or exaggerated their putative impairment might be foiled by VIP results of Irrelevant or Careless, or even, in some circumstances, a finding of Compliant. No doubt a sharp attorney will highlight seemingly contradictory information to counter a clinical assessment which results in the conclusion an examinee has malingered or exaggerated, but examiners who are familiar with the contents of the VIP manual and interpretive report should have no difficulty explaining that there is no inherent conflict in a finding of malingering in light of the totality of the assessment and the classification of Irrelevant, Careless, or even Compliant on the VIP.

Dichotomous Classifications vs. Four-Fold Classifications

The criticism of the VIP by Lees-Haley et al. (1999) was contained within a review of the Victoria Symptom Validity Test (VSVT; Slick, Hopp, Strauss, Hunter, & Pinch, 1994). Lees-Haley et al. claimed the dichotomous classifications of the VSVT and its ilk were more helpful than the four-fold scheme presented by the VIP. Most classification schemes for cognitive/memory malingering tests result in labels of "malingered" and "not malingered" or "compliant" and "non-compliant" (Binder, 1993; Tombaugh, 1997). Frederick and Crosby (2000) identified four problems with the dichotomous classification scheme.

First, the dichotomous classification puts the clinician in danger of making costly classification errors. A false positive classification means a person who is not faking impairment is classified as "faking." A person who is faking is classified as "compliant." Second, most tests designed to detect malingering that use dichotomous classifications provide no demonstrable support for the classification beyond its statistical or clinical atypicality. As Frederick (2000a) noted, one can always argue that scores worse than cut-scores established for individuals with bona fide impairment mean only that the impairment of the examinee is worse than that of the impaired individuals in the research comparison group. When examinees earn compliant scores on such tests, we cannot conclude that they displayed good effort, but only that they did not display bad effort (Faust & Ackley, 1998). Third, dichotomous malingering classifications limit explanations of positive test scores to noncompliance or classification error. A classification scheme should be able to describe a performance as suboptimal (not representative of the individual's maximal capacity to perform well on cognitive tasks) without mechanically concluding that the invalidity was intentional. Fourth, the dichotomous classification scheme makes research into malingering difficult. It has proven difficult, if not nearly impossible, to develop "pure" groups of definite malingerers and fully compliant test takers, even within analog settings (Arbisi & Ben-Porath, 1995; Frederick, 2000b; Frederick et al., 1994; Greiffenstein, Baker, & Gola, 1994, 1996).

Potential Classification Errors

Most members of the Compliant criterion groups in the cross-validation phase were classified as "motivated to perform well." Classification errors for Compliant participants were generally restricted to the classification of Careless and not as "motivated to perform poorly" (i.e., Malingering or Irrelevant). These findings illustrate that potential false positive classifications are mitigated by the four-fold classification scheme. Excessively careless, inconsistent performance will infrequently result in a classification as Irrelevant, but will not result in a classification of Malingering. Such misclassification will accurately reflect the compromised effort that went into generating correct answers, but will incorrectly raise the hypothesis of motivation to perform poorly. Additionally, irrelevant responding will result in false positive classification as Malingering only about 2% of the time (see Table 3).

About half of the noncompliant criterion group members were classified as "motivated to perform poorly." Potential false negative classifications were mitigated by the four-fold classification scheme as well. Truly irrelevant performances were incorrectly categorized as Careless only about 2% of the time (see Table 3). Incorrect classifications of malingering, in which the test taker is making a concerted effort to answer incorrectly, will generally be classified as Irrelevant, which maintains the hypothesis that the test taker did not intend to answer correctly.

Table 3 indicates that some malingerers may be able develop a strategy of correctly answering some easier items so as to generate a classification as Compliant or Careless, false negative classifications. To do so requires *consistent, above-chance* responding for at least the easiest items. Frederick and Crosby (2000) reviewed the nature of the performances of suspected malingerers and coached normals classified as Compliant. These putatively Noncompliant participants clearly generated strong effort to respond correctly on the VIP-NV and VIP-V, with average total correct responses at the same level as Compliant coached normals and with performance curves demonstrating sustained effort to respond correctly. Consequently, it is hard to construe these performances as misclassified Invalid performances, and it is more likely these are instances of criterion group contamination and a source of underestimated VIP sensitivity.

When malingerers answer some items correctly as a means of trying not to be obvious, they run the risk of demonstrating too much ability to generate the gain that impairment would produce or generating performance curves which reveal obvious inconsistency or carelessness. Because the VIP can usually generate an estimate of cognitive capacity for Careless and Compliant performance curves (Crosby & Frederick, 1997; Frederick, 1997), the clinician can also compare that estimate with other estimates obtained during the examination. Such a comparison may shed light on the intentions and effort of the test-taker.

Identifying Potential Classification Errors on the VIP

In reviewing VIP performances, it is useful to review which response styles actually generated which performance curve classifications in the cross-validation phase.

Motivation to Perform Poorly

Malingering. The classification of Malingering was primarily restricted to coached normals asked to feign impairment. Two percent of randomly-generated curves were classified as Malingering.

Irrelevant. The classification of Irrelevant responding was primarily restricted to participants in the Noncompliant group. About one-third of coached normals generated this type of curve. Almost all (96%) of randomly-generated curves resulted in the classification of Irrelevant. A small percentage of suspected malingerers (4%) and Compliant participants with bona fide traumatic brain injury (3%) received a classification of Irrelevant for their performances.

These findings highlight the very high specificity of the VIP with respect to distinguishing between "motivation to perform well" and "motivation to perform poorly." When these categorizations result, the clinician can confidently postulate there was no intention to respond correctly or that severe impairment exists.

Motivation to Perform Well

Compliant. Almost all Compliant normal control participants generated Compliant curves. Most Compliant participants with traumatic brain injury were classified as Compliant, but about one-third generated curves classified as Careless. A large number of Noncompliant participants (about one-fourth of coached normals and over one-half of suspected malingerers) generated strong effort to respond correctly on the VIP-NV and VIP-V, with average total correct responses at the same level as Compliant coached normals and with performance curves demonstrating sustained effort to respond correctly. It is unlikely these individuals were trying to feign impairment.

Careless. Very few Compliant coached normals and about one-third of compliant participants with traumatic brain injury were classified as Careless. About one-half of Noncompliant coached normals and a sizable minority of suspected malingerers were classified as Careless.

COMMENTS

I have three comments. The first two concern questions I routinely receive from consumers of the VIP, and the third comment concerns my belief that research on malingering tests, including my own, is frequently plagued by criterion group contamination.

Careless Curves

As I have just noted in my discussions on classification errors, the Careless categorizations of the cross-validation sample included a mix of Compliant and Noncompliant participants. The nature of these results clearly indicate that the potential for false positive errors on the VIP is highest for this categorization, especially for persons with traumatic brain injury. Users who carefully read the test manual and interpretive reports know that the classification of Careless is the default classification of Invalid performances (i.e., failure of two or more Primary Validity Indicators; PVIs) that cannot be classified as Malingered or Irrelevant. The interpretive report notes that sometimes lucky or unlucky guessing of answers for items beyond the test-taker's ceiling can unduly influence the PVIs to generate a classification of Invalid. This means that curves can receive default classification as Careless if they are classified first as Invalid, *even if the curves have no characteristics associated with careless or inconsistent responding.*

Given that Frederick, Crosby, and Wynkoop (2000) demonstrated that certain features of the performance curve associated with carelessness[2] were associated with other indicators of carelessness, my caveat for inquiries is straightforward. If the curves do not contain either of these features, carelessness or invalidity must be *ruled in* from other sources of information. I urge caution to avoid over-interpreting these curves. If the curves do contain either of these features, however, consider that some sort of inconsistency in responding *is likely*, and should be *ruled out*. Given that a sizeable proportion of individuals with traumatic brain injury generated these sorts of curves, one potential source of inconsistency has nothing to do with motivation to perform poorly, but may reflect unique contributions of certain clinical disorders. Again, I urge clinicians to review the totality of information in making conclusions about VIP performance; I strongly recommend that conclusions about poor effort or motivation to perform poorly reflect a convergence of evidence. Future research on the VIP should attempt to further distinguish among careless categorizations that result from sophisticated malingering, those that result from true carelessness, and those that result from clinical conditions which inhibit concentration or mimic careless responding on the VIP.

Use of the Test with Individuals Who Have Mental Retardation

I am commonly asked whether the test can be used to evaluate individuals *suspected* of mental retardation. My answer is, "Of course." This question primarily arises because of statements on page 4 of the VIP manual:

> The VIP is not recommended for use with individuals with historically demonstrable mental retardation or severe cognitive impairment. Individuals with severe impairment will probably receive a categorization of invalid test performance because of their extremely limited cognitive abilities.

I have evaluated my share of individuals who feign severe mental impairment. Such individuals generally produce Malingered or Irrelevant performance curves. The VIP manual reports a sample of 40 individuals with historically demonstrable mental retardation who were in assisted living in the community. About half of them were fully illiterate. Only

5% of the performances of these individuals resulted in classification as Compliant. Sixty-five percent of the VIP-NV curves and about 50% of the VIP-V curves were classified as Careless, and most of the rest were classified as Irrelevant. One of the 40 individuals produced a VIP-V curve classified as Malingering, consistent with the approximate 2% false positive rate for random responding. The question arises, "How can you distinguish between Irrelevant or Careless curves generated by fakers and those generated by persons with severe impairment?" My answer is, "I can't." I have to make decisions about motivations and effort in light of all the evidence I possess. If I am evaluating an individual with "historically demonstrable mental retardation or [continuing] severe cognitive impairment," I have no use for the VIP or any other instrument which measures response style.

Criterion Group Contamination

In recent research on the VIP (Frederick, Crosby, & Wynkoop, 2000), I have strived to avoid criterion group methodology. Instead, I have focused on comparing performance curve characteristics suggesting different response sets and the accompanying effect on concurrently administered tests of response style. As we noted in that article, it was clear the cross-validation Noncompliant group contained a large proportion of individuals who had completed the VIP compliantly. We had no choice but to include them in our computations of sensitivity, but it was clear to us this resulted in significant underestimations of sensitivity.

In Frederick (2000b), I claimed that traditional criterion group validation of malingering tests is continually seriously flawed by criterion group impurity, resulting in significant underestimations of test diagnostic efficiencies (both sensitivity and specificity). Despite the contention of Rogers (1997) that differential prevalence designs are useless in malingering research, I demonstrated that, with appropriate methodology and analysis, the differential prevalence design overcomes the problem of criterion group impurity and allows for potentially more accurate estimates of sensitivity and specificity. For example, in that paper, I showed that using a differential prevalence design for the Rey 15-Item Test resulted in far superior estimates of sensitivity and specificity than commonly reported in the literature about that procedure. I do not think the problem of criterion group contamination is unique to the VIP, and I would encourage other researchers to attempt validations of validity instruments in ways that do not depend on criterion group designs.

I believe the VIP has made an important contribution in attempting to go beyond simplistic thinking with respect to response style. There are many response styles that contribute to observed performance on cognitive tests. Currently, some response styles cannot be effectively distinguished based solely on test performance; for example, random completion of a test because one refuses to engage in the task cannot currently be distinguished from a random completion because one does not know any answer. The goal for future research will be to identify practical methods for fully distinguishing between cooperative and noncooperative performances on cognitive tests.

NOTES

1. The "Rey malingering tests" refer to the most commonly known of Rey's tools for assessment of malingering, the 15-Item Memory Test, the Word Recognition Test, and the Dot Counting Test (Lezak, 1995; Rey, 1941, 1958).

2. A discussion of these features requires a good deal of explanation beyond the scope of this review. For the interested reader, these characteristics are a large Sector 1 residual and Sector 2 distance greater than or equal to Sector 1 distance (see Frederick, 1997; Frederick & Crosby, 2000; or Frederick, Crosby, & Wynkoop, 2000).

REFERENCES

Arbisi, P. A., & Ben-Porath, Y. S. (1995). An MMPI-2 infrequent response scale for use with psychopathological populations: The Infrequency-Psychopathology Scale, *F(p)*. *Psychological Assessment*, *7*, 424-431.

Binder, L. M. (1993). Assessment of malingering after mild head trauma with the Portland Digit Recognition Test. *Journal of Clinical and Experimental Neuropsychology*, *15*, 170-182.

Brady, P. B., & Lind, D. L. (1961). Experimental analysis of hysterical blindness. *Archives of General Psychiatry*, *4*, 331-339.

Crosby, R., & Frederick, R. I. (1997, August). Predicting IQ ranges from performance curve characteristics. Paper presented at the Annual Convention of the American Psychological Association, Chicago.

Faust, D. & Auckley, M. A. (1998). Did you think it was going to be easy? Some methodological suggestions for the investigation and development of malingering detection techniques (pp. 1-54). In C. R. Reynolds (Ed.). *Detection of Malingering During Head Injury Litigation*. New York: Plenum.

Frederick, R. I. (1997). *Validity Indicator Profile manual*. Minnetonka, MN: NCS Assessments.

Frederick, R. I. (2000a). A personal floor effect strategy to evaluate the validity of performance on memory tests. *Journal of Clinical and Experimental Neuropsychology, 22*, 720-730.

Frederick, R. I. (2000b). Mixed group validation: A method to address the limitations of criterion group validation in research on malingering detection. *Behavioral Sciences and the Law, 18*, 693-718.

Frederick, R. I., & Crosby, R. D. (2000). Development and validation of the Validity Indicator Profile. *Law and Human Behavior, 24*, 59-82.

Frederick, R. I., Crosby, R. D., & Wynkoop, T. F. (2000). Performance curve classification of invalid responding on the Validity Indicator Profile. *Archives of Clinical Neuropsychology, 15*, 281-300.

Frederick, R. I., & Foster, H. G. (1991). Multiple measures of malingering on a forced-choice test of cognitive ability. *Psychological Assessment, 3*, 596-602.

Frederick, R. I., Sarfaty, S. D., Johnston, J. D., & Powel, J. (1994). Validation of a detector of response bias on a forced-choice test of nonverbal ability. *Neuropsychology, 8*, 118-125.

Gamache, M. (1998, Spring). The Validity Indicator Profile: Review of an instrument to assess response style. *American Psychology-Law Society Newsletter, 18(2)*, 11-43.

Gebart-Eaglemont, J. E. (2001). Review of the Validity Indicator Profile. In B. S. Plake and J. C. Impara (Eds.). *The Fourteenth Mental Measurements Yearbook*. Lincoln, NE: Buros Institute of Mental Measurements.

Greiffenstein, M. F., Baker, W. J., & Gola, T. (1994). Validation of malingered amnesia measures in a large clinical sample. *Psychological Assessment, 6*, 218-224.

Greiffenstein, M. F., Baker, W. J., & Gola, T. (1996). Comparison of multiple scoring methods for Rey's malingered amnesia measures. *Archives of Clinical Neuropsychology, 11*, 283-293.

Gudjonsson, G. H., & Shackleton, H. (1986). The pattern of scores on Raven's Matrices during "faking bad" and "non faking" performances. *British Journal of Clinical Psychology, 25*, 35-41.

Ivens, S. H. (2001). Review of the Validity Indicator Profile. In B. S. Plake and J. C. Impara (Eds.). *The Fourteenth Mental Measurements Yearbook*. Lincoln, NE: Buros Institute of Mental Measurements.

Lees-Haley, P. R., Dunn, J. T., & Betz, B. P. (1999, Fall). Test review: The Victoria Symptom Validity Test. *American Psychology-Law Society Newsletter, 19(3)*, 12-16.

Lezak, M. D. (1995). *Neuropsychological assessment* (3rd ed.). New York: Oxford.

McKinzey, R. K., Podd, M. H., Krehbiel, M. A., & Raven, J. (1999). Detection of malingering on the Raven's Standard Progressive Matrices: A cross-validation. *British Journal of Clinical Psychology, 38*, 435-439.

Pankratz, L. (1979). Symptom validity testing and symptom retraining: Procedures for the assessment and treatment of functional sensory deficits. *Journal of Consulting and Clinical Psychology, 47*, 409-410.

Rey, A. (1941). L'examen psychologie dans les cas d'encephalopathie traumatique. *Archives de Psychologie, 28*, 286-340.

Rey, A. (1958). *L'Examen clinique de psychologie.* Paris: Presses Universitaires de France.

Rogers, R. (Ed., 1997). *Clinical assessment of malingering and deception* (2nd ed.). New York: Guilford Press.

Rogers, R., Bagby, R. M., & Dickens, S. E. (1992). *Structured Interview of Reported Symptoms: Professional Manual.* Odessa, FL: Psychological Assessment Resources.

Rogers, R., Harrell, E. H., & Liff, C. D. (1993). Feigning neuropsychological impairment: A critical review of methodological and clinical considerations. *Clinical Psychology Review, 13*, 255-274.

Ross, S. R., & Adams, K. M. (1999). Test review: One more test of malingering? *Clinical Neuropsychologist, 13*, 112-116.

Slick, D., Hopp, G., Strauss, E., Hunter, M., & Pinch, D. (1994). Detecting dissimulation: Profiles of simulated malingerers, traumatic brain-injury patients, and normal controls on a revised version of Hiscock and Hiscock's forced-choice memory test. *Journal of Clinical and Experimental Neuropsychology, 16*, 472-481.

Tatsuoka, K. M., & Tatsuoka, M. M. (1982). Detection of aberrant response patterns and their effect on dimensionality. *Journal of Educational Statistics, 7*, 215-231.

Tatsuoka, K. M., & Tatsuoka, M. M. (1983). Spotting erroneous rules of operation by the Individual Consistency Index. *Journal of Educational Measurement, 20*, 221-230.

Tombaugh, T. N. (1997). The Test of Memory Malingering (TOMM): Normative data from cognitively intact and cognitively impaired individuals. *Psychological Assessment, 9*, 260-268.

Theodor, L. H., & Mandelcorn, M. S. (1973). Hysterical blindness: A case report and study using a modern psychophysical technique. *Journal of Abnormal Psychology, 82*, 552-553.

Vallabhajosula, B., & van Gorp, W. G. (2001). Post-Daubert admissibility of scientific evidence on malingering of cognitive deficits. *Journal of the American Academy of Psychiatry and the Law, 29*, 207-215.

Warrington's Recognition Memory Test in the Detection of Response Bias

Scott R. Millis

Kessler Medical Rehabilitation Research and Education Corporation

SUMMARY. Use of Warrington's Recognition Memory Test (RMT) for the detection of response bias and malingering is evaluated. The RMT's psychometric characteristics are reviewed. A method for using the RMT to detect response bias is presented: determining the probability of obtaining specific RMT scores; comparing the individual patient's RMT scores with group data from patients with established neurologic disorders; combining RMT data with other test data; integrating injury characteristics and psychosocial factors with RMT scores; and use of prevalence rates with the RMT. RMT data from a sample 90 persons with acute traumatic brain injury, stratified by injury severity, are presented to provide clinical benchmarks. The evidentiary reliability of the RMT is also discussed in light of *Daubert* factors. *[Article copies available for a fee from The Haworth Document Delivery Service: 1-800-HAWORTH. E-mail address: <getinfo@haworthpressinc.com> Website: <http://www. HaworthPress.com> © 2002 by The Haworth Press, Inc. All rights reserved.]*

KEYWORDS. Recognition memory test, malingering, psychophysiologic disorders, neuropsychological tests

---

Scott R. Millis is affiliated with the Kessler Medical Rehabilitation Research and Education Corporation, University of Medicine and Dentistry of New Jersey-New Jersey Medical School, West Orange, NJ.

Address correspondence to: Scott R. Millis, Kessler Medical Rehabilitation Research and Education Corporation, Research Department, 1199 Pleasant Valley Way, West Orange, NJ 07052 (E-mail: smillis@kmrrec.org).

[Haworth co-indexing entry note]: "Warrington's Recognition Memory Test in the Detection of Response Bias." Millis, Scott R. Co-published simultaneously in *Journal of Forensic Neuropsychology* (The Haworth Medical Press, an imprint of The Haworth Press, Inc.) Vol. 2, No. 3/4, 2002, pp. 147-166; and: *Detection of Response Bias in Forensic Neuropsychology* (ed: Jim Hom, and Robert L. Denney) The Haworth Medical Press, an imprint of The Haworth Press, Inc., 2002, pp. 147-166. Single or multiple copies of this article are available for a fee from The Haworth Document Delivery Service [1-800-HAWORTH, 9:00 a.m. - 5:00 p.m. (EST). E-mail address: getinfo@haworthpressinc.com].

© 2002 by The Haworth Press, Inc. All rights reserved.

WARRINGTON'S RECOGNITION MEMORY TEST IN THE DETECTION OF RESPONSE BIAS

Forced-choice tests, also known as symptom validity tests (SVTs), are among the most extensively evaluated tests for the detection of response bias in the neuropsychological examination (Slick, Sherman, & Iverson, 1999). A target stimulus is presented and is then followed by a two-choice recognition task with the original target item paired with a distractor item not presented. The individual is then asked to identify the target item that was presented during the acquisition trial. The delay between the exposure and recognition trials varies across tests, ranging from essentially no delay to a delay of several minutes. A wide variety of stimuli have been used in this test paradigm, including words, digits, photographs, line drawings, and tasks modified from the sensory-perceptual examination (e.g., finger-tip number writing and tactile finger recognition).

An individual who has not been exposed to the target items, and, thus, having no prior knowledge or memory of the stimuli, would perform at chance level during the recognition trial. A performance that is significantly below chance from a statistical perspective (e.g., $p < .05$) would imply that an individual did, indeed, remember the target items, i.e., the accurate memory of the target items allows the individual to differentiate the target from the foils. Response bias can thus be assessed by comparing an individual's performance on the two-alternative forced-choice test with the binomial distribution to determine the probability of obtaining a particular score. As scores deviate from chance, it is increasingly likely that the individual was deliberately choosing wrong answers.

Standard neuropsychological measures with a forced-choice format such as the Recognition Memory Test (RMT; Warrington, 1984) have also been used to detect response bias in a manner similar to SVTs (e.g., Iverson & Franzen, 1994; Iverson & Franzen, 1998; Millis, 1992; Millis, 1994; Millis & Putnam, 1994). This paper will examine the RMT and will provide practical guidelines for its use in the assessment of response bias.

TEST DESCRIPTION

The RMT consists of two subtests, Words (RMT-W) and Faces (RMT-F). The RMT-W subtest consists of 50 stimulus words and 50 distractor words, ranging in length from 4 to 6 letters and of A or AA frequency on the Thorndike-Lorge count (Warrington, 1984). The RMT-F consists of 50 photographs of unfamiliar faces and fifty distractor faces. Both subtests follow the same administration procedure with the 50 stimulus items presented at a rate of one item every three seconds. The participant is asked to respond "yes" or "no" to indicate if the item is "pleasant" or "not pleasant," respectively. Retention is then tested by a forced, two-choice recognition paradigm administered immediately after the presentation of the set of 50 test stimuli. Target and distractor are presented side-by-side, and the right/left position of the items is randomized. The order of the stimulus items for both subtests is not maintained in the recognition trial. A clinically attractive feature of the RMT is that it makes minimal motor or verbal response demands, and, hence can be used with patients with paralysis, dysarthria, tracheostomy, or similar conditions that preclude assessment with other memory measures. At the time of this writing, the RMT can be purchased in North America from Psychological Assessment Resources (http://www.parinc.com) and Western Psychological Services (http://www.wpspublish.com).

PSYCHOMETRIC CHARACTERISTICS

The RMT has been used to detect memory impairment in a broad range of neurologic and psychiatric disorders, including probable Alzheimer-type dementia, cerebral vascular disease, Parkinson's disease, neurosyphilis, herpes encephalitis, seizure disorders, aneurysms, traumatic brain injury, tumors, and various psychiatric illnesses in North America and Europe (Aggleton & Shaw, 1996; Baxendale, 1997; Bigler et al., 1996; Dewick et al., 1991; Diesfeldt, 1990; Hermann, Connell, Barr & Wyler, 1995; Kelly, Johnson, & Govern, 1996; Kneeborn, Chelune, & Luders, 1997; Millis & Dijkers, 1993; Morris, Abrahams, & Polkey, 1995; Naugle, Chelune, Schuster, Luders, & Comair, 1994; Rapcsak, Polster, Comer, & Rubens, 1994; Soukup, Bimbela, & Schiess, 1999; Sweet, Demakis, Ricker, & Millis, 2000).

Malina, Bowers, Millis, and Uekert (1998) examined the internal consistency of the RMT in a sample of 72 patients with traumatic brain injuries ranging in severity from complicated mild to severe. The internal consistency reliability coefficient, Cronbach's alpha (Cronbach, 1951), for the RMT-W was .86 and for the RMT-F was .77. In a mixed neurologic disorder sample of 40 participants, Soukup et al. (1999) reported a test-retest reliability coefficient of .81 for the RMT-F (mean retest interval = 7 months). A principal components analysis of RMT and Wechsler Memory Scale data from a mixed clinical sample (Compton, Sherer, & Adams, 1992) found that the RMT subtests loaded on a component separate from the WMS subtests. With regard to demographic factors, Kelly et al. (1996) found statistically nonsignificant relationships between the RMT and age, race, and education in a sample of persons with traumatic brain injury.

Although initially designed to detect material specific memory deficits associated with lateralized brain dysfunction, the RMT's clinical sensitivity in this regard is low (Hermann et al., 1995; Kneebone et al., 1997; Naugle et al., 1994; Sweet et al., 2000). Similarly, the RMT appears to be less sensitive to the effects of brain injury than other memory tests. Millis and Dijkers (1993) found that RMT-W had low sensitivity (.63) to brain injury in a sample of rehabilitation inpatients with complicated mild to severe traumatic brain injuries. When investigated from the perspective of magnetic resonance volumetric image analysis, Bigler et al. (1996) found that both RMT subtests had small, statistically nonsignificant correlations with ventricle-to-brain ratio, third ventricle, and total brain volume in a sample of persons with traumatic brain injury. In addition, the RMT had statistically nonsignificant correlations with left and right hippocampi and temporal horn volume, in contrast to savings scores derived from Logical Memory and Visual Reproduction subtests from the Wechsler Memory Scale-Revised and the Rey Complex Figure. The RMT-W mean score for the group of patients assessed less than 90 days post-injury in Bigler et al. (1996) was 46.6 out of 50–a score well within normal limits. Squire and Shimamura (1986) gave the RMT to a group of 10 amnestic patients: the median scores for the RMT-W and the RMT-F were 36.5 and 38, respectively, and none performed below chance on either subtest. In the same study, the authors constructed a parallel form of the RMT and tested retention after a *24-hour delay*: none of the amnestic patients performed below chance even after 24 hours, and the median scores for the RMT-W and the RMT-F were 28.5 and 33.5, respectively, following the 24-hour delay. Although this ceiling effect for the RMT may be considered undesirable in some respects, it is actually a very useful feature in the detection of response bias when combined with other tests and background data. Put simply, it appears that substantial brain dysfunction is required to disrupt performance on the RMT. As a starting point, low RMT scores in cases of mild traumatic brain injury should raise a red flag.

DETECTION OF RESPONSE BIAS WITH THE RECOGNITION MEMORY TEST

The assessment of response bias with RMT is a multiple step process:

- Determining the probability of obtaining specific RMT subtest scores;
- Comparing the individual patient's RMT scores with group data from patients with established neurologic disorders;
- Putting the RMT scores in perspective with regard to broader contextual factors;
- Combining RMT data with other test data;
- Dealing with prevalence rates.

Chance Level Performance: Determining the Probability of a Test Score

Although not originally designed to detect response bias, the RMT's forced-choice format and ceiling effect led investigators to examine its utility in this regard. As with any other dichotomous forced-choice measure, the normal approximation to the binomial distribution (Altman, 1999) can be used to determine the probability of obtaining a given RMT score, where x is the observed score and n is the total number of items (50) on the each RMT subtest:

$$z = \frac{x - (0.5 \times n)}{\sqrt{0.25 \times n}}$$

A continuity correction is often used when a continuous distribution is used to approximate noncontinuous data, as in the case of the normal and binomial distributions:

$$z = \frac{\left| x - (0.5 \times n) \right| - 0.5}{\sqrt{0.25 \times n}}$$

For example, the probability of obtaining score of less than 19 on either RMT subtest is 0.03. Clinical and analog simulator studies using the RMT to detect response bias did find that presumed malingerers as a group obtained significantly lower scores on the RMT than did persons with brain injury. For example, the RMT differentiated persons with moderate to severe TBI from litigating mild head injury claimants (Millis, 1992; Millis & Putnam, 1994) with overall correct classification ranging from 76% to 83% with associated large effect sizes, Hedges' $g = .90$ to 1.28. Hedges' g is an estimate of the standardized mean difference between two groups (Hedges & Olkin, 1985). Similar patterns were found in an analog malingering study with the RMT by Iverson and Franzen (1998) with even larger effect sizes, $g = 2.80$ to 4.62.

Hence, at the group level, there is substantial separation in group means. Inspection of the group means of the presumed malingerers across studies reveals a performance at chance levels. Yet, as found with other SVTs, the majority of presumed malingerers do not perform significantly below chance on the RMT (Slick et al., 1999). This finding prompted investigators to attempt to find alternative cutoff scores. For example, Millis (1992) found that a cutoff of less than 32 on the RMT-W correctly classified 90% of persons with TBI in his sample and 70% of the litigants with alleged brain injury. Using the same cutoff, Iverson and Franzen (1998) correctly classified 90% of their analog malingerers and 100% of persons with brain dysfunction. Millis (1992) derived this cutoff score empirically, but it is interesting to note that this score falls within the 95% confidence interval for random responding with a 50-item dichotomous-choice test. Attempts to find diagnostically efficient cutoff scores for the RMT-F have been mixed: Millis (1992) was not able to find an acceptable cutoff, but Iverson and Franzen (1998) reported that cutoff scores of less than 28 and 33 yielded acceptable classification rates.

In summary, a score of less than 19 on either RMT subtest would indicate definite response bias. Using additional diagnostic criteria proposed by Slick et al. (1999), a finding of definite response bias ". . . not fully accounted for by psychiatric, neurologic, or developmental factors" (p. 552) along with the presence of "substantial external incentive" (p. 553) warrants diagnostic consideration of malingered neurocognitive dysfunction. In cases in which the RMT score is not significantly below chance but within the 95% confidence interval of random responding (i.e., 19 to 32), probable or possible response bias needs to be considered but cannot be established on the basis of the RMT data alone. Discussion of the additional analytic steps follows.

Comparisons with Group Data of Persons with Established Brain Dysfunction

Because the majority of cases of response bias will not yield scores significantly below chance on the RMT and standard SVTs, it is helpful to know how persons with established neurologic disorders perform on these measures. Moreover, the RMT is fundamentally different from standard SVTs in terms of level of difficulty. Most SVTs were designed to be simple enough to be performed with minimal error by persons with even marked cognitive impairment. Although the RMT has a low ceiling, many persons with brain dysfunction will obtain low scores on the RMT that do not reflect response bias.

To assist the neuropsychologist in determining whether a given RMT score is consistent with various levels of traumatic brain injury severity, RMT data are presented on 90 inpatients from a university-affiliated inpatient rehabilitation hospital, stratified by injury severity (Table 1). All patients completed the RMT-W and 83 completed the RMT-F. Of the sample, 81% were male, mean age was 32.4 years (SD = 13.2), and mean educational level was 11.8 years (SD = 2.2). It should be noted that the mild injury group in this sample was *not* representative of most persons with mild TBI: although having initial GCS scores in the 13 to 15 range, many of these patients had subdural hematomas or related intracranial pathology or other body systems injuries requiring inpatient rehabilitation care. In short, this mild injury sample should be characterized as a "complicated" mild TBI group with likely greater neuropsychological impairment than is typically associated with mild TBI (Williams, Levin, & Eisenberg, 1990).

Violin plots (Hintze & Nelson, 1998) were prepared to portray RMT distributions for this study's sample, stratified by brain injury severity (Figures 1 and 2). Violin plots combine the summary statistics of a box plot with the graphical information given by a local density estimator to show the distributional structure of the RMT scores of the subgroups. The median is the short horizontal line, the interquartile range is the narrow shaded box, the y-axis is labeled at the minimum, median, and maximum scores for each group, and the data are surrounded by mirrored density traces. Figures 3 and 4 are cumulative distribution plots of the RMT scores obtained by this TBI sample. The cumulative probability is plotted on the y-axis with the associated RMT scores appearing on the x-axis.

The neuropsychologist can use Table 1 and Figures 1 through 4 when evaluating an individual patient's performance on the RMT to deter-

TABLE 1. Total Number of Words Correct on the Recognition Memory Test During Inpatient Rehabilitation Hospitalization Stratified by Initial Injury Severity

	Injury severity	N	Mean	SD	25th percentile	Median	75th percentile	Min	Max
Words	Severe	50	40.8	6.7	35.8	41	47.3	28	50
	Moderate	13	42.5	5.7	40	43	47	31	49
	Mild	27	43.5	5.0	42	44	47	27	50
	Total	90	41.9	6.2	38.8	43	47	27	50
Faces	Severe	50	36.0	6.1	31	36	40	26	49
	Moderate	11	37.8	6.9	35	35	45	24	46
	Mild	22	39.2	5.6	36	40.5	43	27	50
	Total	83	37.1	6.2	33	37	42	26	50

mine whether that patient's RMT scores fall within expected levels of performance based on injury severity. These data are from a homogeneous group of patients with regard to acuteness of injury: all were given the RMT within two months of injury, and the mean and median RMT scores are nearly equivalent. Given the acuteness of the injury, it is reasonable to characterize these scores as representing a likely lower bound for the performances of persons with TBI on the RMT. A useful starting point is to use the interquartile range of RMT score distributions (i.e., scores included in the 25th to 75th percentile range) when analyzing an individual patient's score. For example, the interquartile range for the RMT-W for the severe group is 35.8 to 47.3. Hence, if a patient with a history of mild TBI obtains a score of 32 on the RMT-W, additional assessment for response bias is warranted. This is not to imply that the patient is "malingering," but that this particular RMT score in a patient with mild TBI is aberrant and in need of explanation. As described in the following section, evaluation of broader contextual factors can assist the neuropsychologist in interpreting aberrant RMT scores. Neuropsychologists can also consult the studies listed in the Psychometric Characteristics section of this paper for RMT data on other disorders for comparison purposes. For example, it is notable in the Squire and Shimamura (1986) study that none of the amnestic patients performed below chance even after a 24-hour delay and that the median scores for the RMT-W and the RMT-F were 28.5 and 33.5, respectively.

FIGURE 1. Violin plots of total number of words correct on the Recognition Memory Test–Words Subtest during inpatient rehabilitation hospitalization stratified by initial injury severity.

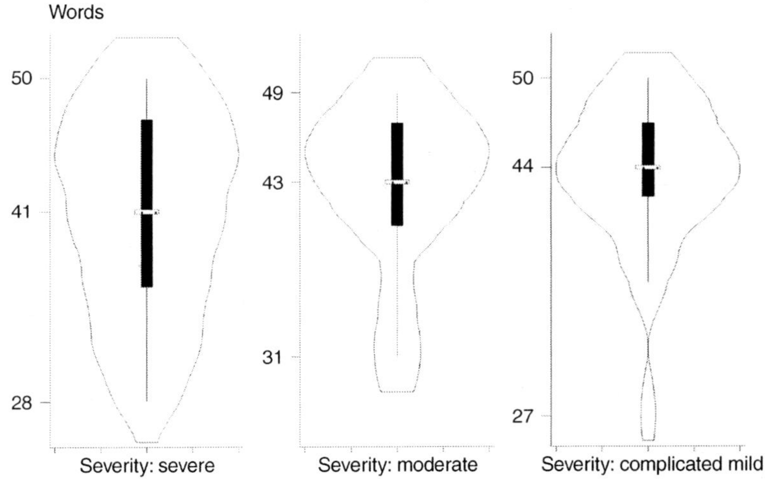

FIGURE 2. Violin plots of total number of words correct on the Recognition Memory Test–Faces Subtest during inpatient rehabilitation hospitalization stratified by initial injury severity.

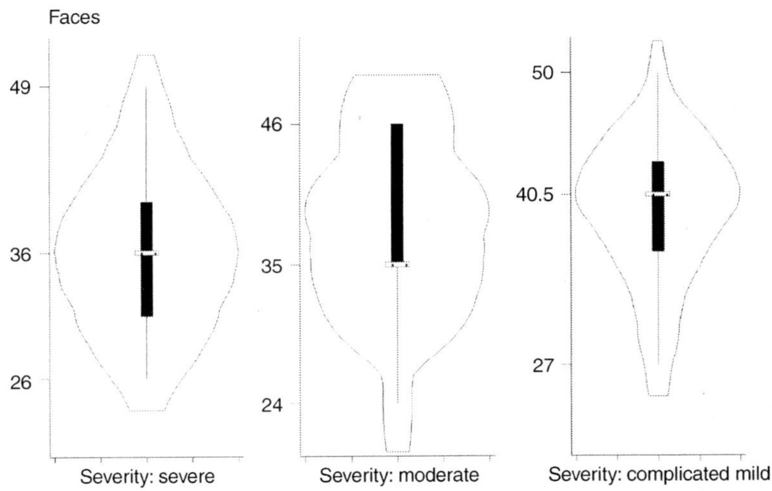

FIGURE 3. Cumulative distribution plot total for number of words correct on the Recognition Memory Test–Words Subtest stratified by initial injury severity.

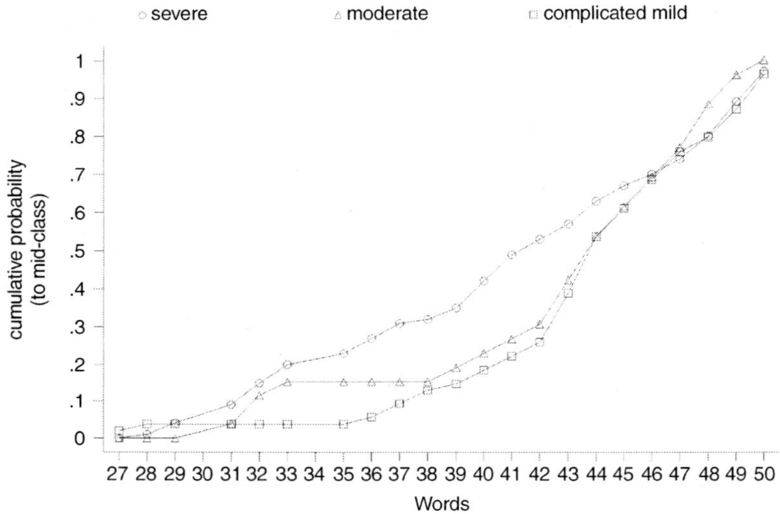

FIGURE 4. Cumulative distribution plot total for number of words correct on the Recognition Memory Test–Faces Subtest stratified by initial injury severity.

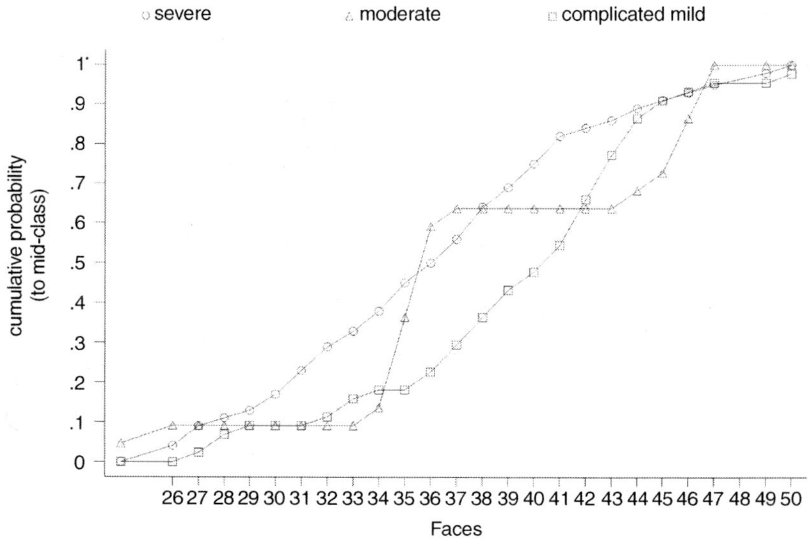

Assessing Contextual Factors

No single test score in isolation can establish a definite diagnosis. Test scores can only provide evidence in support of various diagnoses. A test result must be combined with other information before it can be interpreted meaningfully. Cases of alleged traumatic brain injury (TBI) are common in forensic neuropsychology practice. When evaluating traumatic brain injury claims, it is important to obtain the following information when interpreting all neuropsychological tests performances to determine the degree of consistency between test score and injury:

- Patient's initial injury severity as established by the Glasgow Coma Scale score, Revised Trauma Score, time-to-follow commands (derived from the motor score on the Glasgow Coma Scale), length of posttraumatic amnesia as determined by the Galveston Orientation and Amnesia Scale, or related injury severity measures;
- Amount of time post-injury;
- Admission pupillary response;
- Neuroimaging findings such as presence of mass lesion midline shift;
- Presence of raised intracranial pressure or hypotension shortly after trauma;
- Presence of injuries to organ systems other than the brain;
- Litigation status;
- Quality of the patient's social support system;
- Patient's mean of financial support and disability status;
- Demographic and premorbid factors including age, educational attainment, occupational history, past and current medical, psychiatric and substance abuse disorders, and history of physical or sexual abuse;
- Estimated prevalence of response bias in the particular setting or environment in which the patient is being evaluated.

Two patients can obtain the same score on the RMT, but the diagnostic implications may be vastly different. For illustration, assume that the following patients both achieved scores of 29 correct on the RMT-W (Figure 5). The score of 29 on the RMT-W might reflect response bias in the case of Patient A, whereas the same score in Patient B is probably indicative of brain dysfunction. This obvious scenario is to emphasize the need for the neuropsychologist to gather the necessary contextual

FIGURE 5. Hypothetical cases.

Patient A

- Patient tested at 2 years post-injury
- GCS = 15
- Patient examined and released from emergency department
- Negative CT
- Patient referred by attorney
- Pending litigation
- Patient was in motor vehicle accident in which the other driver was at fault

Patient B

- Patient tested at 2 months post-injury in inpatient rehabilitation unit
- Admission Glasgow Coma Scale = 3
- 24-hour CT scan showed midline shift of 6 mm
- Left pupil nonresponsive in ER
- Time-to-follow command = 20 days
- Patient was an assault victim

data when using the RMT as one element in the assessment of response bias. Although the RMT resembles SVTs in terms of a forced-choice response format, it needs to be stressed from the outset that the RMT should not be used as a sole measure to detect response bias. Some persons with traumatic brain injury, particularly during the acute phase of recovery, will obtain low scores on the RMT that likely reflect brain dysfunction and not response bias.

Combining the RMT with Other Measures

Neuropsychologists will invariably have other test data with which to compare RMT scores. It can be informative to compare the RMT performance with tests explicitly developed to measure effort, such as the Portland Digit Recognition Test (Binder & Willis, 1991), Computerized Assessment of Response Bias (Conder, Allen, & Cox, 1992), Test of Memory Malingering (Tombaugh, 1997), Victoria Symptom Validity Test (Slick, Hopp, Strauss, & Thompson, 1997), or Word Memory Test (Green, Allen, & Astner, 1996).

In addition, the neuropsychologist can combine RMT data with information from other standard measures having a forced-choice format that appear useful in detecting response bias such as the Seashore Rhythm Test (SRT) and Speech-Sounds Perception Test (SSPT) (Gfeller & Cradock, 1998; Goebel, 1983; Heaton, Smith, Lehman, & Vogt, 1978; Millis, Putnam, & Adams, 1996; Mittenberg, Rotholc, Russell, & Heilbronner, 1996; Trueblood & Schmidt, 1993). Comparisons can also be made with single variable and multivariate composite indicators of response bias derived from the California Verbal Learning

Test (Baker, Donders, & Thompson, 2000; Coleman, Rapport, Millis, Ricker, & Farchione, 1998; Millis, Putnam, Adams, & Ricker, 1995; Sweet, Wolfe, Sattlberger, Numan, Rosenfeld, Clingerman, & Nies, 2000; Trueblood & Schmidt, 1993). Convergent evidence from these measures can clarify the meaning of RMT tests scores that appear unusually low yet not significantly below chance.

Prevalence Rates

The issue of prevalence rates of biased responding in a given sample must be considered when the RMT score is not significantly below chance. Estimates of a test's sensitivity and specificity cannot be applied in isolation, but must be used in combination with prevalence (base rates) of the disorder or condition that the test purports to detect. In a modification of the Bayes theorem, Meehl and Rosen (1955) formulated a rule that can be used to determine whether a test adds any incremental accuracy beyond a prediction based on the prevalence rate alone:

$$\frac{Prevalence}{1 - Prevalence} > \frac{1 - Specificity}{Sensitivity}$$

For example, assuming a sensitivity to response bias of .80 and a specificity with regard to TBI of .90, a prevalence of response bias in a given sample would need to exceed 11% in order for the RMT-W to be diagnostically useful in the detection of response bias when using the derived cutoff scores.

OTHER RMT INDICES

Although much of the attention given to the use of the RMT for the detection of response bias has focused on the overall correct score and its degree of departure from chance, there may be other useful indices, such as the longest run of consistently incorrect responses or infrequently missed items. However, there is insufficient empirical data now to recommend use of either index for clinical or forensic use. Nonetheless, preliminary information is presented to encourage future research.

Analysis of the RMT-W performance of a subset of 46 inpatients with TBI from the sample of 90 persons described earlier in Table 1, revealed that the longest run of incorrect responses was four; for RMT-F, five. Hence, it appears that long runs of incorrect responses on the RMT are rare among persons with TBI. Still to be determined, however, is whether malingering behavior on the RMT is associated with longer runs of incorrect responses. That is, malingerers would need to make significantly longer runs of incorrect responses than do persons with brain dysfunction in order for the index to be diagnostically useful.

With regard to infrequently missed items on the RMT, individual item responses on the Words subtest were analyzed from the sample of 72 persons with TBI from the RMT reliability study previously discussed (Malina, Bowers, Millis, & Uekert, 1998). The following RMT-W items were passed by over 90% of the TBI sample: 2, 5, 6, 8, 14, 16, 19, 23, 26, and 29. It should be noted that the item numbers refer to the items as numbered on the answer sheet–not the order of presentation. Usefulness of this index is based on the assumption that some of the RMT items are more easily remembered or have greater salience than other items. However, replication on an independent clinical sample needs to be completed to determine whether the same RMT items are infrequently missed. In addition, it remains to be seen whether malingerers fail these items more frequently than persons with TBI do. With only 10 items, this index may also have insufficient variance to discriminate among groups.

If these indices were found to have favorable diagnostic properties in detecting response bias as single indicators, the next step would be to determine whether they add significant incremental discriminating power above and beyond the total score correct. Substantial collinearity may be present among the indices such that they may provide only redundant information.

DAUBERT AND THE ADMISSIBILITY OF THE RECOGNITION MEMORY TEST

The court decides whether the neuropsychologist and test findings meet the legal criteria for admissibility (Ogloff, 1995). Admissibility of evidence is governed by the Federal Rules of Evidence (FRE) in the federal courts, although many state courts have adopted portions of the FRE in their evidentiary law (Ogloff, 1995). Beginning with *Daubert* (*Daubert v. Merrell Dow Pharmaceuticals, Inc.*, 1993), the United States Supreme Court has clarified evidentiary standards for expert testimony through a series of decisions to help trial judges to separate good science from junk science, i.e., "evidentiary reliability."

A brief discussion follows that examines how the RMT might fare when *Daubert* "factors" are applied to it. That is, does the RMT have sufficient evidentiary reliability as a test of response bias to be admissible under *Daubert*? It should be emphasized that there are no strict *Daubert* "criteria": the court is to evaluate evidence in a flexible manner. Nonetheless, the following guidelines provide a framework for trial judges to evaluate evidence.

Has the RMT Been Tested?

Yes, the RMT's capacity to detect response bias has been evaluated by independent investigators with both clinical and simulator (analog) research designs: Cradock, Gfeller, and Falkenhain (1994), Iverson and Franzen (1994), Iverson and Franzen (1998), Millis (1992), Millis (1994), and Millis and Putnam (1994). The findings from these independent investigations have been consistent with regard to the RMT's diagnostic properties. In addition, the RMT has been tested with a wide variety of neurologic and psychiatric disorders. Hence, an "empirical floor" (Bianchini, Mathias, & Greve, 2001) can be established with the RMT, which is ". . . a norm-referenced, clinically-derived above-chance cutoff which classifies as invalid those cases falling below the lowest score of some confirmed brain-injured, psychiatric, or other cognitively impaired patient sample" (p. 35).

Has the RMT Been Subjected to Peer Review and Publication?

Yes, the RMT has an extensive history of peer review and publication.

What Is the Known or Potential Error Rate in Applying the RMT?

In a review of RMT studies, Bianchini et al. (2001) provide a summary table of sensitivity and specificity values for various cutoff scores for the RMT derived from a number of studies. Sensitivity is defined as the probability of having a positive test result (i.e., positive for response bias) among persons thought to be malingering. The false negative rate is given by (1 − sensitivity). Specificity is the probability of having a negative test result among persons with TBI or other neurologic disorder. The false positive rate is (1 − specificity). Sensitivity for the RMT-W has been found to range from .70 to .95 with specificity ranging from .90 to 1.00. For RMT-F, sensitivity has been reported to range from .78 to .95 and specificity from .78 to 1.00. A linear discriminant function including both the RMT-W and RMT-F was derived (Millis, 1992) and cross-validated (Millis & Putnam, 1994) with a sensitivity of .85 and specificity of .82.

The prevalence of the condition or disorder of interest must be considered along with the test's sensitivity and specificity. For example, assuming a sensitivity of .80 and a specificity of .90, a prevalence of response bias in a given sample would need to exceed 11% in order for the RMT-W to be diagnostically useful in the detection of response bias when using the derived cutoff scores.

To What Extent Has the RMT Received General Acceptance in the Neuropsychological Community?

Use of the RMT in the detection of response bias has undergone extensive review and critique since 1994, e.g., Bianchini et al. (2001), Iverson and Binder (2000), Lezak (1995), Millis and Putnam (1996), Nies and Sweet (1994), Putnam, Millis, and Adams (1996), Spreen and Strauss (1998), and Sweet (1999), and Williams (1998). Although not without limitations, a general consensus is that the RMT can be a useful test in the comprehensive assessment of response bias in the neuropsychological examination.

In summary, it is this author's opinion that the admission of RMT data will make some fact ". . . more probable or less probable than it would be without the evidence" (FRE 401) when used in the context of a comprehensive neuropsychological assessment.

REFERENCES

Aggleton, J. P., & Shaw, C. (1996). Amnesia and recognition memory: A re-analysis of psychometric data. *Neuropsychologia, 34*, 51-62.

Altman, D. G. (1999). *Practical statistics for medical research*. Boca Raton, FL: Chapman and Hall/CRC.

Baker, R., Donders, J., & Thompson, E. (2000). Assessment of incomplete effort with the California Verbal Learning Test. *Applied Neuropsychology, 7*, 111-114.

Baxendale, S. A. (1997). The role of the hippocampus in recognition memory. *Neuropsychologia, 35*, 591-598.

Bianchini, K. J., Mathias, C. W., & Greve, K. W. (2001). Symptom validity testing: A critical review. *The Clinical Neuropsychologist, 15*, 19-45.

Bigler, E. D., Johnson, S. C., Anderson, C. V., Blatter, D. D., Gale, S. D., Russo, A. A., Ryser, D. K., Macnamara, S. E., Bailey, B. J., Hopkins, R. O., & Abildskov, T. J. (1996). Traumatic brain injury and memory: The role of hippocampal atrophy. *Neuropsychology, 10*, 333-342.

Binder, L. M., & Willis, S. C. (1991). Assessment of motivation after financially compensable minor head injury. *Psychological Assessment, 3*, 175-181.

Coleman, R., Rapport, L., Millis, S., Ricker, J., & Farchione, T. (1998). Effects of coaching on the detection of malingering on the California Verbal Learning Test: An analog study of malingered head injury. *The Clinical Neuropsychologist, 20*, 201-210.

Compton, J., M., Sherer, M., & Adams, R. L. (1992). Factor analysis of the Wechsler Memory Scale and the Warrington Recognition Memory Test. *Archives of Clinical Neuropsychology, 7*, 165-173.

Conder, R., Allen, L., & Cox, D. (1992). *Computerized Assessment of Response Bias Test Manual*. Durham, NC: CogniSyst.

Cradock, M., Gfeller, J., & Falkenhain, M. (1994, November). Detecting feigned memory deficits with the Rey Auditory Verbal Learning Test and the Recognition Memory Test. Presented at the Annual Conference of the National Academy of Neuropsychology, Orlando, FL.

Cronbach, L. J. (1951). Coefficient alpha and the internal structure of tests. *Psychometrika, 16*, 297-334.

Daubert v. Merrell Dow Pharmaceuticals, 727 F. Supp. 570 (S.D. Cal. 1989), *aff'd*, 951 F.2d 1128 (9th Cir 1990), *vacated*, 113 S. Ct. 2786 (1993).

Dewick, H. C., Hanley, J. R., Davies, A. D. M., Playfer, J., & Turnbull, C. (1991). Perception and memory for faces in Parkinson's Disease. *Neuropsychologia, 29*, 785-802.

Deisfeldt, H. F. A. (1990). Recognition memory for words and faces in primary degenerative dementia of the Alzheimer type and normal old age. *Journal of Clinical and Experimental Neuropsychology, 12*, 931-945.

Federal Rules of Evidence. (1976). *28 United States Code*. 101-1103.

Gfeller, J. D., & Cradock, M. M. (1998). Detecting feigned neuropsychological impairment with the Seashore Rhythm Test. *Journal of Clinical Psychology, 54*, 431-438.

Goebel R. A. (1983). Detection of faking on the Halstead-Reitan Neuropsychological Test Battery. *Journal of Clinical Psychology, 39*, 731-742.

Green, P., Allen, L. M., & Astner, K. (1996). The Word Memory Test: A user's guide to the oral and computer administered forms, US version 1.1. Durham, NC: CogniSyst.

Heaton, R. K., Smith, H. H., Lehman, R. A. W., & Vogt, A. T. (1978). Prospects for faking believable deficits on neuropsychological testing. *Journal of Consulting and Clinical Psychology, 46*, 892-900.

Hedges, L.V., & Olkin, I. (1985). *Statistical methods for meta-analysis*. New York: Academic Press.

Hermann, B. P., Connell, B., Barr, W. B., & Wyler, A. R. (1995). The utility of the Warrington Recognition Memory Test for temporal lobe epilepsy: Pre-and postoperative results. *Journal of Epilepsy, 8*, 139-145.

Hintze, J. L., & Nelson, R. D. (1998). Violin plots: A box plot-density trace synergism. *The American Statistician, 52*, 181-184.

Iverson, G. L., & Binder, L. M. (2000). Detecting exaggeration and malingering in neuropsychological assessment. *Journal of Head Trauma Rehabilitation, 15(2)*, 829-858.

Iverson, G. L., & Franzen, M. D. (1994). The Recognition Memory Test, Digit Span, and Knox Cube Test as markers of malingered memory impairment. *Assessment, 1*, 323-334.

Iverson, G. L., & Franzen, M. D. (1998). Detecting malingered memory deficits with the Recognition Memory Test. *Brain Injury, 12*, 275-282.

Kelly, M. P., Johnson, C. T., & Govern, J. M. (1996). Recognition memory test: Validity in diffuse traumatic brain injury. *Applied Neuropsychology, 3/4*, 147-154.

Kneeborn, A. C., Chelune, G. J., & Luders, H. O. (1997). Individual patient prediction of seizure lateralization in temporal lobe epilepsy: A comparison between neuropsychological memory measures and the intracarotid amobarbitol procedure. *Journal of the International Neuropsychological Society, 3*, 159-168.

Lezak, M. D. (1995). *Neuropsychological assessment* (3rd ed.). New York: Oxford University Press.

Malina, A. C., Bowers, D. A., Millis, S. R., & Uekert, S. (1998). Internal consistency of the Warrington Recognition Memory Test. *Perceptual and Motor Skills, 86*, 1320-1322.

Meehl, P. E., & Rosen, A. (1955). Antecedent probability and the efficiency of psychometric signs, patterns, or cutting scores. *Psychological Bulletin, 52*, 194-216.

Millis, S. R. (1992). The Recognition Memory Test in the detection of malingered and exaggerated memory deficits. *Clinical Neuropsychologist, 6*, 406-414.

Millis, S. R. (1994). Assessment of motivation and memory with the Recognition Memory Test after financially compensable mild head injury. *Journal of Clinical Psychology, 50*, 601-605.

Millis, S. R., & Dijkers, M. (1993). Use of the Recognition Memory Test in traumatic brain injury. *Brain Injury, 7*, 53-58.

Millis, S. R., & Putnam, S. H. (1994). The Recognition Memory Test in the assessment of memory impairment after financially compensable mild head injury: A replication. *Perceptual and Motor Skills, 79*, 384-386.

Millis, S. R., & Putnam, S. H. (1996). Detection of malingering in postconcussive syndrome. In M. Rizzo & D. Tranel (Eds.), *Head injury and postconcussive syndrome* (pp. 481-498). New York: Churchill Livingstone.

Millis, S. R., Putnam, S. H., & Adams, K. M. (1996). Speech-sounds Perception Test and Seashore Rhythm Test as validity indicators in the neuropsychological evaluation of mild head injury [abstract]. *Archives of Clinical Neuropsychology, 11*, 425.

Millis, S. R., Putnam, S. H., Adams, K. M., & Ricker, J. H. (1995). The California Verbal Learning Test in the detection of incomplete effort in neuropsychological evaluation. *Psychological Assessment, 7*, 463-471.

Mittenberg, W., Rotholc, A., Russell, E., & Heilbronner, R. (1996). Identification of malingered head injury on the Halstead-Reitan Battery. *Archives of Clinical Neuropsychology, 11*, 271-281.

Morris, R. G., Abrahams, & Polkey, C. E. (1995). Recognition memory for words and faces following unilateral temporal lobectomy. *British Journal of Clinical Psychology, 34*, 571-576.

Naugle, R. I., Chelune, G. J., Schuster, J., Luders, H. O., & Comair, Y. (1994). Recognition memory for words and faces before and after temporal lobectomy. *Assessment, 1*, 373-381.

Nies, K. J., & Sweet, J. J. (1994). Neuropsychological assessment and malingering: A critical review of past and present strategies. *Archives of Clinical Neuropsychology, 9*, 501-552.

Ogloff, J. R. (1995). The legal basis of forensic applications of the MMPI-2. In Y. S. Ben-Porath, J. R. Graham, G. C. N. Hall, R. D. Hirschman, & M. S. Zaragoza (Eds.)., *Forensic applications of the MMPI-2* (pp. 18-47). Thousand Oaks, CA: Sage Publications.

Putnam, S. H., Millis, S. R., & Adams, K. M. (1996). Mild traumatic brain injury: Beyond cognitive assessment. In I. Grant & K. M. Adams (Eds.), *Neuropsychological assessment of neuropsychiatric disorders* (2nd ed.) (pp. 529-551). New York: Oxford University Press.

Rapscak, S. Z., Polster, M. R., Comer, J. F., & Rubens, A. B. (1994). False recognition and misidentification of faces following right hemisphere damage. *Cortex, 30*, 565-583.

Slick, D. J., Hopp, G., Strauss, E., & Thompson, G. B. (1997). *Victoria Symptom Validity Test: Professional manual*. Odessa, FL: Psychological Assessment Resources, Inc.

Slick, D. J., Sherman, E. M. S., & Iverson, G. L. (1999). Diagnostic criteria for malingered neurocognitive dysfunction: Proposed standards for clinical practice and research. *The Clinical Neuropsychologist, 13*, 545-561.

Soukup, V. M., Bimbela, A., & Scheiss, M. C. (1999). Recognition Memory for Faces: Reliability and validity of the Warrington Recognition Memory Test (RMT) in a neurological sample. *Journal of Clinical Psychology in Medical Settings, 6*, 287-293.

Spreen, O., & Strauss, E. (1998). *A Compendium of Neuropsychological Tests* (2nd ed.). New York: Oxford University Press.

Squire, L. R., & Shimamura, A. P. (1986). Characterizing amnestic patients for neurobehavioral study. *Behavioral Neuroscience, 100*, 866-877.

Sweet, J. J. (1999). Malingering: Differential diagnosis. In J. J. Sweet (Ed.), *Forensic Neuropsychology* (pp. 255-285). Lisse: Swets & Zeitlinger.

Sweet, J. J., Demakis, G. J., Ricker, J. H., & Millis, S. R. (2000). Diagnostic efficiency and material specificity of the Warrington Recognition Memory Test: A collaborative multisite investigation. *Archives of Clinical Neuropsychology, 15*, 301-309.

Sweet, J. J., Wolf, P., Sattlberger, E., Numan, B., Rosenfeld, J. P., Clingerman, S., & Nies, K. J. (2000). Further investigation of traumatic brain injury versus insufficient effort with the California Verbal Learning Test. *Archives of Clinical Neuropsychology, 15*, 105-113.

Tombaugh, T. N. (1997). The Test of Memory Malingering (TOMM): Normative data from cognitively intact and cognitively impaired individuals. *Psychological Assessment, 9*, 260-268.

Trueblood, W., & Schmidt, M. (1993). Malingering and other validity considerations in the neuropsychological evaluation of mild head injury. *Journal of Clinical and Experimental Neuropsychology, 15*, 578-590.

Warrington, E. K. (1984). *Recognition Memory Test.* Windsor: NFER-Nelson.
Williams, D. H., Levin, H. S., & Eisenberg, H. M. (1990). Mild head injury classification. *Neurosurgery, 27,* 422-428.
Williams, J. M. (1998). The malingering of memory disorder. In C. R. Reynolds (Ed.), *Detection of Malingering During Head Injury Litigation* (pp. 105-132). New York: Plenum Press.

Malingering in Forensic Neuropsychology: *Daubert* and the MMPI-2

Paul R. Lees-Haley

Independent Practice

Grant L. Iverson

University of British Columbia & Riverview Hospital

Rael T. Lange

University of British Columbia

David D. Fox

Consultants in Psychological Assessment

Lyle M. Allen III

CogniSyst, Inc.

Paul R. Lees-Haley is in independent practice, Huntsville, AL.

Grant L. Iverson is affiliated with the University of British Columbia & Riverview Hospital, Vancouver, BC.

Rael T. Lange is affiliated with the University of British Columbia, Vancouver, BC.

David D. Fox is affiliated with Consultants in Psychological Assessment, Glendale, CA.

Lyle M. Allen III is affiliated with CogniSyst, Inc., Durham, NC.

Address correspondence to: Paul R. Lees-Haley, PhD, 3021 Panorama Drive, Huntsville, AL 35801 (E-mail: PaulLH@Lees-Haley.com).

The authors thank Jennifer Bernardo for her assistance with manuscript preparation.

[Haworth co-indexing entry note]: "Malingering in Forensic Neuropsychology: *Daubert* and the MMPI-2." Lees-Haley, Paul R. et al. Co-published simultaneously in *Journal of Forensic Neuropsychology* (The Haworth Medical Press, an imprint of The Haworth Press, Inc.) Vol. 3, No. 1/2, 2002, pp. 167-203; and: *Detection of Response Bias in Forensic Neuropsychology* (ed: Jim Hom, and Robert L. Denney) The Haworth Medical Press, an imprint of The Haworth Press, Inc., 2002, pp. 167-203. Single or multiple copies of this article are available for a fee from The Haworth Document Delivery Service [1-800-HAWORTH, 9:00 a.m. - 5:00 p.m. (EST). E-mail address: getinfo@haworthpressinc.com].

© 2002 by The Haworth Press, Inc. All rights reserved.

SUMMARY. The MMPI-2 is one of the most widely used instruments in forensic neuropsychology. Unlike most tests, it has the advantage of containing validity scales that assist the examiner in determining the level of cooperation of the examinee. Scales that provide information for evaluating the validity of an MMPI-2 profile include VRIN, TRIN, L, F, K, F − K, F_B, F(p), FBS (Fake Bad Scale), Total Obvious − Subtle, Ds, Dsr, and Ego Strength. This article discusses research available when considering the applicability of these procedures in the context of challenges to their scientific reliability and validity in legal proceedings, according to the standards set forth in *Daubert v. Merrell Dow Pharmaceuticals, Inc.* *[Article copies available for a fee from The Haworth Document Delivery Service: 1-800-HAWORTH. E-mail address: <getinfo@haworthpressinc.com> Website: <http://www.HaworthPress.com> © 2002 by The Haworth Press, Inc. All rights reserved.]*

KEYWORDS. Malingering, MMPI-2, neuropsychology, cognitive

The use of a neuropsychologist as an expert witness in personal injury litigation has been accepted as a standard practice for some time. The general purpose of a neuropsychological evaluation in this context is to address those issues pertaining to the possible cognitive and/or psychological sequelae sustained by a claimant, as a result of brain injury (e.g., motor vehicle accident) and/or other neurological inference (e.g., toxic exposure). A neuropsychologist acting as an expert witness is typically required to answer a variety of questions such as: (a) is impairment present? (b) is the impairment exaggerated by the patient? (c) what was the cause of that impairment? (d) if there was more than one cause, how much of the impairment is attributable to the cause in question (the defendant)? (e) is the plaintiff different now than pre-injury (i.e., has there been a loss or was this pre-existing)? (f) how much will the plaintiff recover, and when? and (g) what functional deficits are related to any genuine impairments?

Neuropsychologists attempt to answer these questions through a variety of methods such as the administration of formal tests, clinical interviews, and careful review of medical records. However, it is the results from formal tests that often provide the most weight in establishing cognitive and/or psychological sequelae within the context of litigation. Practitioners have long taken for granted that the tests we use are reliable and valid. This is perhaps due to the inadequate study of these issues by test developers and the limited understanding of psychometric theory on the part of the clinician. Moreover, some psychologists might have a false sense of security about our tests that relates to our training in science (i.e., because we are trained in science, then the tools we use must be scientific). However, over the years, courts have become increasingly skeptical about our techniques and have imposed more rigorous guidelines for the admissibility of neuropsychological testimony at trial. The most recent of these standards, referred to as *Daubert*, requires that testimony provided by an expert witness shall be subject to four nonexclusive factors: "the testability of the expert's theories and methods, whether they had been subjected to review by peers, the error rate in study or test results, and the degree of acceptance of the proponent's theories and methods" (Mack, 1994, p. 24). As a result, it is essential that we examine our tools more closely in an effort to determine whether decisions made based on tests administered in the neuropsychological assessment battery will be admissible in court.

The intention of this paper is to provide a discussion of the use of the Minnesota Multiphasic Personality Inventory-Second Edition (MMPI-2; Butcher, Graham, Dahlstrom, Tellegen, & Kaemmer, 1989) within the context of forensic neuropsychology. In particular, the focus is on the use of the MMPI-2 to provide supporting information for the identification of exaggeration or malingering, and on those issues that may be raised in court with respect to the application of *Daubert* guidelines for the admissibility of expert testimony. This article will discuss the following four broad areas: (a) the role of the MMPI-2 in forensic neuropsychological evaluations, (b) overview of MMPI-2 administration, scoring, interpretation, and psychometrics, (c) research on the MMPI-2 validity scales for malingering detection, and (d) *Daubert* guidelines and the MMPI-2.

ROLE OF THE MMPI-2 IN FORENSIC NEUROPSYCHOLOGICAL EVALUATIONS

The MMPI-2 is one of the most widely used objective personality tests by psychologists and neuropsychologists in clinical practice (Camara, Nathan, & Puente, 2000). This edition of the test was released in 1989 following the revision of the original MMPI, and has replaced its predecessor as the generally accepted version. The MMPI was originally designed for clinical diagnosis. Therefore, most of the research over the years has focused on diagnostic issues and personality description, rather than on some of the questions of primary concern to the courts in forensic neuropsychology cases. Nonetheless, the MMPI-2 is commonly used in the forensic setting, and it is well accepted as a valuable tool for assessing a variety of factors in this context.

The purpose of the MMPI-2 in forensic neuropsychological assessment is varied and generally includes the (a) evaluation of the nature and extent of emotional distress injuries, (b) evaluation of chronic as well as acute psychopathology, (c) documentation of symptom presentation, (d) evaluation of the potential effects of psychological variables (e.g., depression and anxiety) on cognitive test performance, and (e) provision of evidence to support the identification of exaggeration or malingering. It can also aid in the discovery of relevant variables not unearthed by the clinical interview (e.g., susceptibility to substance abuse). The MMPI-2 can shed light on characteristics relevant to assessing the nature and extent of a patient's disability, if any, and the patient's ability to function in society (for example, vocationally or as a member of a family). In addition, it reveals psychological characteristics or problems that might help explain the complaints (e.g., somatoform tendencies or bizarre thinking).

Although the MMPI-2 is well accepted and is considered to have high clinical utility, attorneys and consumers sometimes have two misconceptions about what the MMPI-2 can and cannot do. First, the MMPI-2 will not pass a *Daubert* challenge if offered as evidence of brain injury; it does not measure neuropsychological impairment. There is no unique profile distinguishing patients with traumatic brain injuries or toxic injuries. Second, claims that the MMPI-2 indicates specific causation are indefensible under *Daubert*. A valid MMPI-2 provided by a cooperative patient provides evidence related to the condition of the patient but not the cause of that condition. However, the test is relevant to causation arguments in an indirect fashion. For example, a normal MMPI-2 might serve as evidence that event X has not caused the patient to be severely mentally ill or depressed. Similarly, an MMPI-2 indicative of chronic problems (e.g., Borderline Personality Disorder) may be suggestive that some problems, at least, were pre-existing, and thus not simply produced *de novo* by a recent causal agent. However, causation of an MMPI-2 profile indicative of minor psychological distress (e.g., anxiety or depression) cannot be made simply by the results of the test alone. Judgments of causation in this case can only be made through a careful review of pertinent background history.

With respect to malingering detection, a number of validity scales can be used on the MMPI-2 to assist clinicians in formulating hypotheses regarding possible exaggeration. Most validity scales on the MMPI-2 originally were designed to assess a client's test-taking attitude (i.e., to determine whether the test protocol could be reliably interpreted). However, many of these validity scales have also been used to provide support for the identification of malingering. Although these scales cannot be used as an indicator of *cognitive* exaggeration, they are often helpful in providing supporting evidence for the exaggeration of psychological distress. Virtually all forensic neuropsychology personal injury cases involve claims for emotional distress, which is known to elevate some of these scales. Part of a competent forensic neuropsychological evaluation is to assess the nature and extent of emotional distress injury. In these patients, psychopathology must also be evaluated to rule out its confounding effects. For example, a neuropsychologist who failed to account for conditions such as schizophrenia, depression, or anxiety would be overlooking essential differential diagnostic questions. In the context of interpreting neuropsychological test data, it is important to be able to conclude that the claimant's test performance has not been influenced as a result of some other confounding variable (e.g., depression, anxiety, or malingering).

OVERVIEW OF MMPI-2 ADMINISTRATION, SCORING, INTERPRETATION, AND PSYCHOMETRICS

For all tests used in a neuropsychological assessment, it is important to be aware of the psychometric properties of the tests. In a forensic neuropsychological setting, this knowledge is especially crucial when the testimony of an expert witness will be potentially challenged by *Daubert* standards. With regard to the *general* use of the MMPI-2, it is anticipated that the most basic area of challenge will relate to whether the test protocol has been appropriately administered, scored, and interpreted. Although a comprehensive discussion of this topic is well beyond the scope of this paper, presented below is a brief discussion of some issues all expert witnesses should be familiar with when MMPI-2 testimony comes under scrutiny by *Daubert* standards.

Administration and Scoring

Standard administration of the MMPI-2 is in paper-pencil format. Other administration methods include listening to a tape recorder for the questions or taking the test on the computer. Although there is a good correlation between the different formats for administering the test (e.g., booklet vs. tape-recorded vs. computer administered), they cannot automatically be assumed to yield identical scores.

Dozens of scales can be derived from the MMPI-2 with standard scoring programs yielding a bewildering number of scores. However, scoring procedures are vulnerable to attack. Hand scoring is often inaccurate and not recommended (Greene, 2000). In particular, the TRIN and VRIN validity scales are two of the scales most vulnerable to such errors, especially VRIN (Iverson & Barton, 1999). Even automated scoring services can contain scoring errors (Greene, 2000; Lees-Haley, 1991). When attempting to interpret reports generated by computer interpretive programs, special precautions are needed. For example, if demographic data are omitted when entering the raw data, the computer program may interpret the data based on a default option. In one widely used program, when demographic data are omitted, the computer treats all individuals as 18 year olds with 12 years of education, never married, in an outpatient setting. Participants in *Daubert* hearings can anticipate exhibits and cross-examination on alternative test interpretation services, showing contradictory conclusions, and should be actively aware of such discrepancies.

Interpretation

Although there are generally accepted references that provide, more or less, similar interpretations of scores and patterns of scores (i.e., profiles) on the MMPI-2, there remains controversy among experts regarding test interpretation. Some major concerns relate to the efficacy of traditional codetype analyses, the accuracy of the MMPI-2 to discriminate between diagnostic classes (e.g., Senior & Douglas, in press), and the usefulness of the MMPI-2 at predicting functioning in real world settings relevant to the courts. For example, for many years, elevations on MMPI-2 scales have been widely used in disability evaluations. Such data have been accepted in numerous cases in state and federal courts in the United States and several other countries–often based on the testimony of experts. However, when MMPI-2 scores were analyzed in a recent study, to determine which scales best predicted employment status, *none* of the scales were associated with employment (Fox & Lees-Haley, 2001).

There is no generally accepted method for interpreting the MMPI-2 that is unique to neuropsychology cases. There have been suggestions that correction factors that take into account neurological face-valid items are appropriate for patients with brain injuries (e.g., Gass, 1991;

Gass & Wald, 1997); however, other authors have concluded that they are inappropriate for forensic cases (Arbisi & Ben-Porath, 1999; Dunn & Lees-Haley, 1995; Hoffman, Scott, Emick, & Adams, 1999; Rayls, Mittenberg, Burns, & Theroux, 2000). Strategies of interpretation are open to considerable debate and often have limited empirical basis. At times even relatively elementary questions yield different answers in depositions of experts. Thus, there are many points of potential controversy for *Daubert* hearings.

Non-Test Taking Factors

The accuracy of MMPI-2 interpretations can be affected by non-test factors that have received only limited attention in the literature. In general, education and socio-economic history appear to account for more variance than race or ethnic background, neither of which appears to produce large effects on MMPI-2 findings. However, the research is limited for many of these issues (Graham, 2000; Greene, 1987, 2000; Gynther & Green, 1980; Hall, Bansal, & Lopez, 1999; Long, Graham, & Timbrook, 1994; Pritchard & Rosenblatt, 1980; Schinka & LaLone, 1997; Timbrook & Graham, 1994).

Norms and Test Manual

The MMPI-2 normative sample is composed of 1,138 men and 1,462 women, ages 18 to 80, from several geographic regions of the United States. Data concerning age distributions, geographic and ethnic composition, education, marital status, occupation, and income are provided in the manual. The generally accepted test manual for the MMPI-2 is by Butcher et al. (1989). However, the reader should be aware that there are errors in this manual (for details, see Greene, 2000), and a revised version is expected soon.

Concerns have been expressed about whether the standardization sample reasonably reflects the general population, arising especially because the level of education in the restandardization sample was higher. This was a reasonable and important question since there is reason to believe that socio-economic factors including education are more important contributors to MMPI-2 variance than other common concerns (e.g., ethnicity). However, Schinka and LaLone (1997) addressed these concerns by comparing the validity, clinical, content, and supplementary scales of the standardization sample and a census-matched subsample and found a difference of three T score points on only one scale.

Reliability

Test-retest reliability for the most commonly used MMPI-2 scales is relatively good. Test-retest reliability coefficients for the basic clinical scales and L, F, and K are almost all between .70 and .90 and the exceptions are close (Pa is r = .67 for men, F r = .58 for women, Si r = .92 for men, and Si r = .91 for women). Group means on retesting are quite similar, within approximately one or two points, and the standard error of measurement for the basic clinical scales generally are approximately 2 points (range = 1.00 to 2.42; Butcher et al., 1989). However, when standard errors of estimate are calculated around regressed true T scores, the confidence intervals can be surprisingly distant from the obtained scores. Moreover, as noted in the studies by Senior and colleagues referred to in the *Daubert* section of this article, reliability of the diagnoses suggested by MMPI-2 profiles appears to be in need of careful examination.

REVIEW OF THE MMPI-2 VALIDITY SCALE MALINGERING RESEARCH

There is more research on exaggeration and malingering on the MMPI-2 and its predecessor, the MMPI, than for any other test in the history of psychology. Scales that provide information for evaluating the validity of an MMPI-2 profile include VRIN, TRIN, L, F, K, F − K, F_B, F(p), FBS (Fake-Bad Scale), Total Obvious − Subtle, Ds, Dsr, and Ego Strength. To adequately address a *Daubert* challenge regarding the validity scales, it is important for expert witnesses to understand the development of the scales and be familiar with the current research. Thorough knowledge of the strengths and limitations of each scale for providing information concerning the identification of exaggeration is critical for drawing accurate inferences. Research utilizing the validity scales relating to malingering detection is discussed in more detail below.

L Scale

The L Scale was designed to identify persons who were deliberately trying to avoid answering the items of the MMPI in a frank and honest manner. While elevated scores on the L Scale suggest that an individual has tried to create an unusually favorable impression of themselves, examinees who are faking bad or overemphasizing psychopathology on the MMPI-2 often score in the low range on this scale. Greene (2000) notes that low scoring clients (e.g., raw score 0-2), "may be attempting to create an extremely pathological picture of themselves" (p. 94). However, persons who score in this range may also be characterized as normal individuals who are willing to admit to minor social faults (Greene, 2000). The MMPI-2 manual identifies faking bad as one of the possible interpretive implications of scores equal to or below T = 49. Graham (2000) suggests that in some cases scores below T = 50 are indicative of exaggeration of negative characteristics. Other possible interpretations of this score include the hypothesis that the examinee is self-confident and independent, or is cynical and sarcastic. Elevations on this scale, particularly when there are elevations of Dsr and FBS, can also indicate a complex form of malingering in which the person denies having certain problems but over-endorses psychological distress symptoms. Such a pattern is sometimes referred to as "impression management." Although the L Scale has been found to be somewhat useful for the identification of psychological exaggeration, earlier research has demonstrated that this scale has significant limitations for detecting sophisticated persons who have been instructed to falsify their answers on the MMPI (e.g., Vincent, Linsz, & Greene, 1966).

F Scale

The F scale consists of 60 items that are unusually or infrequently answered by either genuinely disturbed patients or members of the normal population. Fewer than 10% of the MMPI-2 normative population answered these items in the scored direction (Greene, 1991, 2000). Butcher (1990) noted that, "The F scale was devised as a measure of the tendency to admit to a wide range of psychological problems or to fake bad. An individual who scores high on the F scale is admitting to a wide range of complaints that are infrequently endorsed by the general population and reflect a tendency to exaggerate problems" (pp. 28-29). The F scale was used from the 1940s on the MMPI and has been used since 1989 on the MMPI-2. Use of the F scale is generally accepted in the field of psychological testing. However, the F scale appears less effective for detecting coached malingerers (Storm & Graham, 2000).

The MMPI-2 manual notes malingering as one of the potential explanations for F scale scores that exceed 70. However, more recently,

Butcher (1998) recommended that T scores of 90-99 are "Exaggerated," T = 100-109 are "Highly Exaggerated," and T ≥ 110 (with VRIN < 79) are "Likely Malingering." Certainly, F scale T scores in excess of 100 are frequently seen in community volunteers, Federal inmates, and psychiatric patients instructed to malinger psychopathology (Bagby, Rogers, Buis, & Kalemba, 1994; Graham, Watts, & Timbrook, 1991; Iverson, Franzen, & Hammond, 1995; Rogers, Sewell, & Ustad, 1995; Wetter, Baer, Berry, Robinson, & Sumpter, 1993). As Greene (2000) noted, elevations of T = 81-110 are associated with a readily apparent level of distress as well as overreporting psychopathology, so mental status observations of the patient are helpful in clarifying the more likely hypothesis. Greene further noted that an elevation of T > 110, if based on accurate responses by the patient, suggest a severely disorganized, floridly psychotic patient. Such a presentation is highly unusual among personal injury plaintiffs, and more likely a product of gross exaggeration if the test has been administered in a standard and appropriate manner.

Personal injury claimants who are malingering emotional distress tend to produce elevated scores on the F scale. However, the content of some items on the F scale includes material they may be reluctant to report, so there is reason to suspect that the F scale may be less sensitive to personal injury malingering than litigants attempting to appear severely mentally ill (especially in criminal forensic evaluations). For example, some of the items that increase F scale scores require the patient to admit being dishonest or in trouble or peculiar in ways that personal injury litigants usually wish to avoid. As a general rule of thumb, personal injury malingerers tend to attempt to present themselves as credible and reasonable or normal, with the exception of the emotional distress they suffer as a result of their injury.

It is important to note, however, that there are other ways by which an F scale may be elevated besides malingering. A patient who is unable to read and thus answers randomly will obtain a high F. While a patient with psychosis might also have a high F scale score, the presence of a severe mental illness can usually be ruled out by clinical observation. Another cause of a high F scale relates to a patient's refusal to cooperate and who is merely answering the questions at random. A review of other portions of the test permits the examiner to rule out this possibility (e.g., VRIN and TRIN). Sometimes examiners interpret F scale elevations as a "cry for help," although this has rarely been studied. Moreover, the examiner should be cautious not to confuse *motive* with *accuracy* (i.e., exaggeration by another name is still exaggeration and thus a false measurement of the true extent of psychological distress). For the clinician to interpret and implicitly approve of the plaintiff's motive for exaggeration (i.e., that the plaintiff needs something) does not make the exaggerated scores real measures of injury.

K Scale

The K scale was originally developed in an effort to help differentiate between persons who were known to have psychopathology yet obtained normal profiles on the MMPI, and normal individuals free from psychopathology who obtained elevated MMPI profiles (Meehl & Hathaway, 1946). Although the K scale serves as a "correction" factor for 5 of the 10 clinical scales to help identify persons with significant psychopathology who have MMPI profiles within the normal range, scores on this scale have also been associated with mental well-being or defensiveness. The K scale is thought to have been further developed from early research that suggested that the L scale was easy for intelligent fakers to bypass because its items were so obvious (e.g., see McKinley, Hathaway, & Meehl, 1948; Meehl & Hathaway, 1946). The K scale was designed to be a more subtle index of attempts to pretend to be healthier ("faking good") or less healthy ("faking bad") than one really is psychologically. A low K score may be associated with deliberate efforts to fake psychopathology. For example, the MMPI-2 manual suggests that K scores of 40 and below may be due to fake-bad responding, and Graham (1993) notes that K scores below 40 may be due to a deliberate attempt to present oneself in an unfavorable light. Greene (2000) notes that clients with markedly low scores on K "probably have either fabricated or greatly exaggerated their problems to create the impression of a severe emotional disturbance" (p. 97). However, it is imperative that the presence of acute psychotic stress and/or severe emotional disturbance be ruled out before such a conclusion is drawn.

Research has consistently supported the ability of the K scale to differentiate between analogue malingerers and control subjects. It has been repeatedly demonstrated that university and college students instructed to "fake bad" have significantly lower K scales compared to individuals instructed to "fake-good" and/or those who received standard instructions (e.g., Brems & Harris, 1996; Graham et al., 1991; Shores & Carstairs, 1998). Similar results have also been demonstrated using various clinical samples, whereby individuals who were instructed to fake borderline personality disorder, PTSD, and/or paranoid schizophrenia had lower scores on the K scale than non-fakers and psychiatric patients

(Wetter, Baer, Berry, & Reynolds, 1994; Wetter et al., 1993). Storm and Graham (2000) further demonstrated that coached and uncoached malingerers had significantly lower scores on the K-scale when compared to a large sample of hospitalized psychiatric patients.

F − K

The F − K (F minus K) index was used with the MMPI from the 1940s (Gough, 1947, 1950) and continued on to the MMPI-2. A variety of cutoffs have been suggested for the F − K index for purposes of detecting malingering in personal injury claimants. An F − K of greater than 0 indicates a need to review the data for possible exaggeration of emotional distress. As Graham (1990) noted, "although a single cutoff score cannot be established for all settings, whenever the F scale raw score is greater than the K scale raw score, the possibility of faking bad should be considered; and as the difference becomes greater, the likelihood of a fake bad profile becomes greater" (p. 42). As a point of comparison, on the MMPI-2, the difference between the average F and K scores for the normative group is −11 (minus 11). In one study of personal injury claimants, 22% had F − K ≥ 0, and 8% were greater than +10 (Fox, Gerson, & Lees-Haley, 1995).

If a cutoff of greater than zero were employed for detecting malingering, 95% of the normal population would be classified as not malingering. Based on data presented by Rothke, Friedman, Dahlstrom, Greene, Arredondo, and Mann (1994), about one in five men and one in four women from a substance dependent sample would be misclassified using this cutoff. It is not clear how many substance abusers exaggerate, but a cutoff of F − K ≥ 5 would classify 90% of the substance dependent sample as not malingering and F − K ≥ 8 would classify 95% as not malingering. Examination of traumatic brain injury samples in this study (50 men and 29 women) suggested that a cutoff of F − K ≥ 0 would classify more than 8 out of 10 men and more than 9 out of 10 women as not malingering. In an analogue malingering study, a cutoff score of F − K ≥ 6 correctly classified 95% of fake-bad simulators (Sivec, Lynn, & Garske, 1994). Practitioners need to examine the literature carefully to identify the most appropriate cutoff scores for specific populations for this index (e.g., Rothke et al., 1994).

F_B

The Back Infrequency Scale [F_B] scale was developed in a manner similar to that used to develop the F scale, i.e., these items were answered in the scored direction by fewer than 10 percent of the subjects on which the MMPI-2 was normed (Greene, 1991). Items for the standard F scale appear early in the test booklet, and there was interest in similar data for validity for the latter part of the test. The F_B is routinely reported in studies relating to over-reporting of symptoms; similar to the F scale, it is typically elevated in these samples. In a recent study, the F_B scale was the most accurate of the validity scales for identifying feigned depression in mental health professionals (Bagby, Nicholson, Buis, & Bacchiochi, 2000).

F_B also appears to be sensitive to random responding (Berry, Wetter, Baer, Widiger et al., 1991; Paolo & Ryan, 1992). Profiles in which the F scale appears valid and F_B is elevated suggest that the patient stopped paying attention to the items in the latter part of the test or shifted to a random response pattern. In this situation, a clinician might interpret the standard scales that are scored with items appearing earlier in the test booklet; however, supplementary and content scales which are based on items that appear later in the test booklet should not be interpreted. (It is also possible that the person intensified his or her exaggeration during the latter part of the test, and thus, this possibility should be considered carefully.) Greene (1991, 2000) suggests that the same interpretive statements be used for both F and F_B.

F(p)

The Infrequency-Psychopathology [F(p)] scale contains 27 items that are usually not endorsed by psychiatric inpatients (Arbisi & Ben-Porath, 1995). No more than 20% of psychiatric inpatients (N = 1,129) or the MMPI-2 normative sample endorsed each item on this scale in the deviant direction (Greene, 2000). The scale taps a number of content areas, including severe psychotic symptoms, very unusual habits, highly amoral attitudes, and identity confusion (Greene, 2000). The commonality, of course, is that these items are usually not endorsed by psychiatric inpatients. Researchers have suggested that the F(p) scale is less sensitive to legitimate psychopathology than the F or F_B scales (e.g., Arbisi & Ben-Parath, 1997; Rothke, Friedman, Jaffe, Greene, Wetter, Cole, & Baker, 2000; Strong, Greene, & Schinka, 2000). Moreover, F(p) was recently shown to be superior to F in identifying malingered PTSD (Elhai, Gold, Sellers, & Dorfman, 2001).

An individual's endorsement of items on this scale can be compared to the MMPI-2 normative subjects, the Caldwell normal subjects, and the Caldwell clinical subjects. The Caldwell clinical sample consists of

50,966 patients, and the Caldwell Personnel sample (i.e., "normals") consists of 6,251 personnel applicants. These samples are presented in Greene (2000). For example, if a person endorsed five items on F(p), this would exceed the endorsement rate of 99% of the MMPI-2 normative sample and 93% of clinical subjects in the Caldwell data set (Greene, 2000). Similar comparisons can be made with other validity scales using the data presented in Table 1. Greene (2000) suggested that F(p) raw scores ranging from 4 to 8 indicate "these clients either are experiencing and reporting a significant level of emotional distress or they may be embellishing the severity and extent of their psychopathology" (p. 76).

It has been argued that the F(p) scale can be used to refine interpretation of the F scale (e.g., was the elevation on the F scale due to real psychopathology?). The following sequence has been proposed: (a) rule out random responding and an acquiescence response set by eliminating profiles with elevated VRIN ($T \geq 100$) or TRIN ($T \geq 80$) scores, (b) rule out malingering or exaggeration by considering whether the F(p) scale is elevated (and whether $F - K$ is elevated), and (c) if steps a and b are negative, then a high F scale might be due to psychopathology (Arbisi & Ben-Porath, 1995; Rothke et al., 2000).

VRIN

The VRIN consists of 67 pairs of items with similar or opposite content (Graham, 1993). Each inconsistent answer counts as one point on the raw score for VRIN. It is important to note that elevations on VRIN render the MMPI-2 protocol meaningless for interpretation. Therefore, it is recommended that VRIN be one of the first scales evaluated. Although the VRIN scale was designed to assess for random responding, certain characteristics of this scale can be used to interpret other validity scales with regards to the issue of malingering. Wetter, Baer, Berry, Smith et al. (1992) found that VRIN was elevated with random responding, but not with malingering. Thus, in the case where a protocol has a high F or F_B, VRIN can help clarify whether these scores are elevated due to inconsistent responding (i.e., high VRIN, high F) or due to exaggeration of psychopathology (i.e., normal VRIN, high F). VRIN scores can be elevated for several reasons, such as a brain injury so severe the patient cannot read the items, or a psychiatric disturbance that is so severe that the patient cannot answer the profile in a coherent manner. However, examinees who are careful to answer consistently while faking emotional distress injuries in an organized manner tend not to produce random scores on the MMPI-2 or highly elevated VRIN scores. A score in the average or below average range suggests that the patient answered the test in a deliberate, consistent fashion, so that if other indicators of faking are elevated, it is not because the patient was answering chaotically due to incapacitation by an emotional distress injury, brain injury, or other impairment.

TRIN

The TRIN scale consists of 23 pairs of items, with contradictory content (14 true-answer pairs and 9 false-answer pairs), designed to assess for the consistency of item responding. The examinee who is faking bad (faking emotional distress or psychological disturbance) by paying attention to the items and answering in a consistent manner, will tend to obtain a TRIN scale that is not extremely high or low, even though obtaining elevations on other scales ostensibly associated with psychopathology (Butcher et al., 1989; Graham, 1990, 1993; Greene, 1991). A useful procedure for evaluating malingering in a case with extremely elevated clinical scales is to examine the VRIN and TRIN scales. Psychopathology scores elevated to an extent suggestive of cognitive disorganization or profound dysfunction, inability to read, or other confounds can be interpreted in the context of the logical consistency of the response style with TRIN and VRIN.

Obvious Minus Subtle Scales

The Obvious minus Subtle scales were used in the MMPI beginning in the 1940s (Wiener, 1948; Wiener & Harmon, 1946) and have been studied with the MMPI-2 since 1989. Wiener and Harmon sorted questions on the MMPI into two categories that they called "obvious" and "subtle." The original concept was that the differential ability of lay people to fake obvious and subtle items provided measures of exaggeration on specific scales. More recent research has suggested that the subtle scales should not be interpreted as independent measures of the same construct as the obvious scales (e.g., Boone, 1994; Nelson, Pham, & Uchiyama, 1996). Moreover, in a meta-analytic review of 24 studies using the MMPI to detect malingering, Berry, Baer, and Harris (1991) cautioned the use of the Obvious minus Subtle scales based on the demonstration of smaller effect sizes of these scales when compared to other validity scales (i.e., F, Ds, and F − K index). Nonetheless, research using the MMPI-2 has provided support for these scales in personal injury evaluations because they are associated with exaggeration (as assessed by other MMPI-2 validity scales) and classifications of valid and invalid claims (e.g., Dush, Simons, Platt, & Nation, 1994; Lees-Haley, 1992, 1997; Lees-Haley & Fox, 1990). Rogers, Sewell, and Salekin (1994) conducted a meta-analysis of the MMPI-2 validity scales and found that Obvious minus Subtle scores had a very strong effect size that was maintained across both nonclinical controls and psychiatric groups. They recommended the combination of using the Obvious minus Subtle score, F, and K in evaluating malingered MMPI-2 profiles. Although noting needs for further research, alternative definitions, and controversies about the nature of the measurement, Greene (2000) reported that these scales show promise for detection of overreporting of symptoms on the MMPI-2.

There are a number of different methods for calculating the Obvious minus Subtle scale, the most common of which is the calculation of the total T score difference between the two scales. Research has been relatively favorable in supporting the clinical utility of the this T-score method, with some research suggesting that these scores might offer valuable additional information about simulators' profiles, beyond that which is provided by other validity scales (e.g., Brems & Harris, 1996). Pensa, Dorfman, Gold, and Schneider (1996) found that Obvious minus Subtle scores contributed to the effectiveness of a discriminant function along with F, F_B, F − K, and BIZ that detected simulators with monetary incentives and training on psychosis. In contrast, Timbrook, Graham, Keiller, and Watts (1993) found that while the Obvious minus Subtle scores correctly classified a high percentage of fake-bad profiles from normal and patient controls, they concluded that the "standard validity scales appear to be more useful than the S-O scales in identifying faked profiles" (p. 53).

From a commonsense perspective, extreme Obvious minus Subtle T scores are not commonly found among persons presenting with approximately normal mental status. Based on the original MMPI, Greene (1991) noted, "When the total T score difference exceeds +200, it should be readily apparent by an interview whether the client is overreporting psychopathology, since if the client's responses were accurate, there is severe psychopathology. Occasionally in an inpatient setting, total T score differences above +200 will be seen in a client who is endorsing the items accurately. In an outpatient setting, it is much less likely for difference scores in this range to reflect actual psychopathology since the client should be so devastated that he or she would be unable to function" (p. 81). Greene (1988) further noted, "in an outpatient setting, it is extremely unlikely for difference scores in this range to reflect actual psychopathology since the patient should be so overwhelmed that he or she would be unable to function" (p. 142). Hedlund and Won Cho (1979) reported data from 8,646 male and 3,743 female psychiatric patients that showed a mean score of 56.5 (SD = 85.1) for the T-score method on the MMPI. Their data indicated that only 28% to 29% of adults who were so disturbed that they required psychiatric hospitalization exceeded the cutoff of 100. With regard to the MMPI-2, Lees-Haley and Fox (1990) found that only 16% of inpatients with psychosis would be misclassified using a T difference of 100. In other words, high scores are not expected from outpatients, and they are improbable. Rogers et al. (1994) recommended using a score greater than 81 as a screening indicator.

Es

The ego strength (Es) scale was originally developed by Barron (1956) as a measure of prognosis for psychotherapy, but it did not prove effective. It has also been applied to the study of healthy, creative persons (Barron, 1968). The Es scale is potentially useful, although it has been underutilized in the assessment of malingering following traumatic injuries including brain injuries. It might be helpful to compare the Es T score with the actual functioning of the patient. Graham (1993) and Greene (2000) have noted that low Es scale scores can be associated with exaggeration or overreporting of symptomatology. Caldwell (1988), referring to the MMPI, noted that patients with a T score of 20 or lower on Es have a "usually urgent if not critical" need to be hospitalized in a mental ward (p. 37). Caldwell (1988) also noted that patients with a T score of 30 and below "consistently need extensive care and support from others and very possibly hospitalization." Although it is acknowledged that MMPI and MMPI-2 T scores are not equivalent, the point is that, because extremely low Es scores are associated with obvious, conspicuous debilitation well in excess of the pathology exhibited by most personal injury claimants, the marked discrepancy between the test data and observable behavior can be dramatic. Cross-validation of this procedure with the MMPI-2 suggests that unrealistically low Es scores are associated with measures of malingering (Lees-Haley, 1991, 1992, 1997).

Ds/Dsr

The Dissimulation Scale (Ds) was created by Gough (1954) and later revised from 74 items to 40 items as the Dsr (Gough, 1957). Gough created this scale by asking normal persons to pretend to be neurotically disturbed. Those items that differentiated normal people faking disturbance from genuinely disturbed patients were then identified. A high score on the dissimulation scale suggests that the person taking the test resembles the fakers as opposed to the truly disturbed patients. During the conversion from MMPI to MMPI-2, a number of items were dropped or changed. The MMPI-2 Ds scale has 58 items and the Dsr scale has 34 items.

As Caldwell (1988) pointed out, a high dissimulation scale score points to malingering and serves as an independent measure not particularly correlated with other validity indicators such as F and F − K (thus, it is useful to examine this score as independent evidence). Berry, Baer et al. (1991) conducted a meta-analysis that showed the Ds scale to have one of the largest effect sizes of the malingering scales on the MMPI. Based on these findings, Greene (2000) noted that ". . . it clearly needs to be used in evaluating whether the person is overreporting psychopathology" (p. 78). An elevation on the Dsr in a personal injury claim raises concern that the patient is simulating or exaggerating psychopathology. The higher the score, the greater the concern.

Researchers examining the clinical utility of the MMPI-2 Ds or Dsr validity scales have repeatedly demonstrated that individuals instructed to fake bad or to fake a specific psychiatric or neurological condition perform significantly higher on the Ds and Dsr scales compared to either healthy control subjects (e.g., Bagby et al., 1994; Rogers et al., 1995; Sivec et al., 1994; Walters & Clopton, 2000; Wetter & Deitsch, 1996) or actual psychiatric patients (e.g., Bagby, Buis, & Nicholson, 1995; Bagby et al., 2000; Bagby et al., 1994; Berry, Adams, Clark, Thacker, Burger, Wetter, Baer, & Bordon, 1996; Elhai, Gold, Frueh, & Gold, 2000; Storm & Graham, 2000; Wetter et al., 1994; Wetter et al., 1993). Notably, the majority of support for the clinical utility of these scales has been established based on group mean analyses. In contrast, research focusing on various classification analyses has been less favorable. Bagby et al. (1995) compared the ability of the Dsr to detect individuals instructed to fake-bad on the MMPI-2 versus honest psychiatric and forensic psychiatric samples. Despite finding significant effect sizes between these groups, based on hierarchical regression analyses, these authors concluded that the Dsr scale does not have "incremental validity to be valuable in the prediction of fake-bad profiles" (p. 91). Similarly, Rogers et al. (1995) examined the ability of both the Ds and Dsr scales to differentiate between psychiatric patients instructed to fake bad versus answering honestly based on cutoff scores. Using a cutoff score of > 35 for the Ds scale and > 22 for the Dsr scale, 81.0% to 83.3% of honest responders were correctly identified, but only 64.3% of malingerers were correctly identified. In contrast, Berry et al. (1996) provided some support for the clinical utility of the Ds scale using cutoff scores. Berry and collegues demonstrated that, by using a similar cutoff score (i.e., > 35), 90% of mildly to moderately disturbed psychiatric outpatients were successfully identified who were instructed to respond on the MMPI-2 in a manner that demonstrated a "cry for help."

Fake Bad Scale (FBS)

The Fake Bad Scale (FBS) was designed to assist in the detection of personal injury malingering (Lees-Haley, English, & Glenn, 1991). Although originally oriented toward emotional distress injuries, research suggests that it is useful in the detection of somatic malingering (i.e., cases reporting physical injuries or pain, including neuropsychological cases; see Larrabee, 1996, 1997, 1998). Larrabee (1997) suggested that, "somatic malingering should be considered whenever elevations on scales 1 and 3 exceed T = 80, accompanied by a significant elevation on the FBS" (p. 203).

Posthuma and Harper (1998) reported that the FBS "already has demonstrated efficacy in discriminating personal injury litigants who are malingering from other groups" and concluded that "in reports or expert testimony, forensic psychologists who use the FBS as one of a number of validity measures have a reasonable scientific basis for doing so" (p. 440).

Millis, Putnam, and Adams (1995) compared 20 mild head injury litigants with external incentives to present impairments associated with their injuries to 20 outpatients with documented moderate and severe traumatic brain injuries. Of the validity scales, the FBS had the best discriminative efficiency. Slick, Hopp, Strauss, and Spellacy (1996) found that Fake Bad Scale scores were correlated positively with response time scores and negatively with the number of items correct on the Victoria Symptom Validity Test (VSVT) for both easy and hard items.

In another known group study applying the FBS to neuropsychological cases, Putnam, Millis, and Adams (1998) found that a cutoff score of 22 resulted in a 92.7% correct classification rate. In a study oriented toward potential utility for detecting invalid emotional distress claims, Lees-Haley (1992) examined data from 119 personal injury claimants. In this emotional distress sample, a cutoff of >23 for men and

>25 for women correctly classified 75% of men and 74% of women with spurious PTSD claims, and 96% of men and 92% of women controls. In this study, patients with presumed spurious PTSD were defined as those who (a) claimed to be suffering a psychological injury so severe that it was disabling, (b) had a "traumatic" experience that was entirely implausible as a candidate for PTSD criterion A in DSM-III-R, and (c) scored T = 65 or higher on the post-traumatic stress disorder subscales of the MMPI-2 (i.e., PK and PS). More recent studies of malingered PTSD have found the standard validity scales to be superior to the FBS for identifying exaggeration (Elhai et al., 2000; Elhai et al., 2001). Exaggeration and malingering of PTSD is a complex clinical issue, especially among combat veterans (Frueh, Hamner, Cahill, Gold, & Hamlin, 2000); it deserves more systematic research.

Rogers et al. (1995) included the FBS in an analogue malingering study using psychiatric outpatients in a within-subjects design. This study found low sensitivity of the FBS to the extreme exaggeration response set (mean F scale score was 109.6) of chronically mentally ill outpatients and a problematic rate of false positive classifications (19%) in the psychiatric patient sample. This, of course, is expected, because the FBS was not designed to detect malingered psychosis.

Tsushima and Tsushima (2001) found that the FBS was the only validity scale that differentiated a large sample of personal injury litigants from a sample of clinical patients. They concluded that high FBS scores could be affected by litigation stress and exaggeration. They further noted that their data were consistent with the growing evidence that personal injury litigants tend to demonstrate somatic preoccupation and symptom over-reporting on the MMPI-2. It should be noted that, based on available cutoff scores and a large data set, the majority of personal injury litigants do not appear to malinger on the FBS (Lees-Haley, 1997). Therefore, elevations, when they occur, likely are clinically meaningful. Greene (2000) recommended additional research with the FBS based on its low correlation with the infrequency scales (thus, its unique contribution to the assessment of validity). The performances of subjects in known groups on the Fake Bad Scale are presented in Table 1.

Examination of Specific Studies and Scores

It is useful for practitioners to have a number of articles relating to the application of the validity scales for specific purposes. Therefore, a list of articles relating to the malingering of depression, PTSD, and severe

TABLE 1. Fake Bad Scale Performances in Known Groups

Group	N	M	SD
Normal Control Subjects			
MMPI-2 Normative Sample–Males[1]	1,138	11.7	3.8
MMPI-2 Normative Sample–Females[1]	1,462	13.8	4.1
Federal Prison Inmates–Minimum Security–Males[2]	25	9.8	4.1
Medical Patients			
Moderate–Severe Traumatic Brain Injury[3]	20	16.1	4.9
Medical Outpatients–Transplant Candidates–Males[4]	20	15.3	7.6
Psychiatric Patients			
MMPI-2 Psychiatric Sample–Estimated Scores for Males[5]	---	16.9	---
MMPI-2 Psychiatric Sample–Estimated Scores for Females[5]	---	19.1	---
Patients with Chronic Psychiatric Problems[6]	42	22.1	5.8
Male Veterans–Inpatient Substance Abuse Unit[4]	25	15.6	6.4
Psychiatric and Medical Patients[7]	208	17.1	5.7
Patients with Depression[8]	48	22.0	5.5
Psychiatric Patients[8]	50	18.5	6.6
Child Custody Litigants[9]			
No Alleged Abuse–Males	---	13.8	3.0
No Alleged Abuse–Females	---	13.8	3.0
Alleged Physical Abuse–Males	---	13.6	3.1
Alleged Physical Abuse–Females	---	15.1	3.6
Alleged Sexual Abuse–Males	---	13.5	3.1
Alleged Sexual Abuse–Females	---	16.0	3.5
Personal Injury Litigants			
Head Trauma, Chronic Pain, or Both[9]	95	22.3	6.9
Unselected, Consecutive Litigants[10]	492	20.8	6.7
Personal Injury Litigants[7]	120	20.7	6.2
Analogue Malingerers			
Medical Outpatients–Simulate Emotional Distress from MVA[5]	16	26	6.7
Medical Outpatients–Simulate Emotional Distress from Toxic Exposure[5]	15	21	9.6
Medical Outpatients–Simulate Emotional Distress from Job Stress[5]	36	27	8.0
Medical Outpatients–Total Analogue Malingerers[5]	67	25	8.5
Patients with Psychiatric Problems–Malinger Severe Psychiatric Problems[6]	42	24.8	5.7
Federal Inmates–Malinger Severe Psychiatric Problems[2]	25	21.6	5.8
Sophisticated Malingerers Faking Depression[8]	23	28.4	4.4
Suspected Malingerers			
Mild Head Injury Litigants[3]	20	29.0	5.1
Personal Injury Litigants[5]	25	27.6	4.7
Litigants with Presumed Spurious PTSD Claims[11]	55	27.1	5.2

[1]Greene (1997)
[2]Iverson, Franzen, & Hammond (1995)
[3]Millis, Putnam, & Adams (1995)
[4]Iverson, Henrichs, Barton, & Allen (in press)
[5]Lees-Haley et al. (1991)
[6]Rogers, Sewell, & Ustad (1995)
[7]Tsushima & Tsushima (2001)
[8]Bagby, Nicholson, Buis, & Bacchiochi (2000)
[9]Posthuma & Harper (1998)
[10]Lees-Haley (1997)
[11]Lees-Haley (1992)

Note: In Posthuma & Harper (1998) there were 188 individuals involved in custody evaluations.

psychiatric illness is presented in Table 2. In addition, articles relating to exaggeration in personal injury claimants also are presented (notably, there is overlap in some of the articles across the categories). This is not meant to be an exhaustive list but is intended to provide the reader with a large amount of the available literature.

It is also useful for practitioners to know which raw scores are rare in the general population or in patients with psychiatric problems. These cutoffs are presented in Table 3 for several large samples. As previously noted, the Caldwell clinical sample referred to in this table consists of 50,966 patients, and the Caldwell Personnel sample (i.e., "normals") consists of 6,251 personnel applicants (Greene, 2000). The MMPI-2 normative sample consists of 2,600 community control subjects. This table can serve as a quick reference for evaluating unusual elevations on the validity scales.

Case Example: Exaggerated Psychopathology

The patient was in a minor automobile accident two years prior to the forensic neuropsychological evaluation. At that time, he was evaluated in the Emergency Department and found to be alert. There was no reported loss of consciousness. There was no evidence in the contemporaneous medical record of retrograde amnesia, post-injury confusion, or post-traumatic amnesia. Therefore, if the patient sustained a concussion in this accident, it would be classified as very mild. As such, his prognosis for rapid and complete recovery would have been excellent. The patient had a history of several non-head injury Workers' Compensation claims prior to the present litigation. In the present case, he was claiming a substantial degree of disability relating to an alleged traumatic brain injury sustained in the accident.

The patient obtained a raw score of 6 on the VRIN scale (T score = 54). This means that he answered only 6 of the 67 item pairs inconsistently. This score definitely does not reflect a random or careless approach to taking the test, but rather this score represents a very consistent approach to answering related items.

The patient obtained a raw score of 31 on the F scale (T score = 120). This is an extreme elevation, indicating that he endorsed a large number of infrequent items. This score is higher than that obtained by 100% of the MMPI-2 normative sample. When compared to the Caldwell dataset, his score was above the 99.9th percentile for the normal subjects and the 99th percentile for the clinical subjects.

TABLE 2. Selected Citations for MMPI-2 Validity Scale Studies Relating to PTSD, Depression, Mental Illness, and Personal Injury Litigation

Citation	Topic
Elhai, Gold, Frueh, & Gold (2000)	PTSD
Elhai, Gold, Sellers, & Dorfman (2001)	PTSD
Lees-Haley (1992)	PTSD
Smith & Frueh (1996)	PTSD
Wetter, Baer, Berry, Robinson, & Sumpter (1993)	PTSD, Mental illness
Wetter & Deitsch (1996)	PTSD, Head injury
Bagby, Nicholson, Buis & Bacchiochi (2000)	Depression
Walters & Clopton (2000)	Depression
Sivec, Lynn, & Garske (1994)	Somatoform Disorder, Paranoid Psychosis, Mental illness
Bagby, Buis, & Nicholson (1995)	Mental illness
Bagby, Rogers, Buis, & Kalemba (1994)	Mental illness
Brems & Harris (1996)	Mental illness
Brunetti, Schlottmann, Scott, & Hollrah (1998)	Mental illness
Cassisi & Workman (1992)	Mental illness
Graham, Watts, & Timbrook (1991)	Mental illness
Iverson, Franzen, & Hammond (1995)	Mental illness
Lim & Butcher (1996)	Mental illness
Nicholson, Mouton, Bagby, Buis, Peterson, & Buigas (1997)	Mental illness
Rogers, Sewell, & Ustad (1995)	Mental illness
Shores & Carstairs (1998)	Mental illness
Sivec, Lynn, & Garske (1994)	Mental illness
Storm & Graham (2000)	Mental illness
Stukenberg, Brady, & Klinetob (2000)	Mental illness
Timbrook, Graham, Keiller, & Watts (1993)	Mental illness
Wetter, Baer, Berry, & Reynolds (1994)	Mental illness
Wetzler & Marlowe (1990)	Mental illness
Berry, Adams, Clark, Thacker, Burger, Wetter, Baer, & Bordon (1996)	Cry for help
Grillo, Brown, Hilsabeck, Price, & Lees-Haley (1994)	Personal injury
Fox, Gerson, & Lees-Haley (1995)	Personal injury
Berry & Butcher (1998)	General
Greene (1997)	General
Greene (2000)	General
Pope, Butcher, Seelen (1993)	General
Rothke, Friedman, Dahlstrom, Greene, Arredondo, & Mann (1994)	General
Rothke, Friedman, Jaffe, Greene, Wetter, Cole, & Baker (2000)	General
Rogers, Sewell, & Salekin (1994)	General
Strong, Greene, & Schinka (2000)	General
Tsushima & Tsushima (2001)	General

Note: This is not meant to be an exhaustive list of the MMPI-2 validity scale literature, but rather a fairly comprehensive list of selected articles.

TABLE 3. Raw Scores Corresponding to the 98% rank (i.e., Two Standard Deviations Above the Mean) for Normal and Clinical Groups

	MMPI-2	Caldwell Data Set	
Scale	Normative	Personnel	Clinical
F Scale	12	7	24
FB-Scale	9	3	20
F − K	3	−5	15
F(p)	4	4	7
Obvious − Subtle T-Difference	135	52	240
Dissimulation Scale	24	16	35

Note: The Caldwell clinical sample consists of 50,966 patients, and the personnel sample (i.e., "normals") consists of 6,251 personnel applicants. The MMPI-2 normative sample consists of 2,600 community control subjects.

On the F_B scale, he obtained a raw score of 18, which corresponds to a T score of 116. This is an extreme elevation, indicating that he endorsed a high number of infrequent items in the latter part of the test. This means that he endorsed more infrequent symptoms than 99% of the MMPI-2 normative subjects. When compared to the Caldwell dataset, he scored higher than 99.9% of normal subjects and between 93% and 98% of clinical subjects.

On the F(p) scale, the patient obtained a raw score of 7. His score exceeded the 99th percentile for the MMPI-2 normative subjects and the Caldwell normal subjects, and was at the 98th percentile for Caldwell's clinical subjects. These results suggest that this client may be "experiencing and reporting a significant level of emotional distress or they may be embellishing the severity and extent of their psychopathology" (p. 76, Greene, 2000).

The patient obtained a raw score of 29 on the Fake Bad Scale. Greene (1997) reported that the average score on the FBS for men in the MMPI-2 normative sample was 11.7 (SD = 3.8). Medical outpatients have been instructed to simulate emotional distress under a variety of circumstances, such as in relation to a motor vehicle accident, toxic exposure, and on-the-job stress (Lees-Haley et al., 1991). For these three combined groups of analogue malingerers (N = 67), the average score on the FBS was 25 (SD = 8.5). In a sample of 20 mild head injury litigants who obtained below chance performance on a two-alternative forced-choice test (presumed exaggerators or malingerers), the average FBS score was 29 (SD = 5.1; Millis et al., 1995). All of the aforementioned samples and scores are presented in Table 1.

For comparison purposes, average scores on three validity scales for multiple groups are reported in Table 4. The table contains six samples of subjects instructed to fake severe mental problems and six samples of subjects with legitimate mental problems. As seen in this table, the patient's scores on the validity measures are much more similar to those obtained by persons instructed to fake mental illness than to those obtained by patients with mental and emotional problems.

A summary of the patient's MMPI-2 findings is presented below.

- He obtained extreme elevations on several validity scales. These scores are uncommon in persons who are being honest and forthright and may reflect exaggerated psychiatric problems.
- He obtained an average score on the VRIN scale. This means that he did not respond inconsistently to pairs of items that have similar content. It is apparent that his approach to completing the MMPI-2 was not random or careless.
- He obtained an elevated score on the Fake Bad Scale (FBS), a scale designed to detect a blended fake-good and fake-bad response set believed to be associated with personal injury malingering.

TABLE 4. Average Scores on the F, F_B, and F − K Scale for Multiple Groups Reported in the Literature

Sample	Number of Subjects	F Scale	F_B Scale	F − K
Community volunteers faking PTSD[1]	20	111.3	110.1	27.4
Community volunteers faking paranoid schizophrenia[1]	22	119.4	119.3	36
University students instructed to fake bad[2]	58	114.8	109.3	25.1
Male university students instructed to fake bad[3]	57	117.5	117.2	--
Male inmates instructed to malinger psychopathology[4]	28	112.9	104.8	24.8
Chronic psychiatric patients instructed to fake bad[5]	42	109.6	--	31.6
Patients with PTSD[1]	20	79.8	85.2	4.4
Patients with paranoid schizophrenia[1]	20	80.8	74.3	0
Psychiatric inpatients[2]	95	71.8	73.8	−2.1
Male psychiatric inpatients[3]	30	79.7	83.9	--
Male psychiatric inpatients[4]	51	60.8	69.2	−4.5
Chronic psychiatric patients[5]	42	82.1	--	5.8
The patient's scores	--	120	116	21

[1]Wetter et al. (1993)
[2]Bagby et al. (1994)
[3]Graham et al. (1991)
[4]Iverson et al. (1995)
[5]Rogers et al. (1995)

After a careful review of his MMPI-2 profile, it would be reasonable to conclude that there is considerable evidence of distortion and exaggeration of his psychiatric problems, physical problems, and level of disability.

DAUBERT V. MMPI-2 IN FORENSIC NEUROPSYCHOLOGY

The essential issue in regard to *Daubert* concerns how accurately we can answer questions. Assuming we can answer questions accurately, the next threshold is whether our tests and other assessment procedures improve decision making by the courts (e.g., are our opinions relevant and helpful?). We can anticipate several potential questions in *Daubert* challenges regarding the admissibility of opinions based on the MMPI-2. These include: (a) Is the test grounded in scientific methodology? (b) Is the test reliable and valid in general? If so, is the particular application in the specific case reliable and valid? (c) What is the error rate? (d) Has the test in general and the particular application of the test in the case at hand been subjected to peer-review in quality scientific journals? (e) Is the procedure generally accepted in the scientific community? (f) Is the expert's opinion (conclusion, allegation, or theory) subject to falsification? These questions will be discussed in more detail below.

Is the MMPI-2 Grounded in Scientific Methodology?

The critical element of grounding in scientific methodology is empirical verification. We should have repeatedly demonstrated that our procedures perform the way we claim they do (i.e., research replication). In order to testify that an expert opinion based on a test is grounded in science, one usually needs controlled studies on samples similar to the issues relevant to the case at hand. Granted, some types of scientific research are not subject to studies with control groups or experimental manipulation. However, forensic neuropsychology testimony relating to test results is generally focused on conclusions such as diagnostic decisions, impairment levels, and predictions that are appropriate subject matter for controlled research.

As discussed in the previous section of this paper, the MMPI-2 validity scales have been subjected to extensive scientific research. There have been an impressive number of studies that have verified some general conclusions relating to exaggeration of symptoms and disability on the MMPI-2. These studies have laid a reasonably solid foundation of scientific credibility. One of the challenges faced by practitioners is selecting from the almost bewildering number of cutoff scores proposed for the various validity scales. In addition, experienced clinicians know that no single scale should be expected to be sensitive to all forms of malingering (e.g., feigned psychosis, emotional distress, or cognitive dysfunction). Therefore, it is important to select validity scales most appropriate for the specific assessment situation.

It is notable that the vast majority of the research on the MMPI-2 and malingering has employed known groups or other experimental designs, and very little research has attempted to cross-validate these findings in large clinical samples against other methods of detecting symptom invalidity. A clear limitation of this research relates to the validity of generalizing from research that has employed experimental volunteers to examinees in applied settings.

Is the Procedure Reliable and Valid?

It is important to use proper scientific language. For example, judges and lawyers often ask "Is this test reliable?" or "Is this a valid test?" There is no such thing as a neuropsychological test (or any other test) that is valid in the abstract. Tests are not reliable or valid. They possess varying degrees of reliability and validity for specific purposes, in specific groups, under specific circumstances (Franzen, 1989, 2000).

Judges and lawyers often use the word "reliability" interchangeably with the word "validity" and with vague concepts such as dependability, soundness, or goodness. Even if legal professionals eschew details about types of reliability and validity, it is important to communicate the general idea that scientific psychologists define reliability as consistency of measurement, regardless of accuracy, and they define validity as accuracy. When the judge and jury need to know whether a procedure is valid, in most cases their concerns lie in areas associated with criterion-related validity.

Surveys of judges and attorneys have identified advocacy by experts as a leading point of criticism of experts (Johnson, Krafka, & Cecil, 2000). There is a clear need for neuropsychologists to use explicit statements of decision criteria in answering fundamental forensic questions. Explicit decision criteria might help reduce the bias inevitable to subjective evaluations. In terms of the MMPI-2 validity scales, these decision criteria might relate to specific cutoff scores applicable to specific groups under specific circumstances, with a careful description of the accuracy of the cutoffs based on the literature.

What Is the Error Rate?

Calculation of error rates requires reliable definitions and gold standards. The general concept of malingering is applied to behaviors with which the plaintiff portrays an inaccurate degree of impairment for the purpose of achieving an identifiable external incentive. However, the specific manifestations of malingering are diverse. One claimant may pretend to have headaches, while another may present with false memory deficits or nonexistent psychopathology. A reliable definition of malingering must be tailored to the behavior relevant to a particular claim. Like validity, error rate is not a general characteristic applicable to all uses of a test. The error rate varies with the nature of the decision or conclusion. A test is more accurate for some purposes than others. Determining the error rate of a test designed to identify exaggeration presents a special problem because of the inherently unreliable entity being measured. Many tests measure varying conditions (e.g., tests of mood or educational achievement), but malingering tests are designed to measure a form of behavior about which the behaving person is seeking to escape detection. If a malingering detection test is 100% accurate in a first examination, the malingerer could stop engaging in the behavior in a second evaluation. Reliability studies have to take into account the potentially varying nature of the phenomenon. In fact, we believe that intra-and inter-test inconsistency is one of the chief characteristics of malingerers. This is easily observed in a large clinical population given a large battery of tests that includes several malingering tests. Poor performance on any of these instruments can often explain the majority of variance in the battery as a whole (Green, Rohling, Lees-Haley, & Allen, in press).

Has the Procedure Been Subjected to Peer Review?

Research relating to the MMPI-2 validity scales has undergone extensive peer review. Peer review is an invaluable asset to the progress of the scientific enterprise, and there is a seemingly endless list of research articles relating to the MMPI-2. So, in a general sense, it is quite easy to put forward considerable evidence to address this criterion. Of course, there are major differences in the quality of studies, reviewers, and journals. In order to meet *Daubert* standards, we must determine whether the methodology in question is a reliable, valid procedure, grounded in good science, as applied to one unique case. It is inadequate for the methodology to be useful in general or in many cases; it must be valid for the particular case, and every step in the reasoning process in this unique case must be valid and reliable.

Is the Procedure Generally Accepted in the Scientific Community?

The MMPI-2 had a great advantage toward admissibility under the old evidentiary standard, the *Frye* test of general acceptance, because it is the most widely used psychological test in general and is one of the most widely used in forensic neuropsychological evaluations. As attorneys challenge the MMPI-2 with *Daubert* standards, many inadmissabilities can be expected, but for the moment, a rejection of the MMPI-2 will not be based on lack of widespread use. Despite the serious emerging criticisms of the test, it is still widely used among psychologists. At present, the test is so widely used and so aggressively defended that relatively few dare question it. Given this inertia, judges usually expect the MMPI-2 to be included in any forensic assessment, with the effect that they might tolerate its admissibility beyond the test's actual scientific validity and predictive power.

Despite its extraordinarily wide use in the psychological community, the MMPI-2 will likely be subjected to many attacks in *Daubert* hearings in years to come when judges begin to realize the serious doubts about the validity of the test that are being suggested by recent researchers. For example, based on a large-scale Australian study, Senior and colleagues strongly suggest that the traditional approach to MMPI-2 interpretation cannot be empirically supported in the forensic context. These researchers are particularly critical of code type interpretations and the use of the MMPI-2 as a basis for diagnostic decisions (for example, see Baker, Senior, & Douglas, 1999; Henry & Senior, 2001; Senior & Douglas, 2000; Senior & Douglas, in press; Senior, Vlahov, & Shapcott, 1999).

Falsification

Can the expert's opinion, conclusion, or theory be tested? Tautological claims and vague definitions are sometimes put forward as scientific arguments. Consider the assertion by the expert who said that the plaintiff was suffering intense subjective emotional pain despite her claim that she had recovered and was feeling happy again, because she was in a state of denial. Because the relevant DSM diagnosis was by definition based on the subjective experience of the patient, the expert's claim that the patient was in denial resulted in an opinion that, for the most part, could not be tested.

Experts frequently confuse DSM definitions with empirical facts. It is true that someone with dysthymia has been depressed most of the day, more days than not, for at least two years *by definition*. But testimony that dysthymia "causes" depressive phenomena like fatigue, poor concentration, or hopelessness is analogous to saying bodies cause arms and legs. Whether a particular patient has specific symptoms is an empirical, not a definitional, question. It is important to identify circular reasoning like that of an expert who diagnosed dysthymia and then claimed the patient had to have various symptoms even if the patient did not admit them, on the grounds that all dysthymic patients have those symptoms.

With MMPI-2 validity scales, the test of falsification does not relate to lie detection. Instead, it relates to the spectrum of statistical probability. The goal is to test (falsify) the probability with which the scales are associated with malingering behavior such as highly improbable claims, contradictory claims, and exaggeration.

CONCLUSIONS

We hope this review has illustrated how a test such as the MMPI-2 does not pass or fail the *Daubert* challenge on its own. Instead, particular components can come under sharp scrutiny, and the specific methods of utilizing its data may be unscientific and hence inadmissible. It is ironic that it may be the legal profession, not psychologists, that finally forces the field to confront the inadequacies of one of its most cherished instruments. However, a profession that does not police itself will surely fall in the courtroom when subjected to rigorous scientific scrutiny in *Daubert* challenges. As Paul Meehl (1993) advised, psychologists should pursue what Bertrand Russell called "the dominant passion of the true scientist–the passion not to be fooled and not to fool anybody else" and should continue to raise "the two searching questions of positivism: 'What do you mean?' 'How do you know?' If we clinicians lose that passion and forget those questions, we are little more than be-doctored, well-paid soothsayers. I see disturbing signs that this is happening and I predict that, if we do not clean up our clinical act and provide our students with role models of scientific thinking, outsiders will do it for us" (pp. 728-729).

REFERENCES

Arbisi, P. A., & Ben-Porath, Y. S. (1995). An MMPI-2 infrequent response scale for use with psychopathological populations: The infrequency-psychopathology scale, F(p). *Psychological Assessment, 7*, 424-431.

Arbisi, P. A., & Ben-Porath, Y. S. (1997). Characteristics of the MMPI-2 F(p) scale as a function of diagnosis in an inpatient sample of veterans. *Psychological Assessment, 9*, 102-105.

Arbisi, P. A., & Ben-Porath, Y. S. (1999). The use of the Minnesota Multiphasic Personality Inventory-2 in the psychological assessment of persons with TBI: Correction factors and other clinical caveats and conundrums. *NeuroRehabilitation, 13*, 117-125.

Bagby, R. M., Buis, T. & Nicholson, R. A. (1995). Relative effectiveness of the standard validity scales in detecting fake-bad and fake-good responding: Replication and extension. *Psychological Assessment, 7*, 84-92.

Bagby, R. M., Nicholson, R. A., Buis, T., & Bacchiochi, J. R. (2000). Can the MMPI-2 validity scales detect depression feigned by experts? *Assessment, 7*, 55-62.

Bagby, R. M., Rogers, R., Buis, T., & Kalemba, V. (1994). Malingered and defensive response styles on the MMPI-2: An examination of validity scales. *Assessment, 1*, 31-38.

Baker, W., Senior, G., & Douglas, L. (1999, November). Difficulty in classifying medicolegal groups with the MMPI-2. Poster presented at the 19th Annual Conference of the National Academy of Neuropsychology. San Antonio, TX.

Barron, F. (1956). An ego strength scale which predicts response to psychotherapy. *Journal of Consulting Psychology, 19*, 239-245.

Barron, F. (1968). *Creativity and Personal Freedom.* New York: Van Nostrand Co., Inc.

Berry, D. T. R., Adams, J. J., Clark, C. D., Thacker, S. R., Burger, T. L., Wetter, M. W., Baer, R. A., & Bordon, J. W. (1996). Detection of a cry for help on the MMPI-2: An analog investigation. *Journal of Personality Assessment, 67*, 26-36.

Berry, D. T. R., Baer, R. A., & Harris, M. J. (1991). Detection of malingering on the MMPI: A meta-analysis. *Clinical Psychology Review, 11*, 585-598.

Berry, D. T. R., & Butcher, J. N. (1998). Detection of feigning of head injury symptoms on the MMPI-2. In C. R. Reynolds (Ed.), *Detection of Malingering During Head Injury Litigation* (pp. 209-238). New York: Plenum Press.

Berry, D. T., Wetter, M. W., Baer, R. A., Widiger, T. A., et al. (1991). Detection of random responding on the MMPI-2: Utility of F, back F, and VRIN scales. *Psychological Assessment, 3*, 418-423.

Boone, D. (1994). Reliability of the MMPI-2 subtle and obvious scales with psychiatric inpatients. *Journal of Personality Assessment, 62*, 346-351.

Brems, C., & Harris, K. (1996). Faking the MMPI-2: Utility of the Subtle-Obvious scales. *Journal of Clinical Psychology 52*, 525-533.

Brunetti, D. G., Schlottmann, R. S., Scott, A. B., & Hollrah, J. L. (1998). Instructed faking and MMPI-2 response latencies: The potential for assessing response validity. *Journal of Clinical Psychology, 54*, 143-153.

Butcher, J. (1990). *The MMPI-2 in Psychological Treatment*. New York: Oxford University Press.

Butcher, J. N. (1998). *Users Guide for the Minnesota Report: Reports for Forensic Settings*. Minneapolis, MN: National Computer Systems.

Butcher, J., Graham, J., Dahlstrom, W., Tellegen, A., & Kaemmer, B. (1989). *Minnesota Multiphasic Personality Inventory-2: Manual for administration and scoring*. Minneapolis, MN: University of Minnesota Press.

Caldwell, A. B. (1988). *MMPI Supplemental Scale Manual*. Los Angeles: Caldwell Report.

Camara, W. J., Nathan, J. S., & Puente, A. E. (2000). Psychological test usage: Implications in professional psychology. *Professional Psychology: Research and Practice*, *31*, 141-154.

Cassisi, J. E., & Workman, D. E. (1992). The detection of malingering and deception with a short form of the MMPI-2 based on the L, F, and K scales. *Journal of Clinical Psychology*, *48*, 54-58.

Dunn, J. T., & Lees-Haley, P. R. (1995). The MMPI-2 correction factor for closed head injury: A caveat for forensic cases. *Assessment*, *2*, 47-51.

Dush, D. M., Simons, L. E., Platt, M., & Nation, P. C. (1994). Psychological profiles distinguishing litigating and nonlitigating pain patients: Subtle, and not so subtle. *Journal of Personality Assessment*, *62*, 299-313.

Elhai, J. D., Gold, P. B., Frueh, B. C., & Gold, S. N. (2000). Cross-validation of the MMPI-2 in detecting malingered posttraumatic stress disorder. *Journal of Personality Assessment*, *75*, 449-463.

Elhai, J. D., Gold, P. B., Sellers, A. H., & Dorfman, W. I. (2001). The detection of malingered posttraumatic stress disorder with the MMPI-2 fake bad indices. *Assessment*, *8*, 221-236.

Fox, D., Gerson, A., & Lees-Haley, P. (1995). Interrelationship of MMPI-2 validity scales in personal injury claims. *Journal of Clinical Psychology*, *51*, 42-47.

Fox, D. D., & Lees-Haley, P. R. (2001). MMPI-2 scores fail to correlate with employment status. *Journal of Forensic Neuropsychology*, *2* (2), 53-56.

Franzen, M. D. (1989). *Reliability and Validity in Neuropsychological Assessment*. New York: Plenum Press.

Franzen, M. D. (2000). *Reliability and Validity in Neuropsychological Assessment*, 2nd Edition. New York: Kluwer Academic/Plenum Publishers.

Frueh, B. C., Hamner, M. B., Cahill, S. P., Gold, P. B., & Hamlin, K. L. (2000). Apparent symptom overreporting among combat veterans evaluated for PTSD. *Clinical Psychology Review*, *20*, 853-885.

Gass, C. S. (1991). MMPI-2 interpretation and closed head injury: A correction factor. *Psychological Assessment*, *3*, 27-31.

Gass, C. S., & Wald, H. S. (1997). MMPI-2 interpretation and closed-head trauma: Cross-validation of a correction factor. *Archives of Clinical Neuropsychology*, *12*, 199-205.

Gough, H. G. (1947). Simulated patterns on the MMPI. *Journal of Abnormal and Social Psychology*, *42*, 215-225.

Gough, H. G. (1950). The F minus K dissimulation index for the MMPI. *Journal of Consulting Psychology*, *14*, 408-413.

Gough, H. G. (1954). Some common misconceptions about neuroticism. *Journal of Consulting Psychology, 18*, 287-292.

Gough, H. G. (1957). *California Psychological Inventory manual*. Palo Alto, CA: Consulting Psychologists Press.

Graham, J. (1990). *MMPI-2: Assessing Personality and Psychopathology*. New York: Oxford Press.

Graham, J. R. (1993). *MMPI-2: Assessing Personality and Psychopathology* (2nd ed.). New York: Oxford University Press.

Graham, J. R. (2000). *MMPI-2: Assessing Personality and Psychopathology* (3rd ed.). New York: Oxford University Press.

Graham, J. R., Watts, D., & Timbrook, R. E. (1991). Detecting fake-good and fake-bad MMPI-2 profiles. *Journal of Personality Assessment, 57*, 264-277.

Green, P., Rohling, M. L., Lees-Haley, P. R., & Allen III, L. M. (in press). Effort has a greater effect on test scores than severe brain injury in compensation claimants. *Brain Injury*.

Greene, R. L. (1987). Ethnicity and MMPI performance: A review. *Journal of Consulting and Clinical Psychology, 55*, 497-512.

Greene, R. (1988). The relative efficacy of F-K and the obvious and subtle scales to detect overreporting of psychopathology on the MMPI. *Journal of Clinical Psychology, 44*, 152-159.

Greene, R. (1991). *The MMPI-2/MMPI: An Interpretive Manual*. New York: Grune & Stratton.

Greene, R. L. (1997). Assessment of malingering and defensiveness by multiscale personality inventories. In R. Rogers (Ed.), *Clinical Assessment of Malingering and Deception* (pp. 169-207). New York: The Guilford Press.

Greene, R. (2000). *The MMPI-2/MMPI: An Interpretive Manual*, 2nd ed. New York: Grune & Stratton.

Grillo, J., Brown, R. S., Hilsabeck, R., Price, J. R., & Lees-Haley, P. R. (1994). Raising doubts about claims of malingering: Implications of relationships between MCMI-II and MMPI-2 performances. *Journal of Clinical Psychology, 50*, 651-655.

Gynther, M.D., & Green, S. B. (1980). Accuracy may make a difference, but does a difference make for accuracy? A response to Pritchard and Rosenblatt. *Journal of Consulting and Clinical Psychology, 48*, 268-272.

Hall, G. C. N., Bansal, A., & Lopez, I. R. (1999). Ethnicity and psychopathology: A meta-analytic review of 31 years of comparative MMPI/MMPI-2 research. *Psychological Assessment, 11*, 186-197.

Hedlund, J. L., & Won Cho, D. (1979). [MMPI data research tape for Missouri Department of Mental Health patients.] Unpublished raw data. Cited in Greene, R. (1991). *The MMPI-2/MMPI: An Interpretive Manual*. New York: Grune & Stratton.

Henry, J. R., & Senior, G. (2001, February). Examining the diagnostic utility of MMPI-2 scales in personal injury cases. Poster presented at the 1st Annual Conference of the APS College of Forensic Psychologists. Sydney, NSW, Australia.

Hoffman, R. G., Scott, J. G. Emick, M. A. & Adams, R. L. (1999). The MMPI-2 and closed head injury: Effects of litigation and head injury severity. *Journal of Forensic Neuropsychology, 1*, 3-13.

Iverson, G. L., & Barton, E. A. (1999). Interscorer reliability of the MMPI-2: Should TRIN and VRIN be computer scored? *Journal of Clinical Psychology*, *55*, 65-69.

Iverson, G. L., Franzen, M. F., & Hammond, J. A. (1995). Examination of inmates' ability to malinger on the MMPI-2. *Psychological Assessment*, *7*, 118-121.

Iverson, G. L., Henrichs, T. F., Barton, E. A., & Allen, S. (in press). Specificity of the MMPI-2 Fake Bad Scale as a marker for personal injury malingering. *Psychological Reports*.

Johnson, M. T., Krafka, C., & Cecil, J. S. (2000). *Expert Testimony in Federal Civil Trials: A Preliminary Analysis*. Washington, DC: Federal Judicial Center.

Larrabee, G. J. (1996, November). Somatic malingering on the MMPI/MMPI-2 in litigating subjects. Presented to the National Academy of Neuropsychology annual conference, New Orleans, LA.

Larrabee, G. J. (1997). Neuropsychological outcome, post concussion symptoms, and forensic considerations in mild closed head trauma. *Seminars in Clinical Neuropsychiatry*, *2*, 196-206.

Larrabee, G. J. (1998). Somatic malingering on the MMPI and MMPI-2 in personal injury litigants. *The Clinical Neuropsychologist*, *12*, 179-188.

Lees-Haley, P. R. (1991). Ego strength denial on the MMPI-2 as a clue to simulation of personal injury in vocational neuropsychological and emotional distress evaluations. *Perceptual and Motor Skills*, *72*, 815-819.

Lees-Haley P. R. (1992). Efficacy of MMPI-2 validity scales and MCMI-II modifier scales for detecting spurious PTSD claims: F, F-K, Fake Bad Scale, ego strength, subtle-obvious subscales, DIS, and DEB. *Journal of Clinical Psychology*, *48*, 681-689.

Lees-Haley P. R. (1997). MMPI-2 base rates for 492 personal injury plaintiffs: Implications and challenges for forensic assessment. *Journal of Clinical Psychology*, *53*, 745-755.

Lees-Haley P. R., English L.T., & Glenn W. J. (1991). A Fake Bad Scale on the MMPI-2 for personal injury claimants. *Psychological Reports*, *68*, 203-210.

Lees-Haley, P. R., & Fox, D. D. (1990). MMPI Subtle-Obvious scales and malingering: Clinical versus simulated scores. *Psychological Reports*, *66*, 907-911.

Lim, J., & Butcher, J. N. (1996). Detection of faking on the MMPI-2: Differentiation among faking-bad, denial, and claiming extreme virtue. *Journal of Personality Assessment*, *67*, 1-25.

Long, K.A., Graham, J. R., & Timbrook, R. E. (1994). Socioeconomic status and MMPI-2 interpretation. *Measurement and Evaluation in Counseling and Development*, *27*, 158-177.

Mack, T. J. (1994). Scientific Testimony after Daubert: Some early returns from lower courts. *Science and the Law*, August, pp. 23-31.

McKinley, J. C., Hathaway, S. R., & Meehl, P. E. (1948). The MMPI: VI. The K scale. *Journal of Consulting Psychology*, *12*, 20-31.

Meehl, P. E. (1993). Philosophy of science: Help or hindrance? *Psychological Reports*, *72*, 707-733.

Meehl, P. E., & Hathaway, S. R. (1946). The K factor as a suppressor variable in the MMPI. *Journal of Applied Psychology*, *30*, 525-564.

Millis, S. R., Putnam, S. H., & Adams, K.M. (1995, March). Neuropsychological malingering and the MMPI-2: Old and new indicators. Paper presented at the 30th Annual Symposium on Recent Developments in the Use of the MMPI, MMPI-2 and MMPI-A, St. Petersburg Beach, FL.

Nelson, L. D., Pham, D., & Uchiyama, C. (1996). Subtlety of the MMPI-2 Depression Scale: A subject laid to rest? *Psychological Assessment, 8*, 331-333.

Nicholson, R. A., Mouton, G. J., Bagby, R. M., Buis, T., Peterson, S. A., & Buigas, R. A. (1997). Utility of MMPI-2 indicators of response distortion: Receiver operating characteristic analysis. *Psychological Assessment, 9*, 471-479.

Paolo, A. M., & Ryan, J. J. (1992). Detection of random response sets on the MMPI-2. *Psychotherapy in Private Practice, 11*, 1-8.

Pensa, R., Dorfman, W., Gold, S. N., & Schneider, B. (1996). Detection of malingered psychosis with the MMPI-2. *Psychotherapy in Private Practice, 14*, 47-64.

Pope, K. S., Butcher, J. N., & Seelen, J. (1993). *The MMPI, MMPI-2 & MMPI-A in Court: A Practical Guide for Expert Witnesses and Attorneys.* Washington, DC: American Psychological Association.

Posthuma, A. B. & Harper, J. F. (1998). Comparison of MMPI-2 responses of child custody and personal injury litigants. *Professional Psychology: Research and Practice, 29*, 437-443.

Pritchard, D. A., & Rosenblatt, A. (1980). Racial bias in the MMPI: A methodological review. *Journal of Consulting and Clinical Psychology, 48*, 263-267.

Putnam, S. H., Millis, S. R., & Adams, K. M. (1998, August). Consideration of impression management in the neuropsychological examination with the MMPI-2. Paper presented at the Annual Meeting of the American Psychological Association, San Francisco, CA.

Rayls, K. R., Mittenberg, W., Burns, W. J., Theroux, S. (2000). Prospective study of the MMPI-2 correction factor after mild head injury. *The Clinical Neuropsychologist, 14*, 546-550.

Rogers, R., Sewell, K. W., & Salekin, R. T. (1994). A meta-analysis of malingering on the MMPI-2. *Assessment, 1*, 227-237.

Rogers, R., Sewell, K. W., & Ustad, K. L. (1995). Feigning among chronic outpatients on the MMPI-2: A systematic examination of fake-bad indicators. *Assessment, 2*, 81-89.

Rothke, S. E., Friedman, A., Dahlstrom, W., Greene, R., Arredondo, R., & Mann, A. (1994). MMPI-2 Normative data for the F-K Index: Implications for clinical, neuropsychological, and forensic practice. *Assessment, 1*, 1-15.

Rothke, S. E., Friedman, A. F., Jaffe, A. M., Greene, R. L., Wetter, M. W., Cole, P., & Baker, K. (2000). Normative data for the F(p) scale of the MMPI-2: Implications for clinical and forensic assessment of malingering. *Psychological Assessment, 12*, 335-340.

Schinka, J. A., & LaLone, L. (1997). MMPI-2 norms: Comparisons with a census-matched subsample. *Psychological Assessment, 9*, 307-311.

Senior, G., & Douglas, L. (2000, November). Personal injury base rates and interpretative guidelines for the MMPI-2. Special Topic Presentation at the 20th Annual Conference of the National Academy of Neuropsychology. Orlando, FL.

Senior, G., & Douglas, L. (in press). Misconceptions and misuse of the MMPI-2 in assessing personal injury claimants. *Neurorehabilitation.*

Senior, G., Vlahov, J., & Shapcott, R. (1999). The trouble with codetypes: Concerns regarding traditional MMPI-2 interpretative strategies in the medicolegal context. Paper presented at the 5th Annual Conference of the College of Clinical Neuropsychologists. Leura, NSW, Australia. *Australian Journal of Psychology, 5*, 159.

Shores, E. A., & Carstairs, J. C. (1998). Accuracy of the MMPI-2 computerized report in identifying fake-good and fake-bad response sets. *The Clinical Neuropsychologist, 12*, 101-106.

Sivec, H. J., Lynn, S., & Garske, J. P. (1994). The effect of somatoform disorder and paranoid psychotic role-related dissimulations as a response set on the MMPI-2. *Assessment, 1*, 69-81.

Slick, D. J., Hopp, G., Strauss, E., & Spellacy, F. J. (1996). Victoria Symptom Validity Test: Efficiency for detecting feigned memory impairment and relationship to neuropsychological tests and MMPI-2 validity scales. *Journal of Clinical and Experimental Neuropsychology, 18*, 911-922.

Smith, D. W., & Frueh, B. C. (1996). Compensation seeking, comorbidity, and apparent exaggeration of PTSD symptoms among Vietnam combat veterans. *Psychological Assessment, 8*, 3-6.

Storm, J., & Graham, J. R. (2000). Detection of coached general malingering on the MMPI-2. *Psychological-Assessment, 12*, 158-165.

Strong, D. R., Greene, R. L., Schinka, J. A. (2000). A taxometric analysis of MMPI-2 infrequency scales [F and F(p)] in clinical settings. *Psychological Assessment, 12*, 166-173.

Stukenberg, K., Brady, C., & Klinetob, N. (2000). Use of the MMPI-2's VRIN scale with severely disturbed populations: Consistent responding may be more problematic than inconsistent responding. *Psychological Reports, 86*, 3-14.

Timbrook, R. E., & Graham, J. R. (1994). Ethnic differences on the MMPI-2? *Psychological Assessment, 6*, 212-217.

Timbrook, R. E., Graham, J. R., Keiller, S. W., & Watts, D. (1993). Comparison of the Wiener-Harmon Subtle-Obvious scales and the standard validity scales in detecting valid and invalid MMPI-2 profiles. *Psychological Assessment, 5*, 53-61.

Tsushima, W. T., & Tsushima, V. G. (2001). Comparison of the Fake Bad Scale and other MMPI-2 validity scales with personal injury litigants. *Assessment, 8*, 205-212.

Vincent, N. M., Linsz, N. L., & Greene, M. I. (1966). The L scale of the MMPI as an index of falsification. *Journal of Clinical Psychology, 22*, 211-216.

Walters, G. L., & Clopton, J. R. (2000). Effect of symptom information and validity scale information on the malingering of depression on the MMPI-2. *Journal of Personality Assessment, 75*, 183-199.

Wetter, M. W., Baer, R. A., Berry, D. T. R., & Reynolds, S. K. (1994). The effect of symptom information on faking on the MMPI-2. *Assessment, 1*, 199-207.

Wetter, M. W., Baer, R. A., Berry, D. T. R., Robison, L. H., & Sumpter, J. (1993). MMPI-2 profiles of motivated fakers given specific symptom information: A comparison to matched patients. *Psychological Assessment, 5*, 317-323.

Wetter, M. W., Baer, R. A., Berry, D. T., Smith, G. T., et al. (1992). Sensitivity of MMPI-2 validity scales to random responding and malingering. *Psychological Assessment, 4*, 369-374.

Wetter, M. W., & Deitsch, S. E. (1996). Faking specific disorders and temporal response consistency on the MMPI-2. *Psychological Assessment, 8*, 39-47

Wetzler, S., & Marlowe, D. (1990). "Faking bad" on the MMPI, MMPI-2, and Millon-II. *Psychological Reports*, *67*, 1117-1118.
Wiener, D. N. (1948). Subtle and obvious keys for the MMPI. *Journal of Consulting Psychology*, *12*, 164-170.
Wiener, D., & Harmon, L. (1946). *Subtle and obvious keys for the MMPI: Their development* (Advisement Bulletin No. 16). Minneapolis, MN: Regional Veterans Administration Office.

Computerized Assessment of Response Bias in Forensic Neuropsychology

Lyle M. Allen III

CogniSyst, Inc.

Grant L. Iverson

University of British Columbia & Riverview Hospital

Paul Green

Independent Practice

SUMMARY. The Computerized Assessment of Response Bias (CARB) is a forced-choice digit recognition test designed to detect suboptimal performance during a psychological or neuropsychological evaluation. First developed in 1992, CARB has incorporated a number of refinements such as early termination for excellent early performance and analysis of response times and patterns. Patients with moderate or severe brain injury, or neurological disease, easily pass CARB. These groups provide primary validation for the test, along with more recent analogue malingering studies. CARB is sensitive to poor effort or suboptimal performance in patients with a wide variety of diagnoses, including outpa-

---

Lyle M. Allen III is affiliated with CogniSyst, Inc., Durham, NC.

Grant L. Iverson is affiliated with the University of British Columbia & Riverview Hospital, Vancouver, BC.

Paul Green is in independent practice, Edmonton, AB.

Address correspondence to: Lyle M. Allen III, MS, 3937 Nottaway Road, Durham, NC 27707.

[Haworth co-indexing entry note]: "Computerized Assessment of Response Bias in Forensic Neuropsychology." Allen, Lyle M. III, Grant L. Iverson, and Paul Green. Co-published simultaneously in *Journal of Forensic Neuropsychology* (The Haworth Medical Press, an imprint of The Haworth Press, Inc.) Vol. 3, No. 1/2, 2002, pp. 205-225; and: *Detection of Response Bias in Forensic Neuropsychology* (ed: Jim Hom, and Robert L. Denney) The Haworth Medical Press, an imprint of The Haworth Press, Inc., 2002, pp. 205-225. Single or multiple copies of this article are available for a fee from The Haworth Document Delivery Service [1-800-HAWORTH, 9:00 a.m. - 5:00 p.m. (EST). E-mail address: getinfo@haworthpressinc.com].

© 2002 by The Haworth Press, Inc. All rights reserved.

tients with mild traumatic brain injuries, pain disorders, fibromyalgia, and depression. When used properly, CARB will likely hold up under *Daubert* challenges due to its specific focus and purpose, and extensive validation research. *[Article copies available for a fee from The Haworth Document Delivery Service: 1-800-HAWORTH. E-mail address: <getinfo@haworthpressinc.com> Website: <http://www.HaworthPress.com> © 2002 by The Haworth Press, Inc. All rights reserved.]*

KEYWORDS. CARB, malingering, effort, symptom validity

HISTORY AND DEVELOPMENT OF KEY FEATURES

The Computerized Assessment of Response Bias (CARB) is a classic, forced-choice digit recognition test that closely follows the paradigm advanced by Hiscock and Hiscock (1989). CARB is based on the forced-choice paradigm, which has been used extensively (and almost exclusively) in symptom validity tests, many of which also involve the presentation and subsequent recognition of digit strings. Popular examples of forced-choice tests include the Digit Memory Test (Hiscock & Hiscock, 1989), Portland Digit Recognition Test (Binder 1993; Binder & Kelly, 1996; Binder & Willis, 1991), and the Victoria Symptom Validity Test (Slick, Hopp, Strauss, Hunter, & Pinch, 1994; Slick, Hopp, Strauss, & Spellacy, 1996; Slick, Hopp, Strauss, & Thompson, 1997). There is no oral or face-to-face administration form of CARB. The test was designed to be computer-administered. Besides eliminating examiner tedium, this form of administration allows additional data on response times and patterns to be gathered painlessly and analyzed quickly.

Version 1.0 of CARB (Conder, Allen, & Cox, 1992) was offered in late 1992. The original version consisted of 111 trials arranged in three blocks of 37 items each, with distraction delays of 5, 10, and 15 seconds per block. In all versions, unqualified positive feedback is given to the examinee before the second and third CARB blocks indicating "excellent" performance and that the next block will be more difficult than the previous one. In each trial, five-digit stimuli are presented briefly (3-5 seconds), followed by a distracter task in which the subject is asked to count backwards. Following the distraction delays (which increase in duration across the three blocks), the target and a foil stimulus are displayed in the lower corners of the screen. The subject must then use either the left or right shift key to identify the target. The overwhelming majority of the foil and target numeric pairs used in the test are readily discernible by a different leading or terminal digit. Only 13 of the 111 stimulus choices (11%) do *not* begin with the same digit and could therefore be described as faintly difficult, requiring at least a slight amount of subject effort.

Paul Green and other early customers supported and then helped validate two optional and independently specified enhancements that were quickly added to version 1.0: omission of item feedback and shortened distraction delays to 3, 6, and 9 seconds per block. CARB versions 1.5 and 1.6 (essentially identical to the original version) were offered in 1995 and 1996. The CARB manual was expanded with additional case examples and interpretive text, and additional performance details were added to the report. In addition, Spanish language instructions were devised and included in the standard package, and more robust third party timing routines were added to the software to ensure consistent administration across 286, 386, and 486 PC-compatible platforms.

CARB '97 contained a number of important innovations and was officially released in 1997 (Allen, Conder, Green, & Cox, 1997). This version is substantially the same as the program sold today (January, 2002). By that time, Allen had obtained sole copyright ownership, but continued to receive substantial collaborative input from the other authors. Paul Green had purchased version 1.0 and led the first largely independent clinical research on CARB. Green and his colleagues produced data on the utility of CARB in several diagnostic groups (Green, Gervais, Astner, Kiss, & Allen, 1993). Green and Allen began collaborating closely in 1995, creating the Word Memory Test (WMT; Green, Allen, & Astner, 1996), and then using both instruments simultaneously in their ongoing clinical research on suboptimal effort/performance. In the CARB '97 manual and scoring software, passing CARB is defined for normative and comparison purposes as achieving a total score of greater than or equal to 89% correct, with all three blocks administered. The computer-generated reports in CARB '97 contained numerous performance comparisons to several compensation-related clinical reference groups. These include the following groups (a) patients with severe traumatic brain injury (Allen & Green, 1999), (b) patients with neurological disease (Green & Allen, 1999), (c) patients with TBI-related claims who passed CARB and the WMT, (d) patients with heterogeneous non-TBI diagnoses who passed CARB and the WMT, and (e) patients with heterogeneous diagnoses (including TBI) demonstrating impaired memory and passing CARB and the WMT. These reports also contained analyses of statistically unlikely response patterns for sequences of left, right, and incorrect key presses using the binomial theorem. To reduce false positive identification of left and right response patterns, the order of the trials in CARB '97 was rearranged so that the number of consecutive left-or right-sided correct responses never exceeded two. The standard administration procedure of CARB '97 offered dramatically shortened distraction delays (1.5, 2.5, and 3.5 seconds per block). Paul Green and his colleague Roger Gervais validated these during 1996 using their clinical practice patients (this validation is described in the test manual). Patients with moderate to severe brain injuries have always served as the most important CARB reference group; their performances were unaffected by the shortened delays. In fact, the available data show a slight nonsignificant improvement with the shortened delays for these patients.

In CARB '97, optional item time-outs were added because some customers complained about patients with trivial injuries performing very slowly. A series of setup screens supported the creation of customized CARB administration protocols. These allowed users to include or omit the early termination (discussed in detail below) and trial time-out options, reduce the number of items per block to 25, control the form (auditory and/or visual) and availability of trial feedback, precisely manipulate stimulus presentation and distraction/interference delay times, and choose between two different distraction suggestions. One option was to "Count backwards *silently* from 20" and the other asked the patient to count backwards silently from a number that varied randomly between 20 and 60 for each trial. Periodic data analyses by Allen and Green led to incremental enhancements in reporting, including response time analyses that both exclude and include omitted responses (substituting the maximum trial window time). The CARB report was further revised in 1999 to include larger and closely studied reference samples of 57 patients with moderate to severe TBI (Allen & Green, 1999) and 40 patients with heterogeneous neurological diseases (Green & Allen, 1999).

Early Termination Feature. For the CARB '97 release, Allen also analyzed block performance patterns in CARB data from serial compensation cases drawn from 13 practices in the US and Canada (Allen et al., 1997). Using 1,752 electronically collected records from these practices. an early termination feature was devised based on excellent first block, or first and second block, performance. Implementing this as part of the standardized administration further shortened average CARB administration times to between 5 and 12 minutes, depending upon how patients performed early on and how many items were administered per block. Back testing predicted that approximately 45% of patients would discontinue CARB after the first block, and approximately two-thirds of all patients would discontinue CARB by the end of the second block. The false negative rate for implementing this time saving option was estimated to be only 3%, compared with administration of all three CARB blocks (Allen et al., 1997).

The research on CARB summarized below has almost exclusively utilized CARB '97 with its standard administration features: early termination enabled, 37 items per block with distraction delays of 1.5, 2.5, and 3.5 seconds per block, and patients asked to count backwards silently from 20 during the distraction intervals. Most of this research has also been conducted in parallel with studies of the Word Memory Test, with CARB administered in a computerized battery between the WMT immediate and 30-minute delayed recognition subtests.

CARB SOFTWARE DESCRIPTION AND TECHNICAL INFORMATION

CARB can be installed automatically and run on most Windows computers, although Windows 95 and 98 may require minor editing of two system configuration files. Windows 2000 and Millennium Edition (Me) are generally running on newer and much faster machines, and these operating systems now include special features designed to support older MS-DOS programs that may not function properly under Windows 95 and 98. To achieve accurate timing for stimulus presentation, inter-stimulus delays, and response times, CARB reprograms a spare channel on the timer chip found in IBM compatible computers to provide one-millisecond accuracy. This is much harder to achieve under Windows due to the fact that it is a cooperative multi-tasking system that will not relinquish complete control to any application. CARB cannot be administered (and thus should not be installed) on Windows NT 3.0, 3.5, or 4.0 because direct access to the timer hardware is prohibited. Windows 2000 Professional has superceded these operating systems, and it can accurately and reliably emulate hardware timer functions called by MS-DOS programs in a way that was not possible in earlier versions of Windows. Windows Me is an outgrowth of Windows 98 and appears to offer support for DOS programs that is similar to that in Windows 2000. However, Windows Me is not nearly as robust or stable as Windows 2000, which is built on Microsoft's NT technology and offers superior memory isolation and management. The operation of CARB under Windows XP has not been thoroughly tested and documented as of this writing. CogniSyst, Inc. is expected to release a Windows version of CARB in the second quarter of 2002.

RELIABILITY

Distribution of Scores

The pattern of CARB scores in all populations studied to date is highly skewed in that the overwhelming majority of patients obtain perfect or nearly perfect scores. Rogers, Harrell, and Liff (1993) and Frederick (2000) have described this as a "floor effect," suggesting that such tasks can be performed by almost anyone. Other authors (Conder, Allen, & Cox, 1992; Iverson & Franzen, 1996; Slick, Iverson, & Green, 2000) have focused on the score distribution itself and used the term "ceiling effect" to describe the massive clumping of scores at or close to 100% correct. This type of non-normal score distribution characterizes the majority of symptom validity tests. CARB scores are always expressed as the percentage correct of all the trials administered in a block or for the entire test (total CARB score)–which often includes only one block (due to the early termination feature). The effect of item "difficulty" in CARB has not been systematically studied, but is likely to reveal more about the test's overall face validity than actual trial difficulty.

Internal Consistency and Stability

"Classical Test Theory" measures of reliability have limited application to the CARB, and many other symptom validity tests. For example, the internal consistency of the CARB for measuring the construct of "biased responding" is (a) influenced by the item-level characteristics of the test (e.g., most subjects trying their best get nearly every item on the test correct), and (b) affected by the construct itself (i.e., we do not assume that biased responding can be measured in a uniform fashion across test items). The internal consistency of CARB performance is very high in patients who are trying their best on the test, but variable in patients who are providing less than optimal effort. In a sample of 1,752 patient records for CARB version 1.0, the range of average block scores in 1,220 patients who were administered and passed CARB was only 96.6% to 97.6%, while average scores for blocks 1 and 3 in the 532 patients failing CARB ranged from 74.6% to 62.4% correct, respectively (Allen et al., 1997; Allen, Richards, Green, Iverson, & Condor, 1998).

These researchers also determined that a difference of 10% between any two blocks of CARB was statistically significant ($p < 0.01$). Using this as a criterion for inconsistent performance, only 11% of passers evidenced inter-block variability, compared with 75% of those who failed CARB. This method of quantifying inconsistency correlated highly "with overall CARB failure ($r = .66, p < 0.0001$) and with the total number of CARB blocks failed ($r = .67, p < 0.0001$)" (Allen et al., 1997, p. 40).

Test-retest reliability in CARB was assessed by de Armas (1996) in a sample of male volunteer court-adjudicated domestic violence offenders attending a court-ordered group psychoeducational intervention program. A one-week test-retest of CARB with participants instructed to do their best each time produced a nearly perfect Pearson reliability coefficient ($r = .97$).

VALIDATION RESEARCH

Moderate and Severe Traumatic Brain Injury

In the original validation study, eight patients with severe TBI who were an average of 16.5 months post injury ($SD = 18.8$) and who evidenced good recovery obtained a mean total CARB score of 96.8% ($SD = 3.6$) correct (Conder et al., 1992). In the CARB '97 manual, similar results were obtained from a separate sample of 26 outpatients with severe traumatic brain injuries who were tested by Paul Green in routine compensation-related neuropsychological evaluations. Total CARB scores in this group were based on all three blocks and averaged 97.4% ($SD = 3.9$) correct (Allen et al., 1997).

In the 1999 Supplement to the CARB and the WMT, this sample had grown to 57 patients with moderate to severe TBI (Allen & Green, 1999). The condition of these patients was carefully studied and summarized. Five other patients were excluded from this sample due to independent evidence of marked symptom exaggeration, and one patient who was considered "untestable" was not given CARB although he passed the orally administered WMT. For approximately 40 patients in this sample, CARB was administered with its early termination option for good performance enabled. Total CARB scores were then computed from all available data (1, 2, or 3 blocks). The 56 patients with severe TBI obtained a mean total CARB score that averaged 98.3% correct ($SD = 2.6$). Fifteen of these patients completed CARB after the first block, another 12 required two CARB blocks, and the remaining 32 patients either required or were given all three blocks of CARB without the early termination. It is possible that the slight increase in mean score over earlier severe TBI samples was due in part to the use of the CARB early termination feature, which may have reduced the tedium and minimal concentration and attention required to perform well on the test. Due to the time span covered in collecting this sample it is also possible that the shortened distraction delays that were introduced in 1996 as part of the standardized administration reduced attentional demands and therefore improved scores.

In this work, the authors also studied the relationship between several objective variables (e.g., loss of consciousness [LOC], Glasgow Coma Scale scores [GCS], post-traumatic amnesia [PTA]) commonly used to quantify head injury severity and the performance of these patients on CARB and the WMT. Several comparison subgroups were defined using median splits on these independent variables, with subsequent comparisons then undertaken on the other indices. To assess potential confounds in this clinical sample, patients with missing data on the criterion variable comprised a third group in every comparison that was undertaken. Effect size differences (*g*) in head injury severity measures between the groups, defined using median splits, ranged from 0.57 to 0.66 for groups defined by PTA, from 0.38 to 0.72 for groups defined by LOC, and from 0.31 to 0.89 for groups defined by GCS. In spite of these variations in head injury severity, there were no significant differences between any of these groups on any CARB total or individual block scores (Allen & Green, 1999). None of the analyses suggested that missing data had biased these findings concerning the insensitivity of CARB to brain injury. Patients with missing data on the independent variable were intermediate between the main comparison groups on the other variables of head injury severity and CARB performance.

Allen and Green (1999) also compared the CARB performance of these patients on measures of verbal learning and memory. Fifty-one of the patients with severe TBIs had been given the California Verbal Learning Test (CVLT; Delis, Kramer, Kaplan, & Ober, 1987), which was scored relative to normal controls based on age, gender, and VIQ (Wiens, Tindall, & Crossen, 1996). Patients were then stratified at the median using an average CVLT Z-score computed for total words learned, short delay free recall, and long delay free recall. While the effect size differences (*g*) between these two groups with normal or impaired verbal memory ranged from .59 to .71 on these CVLT variables, the disparity in total CARB score only varied 1.1% ($p = 0.17$), with the combined group averaging 98.2% correct ($SD = 2.5$).

Green and Iverson (2001) examined CARB performance in 119 TBI patients assessed for compensation-related disability claims. These groups consisted of 25 patients with either moderate ($N = 8$) or severe ($N = 17$) brain injuries verified by radiological findings, 49 mild head injury patients with negative radiological findings and LOC less than 20 minutes, and 45 patients with alleged mild head injuries who reported no LOC. Comparing CARB performances in each of these three groups, the authors found a paradoxical severity effect, wherein mild head injury and alleged mild head injury patient groups scored significantly worse than the 25 patients classified with moderate to severe TBI. While only one TBI patient (4%) scored below the CARB cutoff in this study, 24% of the mild head injury patients and 29% of the alleged mild head injury patients failed CARB. Parallel findings were reported for average response latencies, with the TBI group evidencing significantly faster times than the other two groups. A significant negative correlation was observed between response latencies and total CARB scores, such that faster times were associated with better CARB performance. The authors ascribed the observed group differences in CARB percent correct and response times to a higher prevalence of symptom exaggeration in the mild head injury and alleged mild head injury groups.

Green, Rohling, Lees-Haley, and Allen (2001) replicated and extended the main findings of the two previous studies. These researchers demonstrated the profound effect of patient effort on patients' corresponding neuropsychological test battery results in compensation-related evaluations. A total of 904 cases with heterogeneous diagnoses were studied, along with a subset of 470 TBI patients (52%) that were separately analyzed based on head injury severity. The primary measures consisted of an overall test battery mean Z-score (OTBM) computed from an average of 37 individual measures of cognitive ability, and a symptom validity test (SVT) composite Z-score variable calculated from patients' average CARB score, the three WMT effort measures, and the CVLT Logit formula (Millis, Putnam, Adams, & Ricker, 1995). The paradoxical severity effects related to head injury severity reported by Green and Iverson (2001) were replicated using this expanded sample. Patients with mild or questionable head injuries who demonstrated suboptimal performance by virtue of SVT failure performed 1.26 standard deviations worse on the OTBM than a combined group of patients with neurological disease and moderate to severe TBI who evidenced good effort. In the entire sample, the SVT composite score accounted for 51% of the variance in the OTBM, or approximately 4.5 times the variance that could be related to the demographic variables of age, gender, or years of education. CARB total scores were significantly correlated with the OTBM (Spearman's Rho = .44 and Pearson's product moment [$r = .57$]). There was also a highly significant difference on the OTBM mean score between patients who passed CARB ($M = -.31$, $SD = .70$, $n = 701$) and those who failed ($M = -1.29$; $SD = 1.00$, $n = 185$; F [1, 884] = 221, $p < .0005$).

Neurological Disease

In the 1999 Supplement to the CARB and WMT manuals, 40 patients with heterogeneous neurological diseases were individually described and thoroughly studied in their performances on CARB and the WMT. Patients were identified as having a primary neurological diagnosis, such as brain tumor, ruptured aneurysm, stroke, or multiple sclerosis. CARB, WMT, the CVLT, and Warrington's Recognition Memory Test for words and faces (Warrington, 1984) were administered in all cases, along with a comprehensive neuropsychological test battery. All assessments were undertaken for compensation or disability related claims and the results were made available to lawyers or the benefit funding agencies, such as insurance companies and the Workers' Compensation Board in Edmonton, Alberta, Canada (Green & Allen, 1999, p. 19).

Total CARB scores in these 40 patients with neurological disease averaged 97.2% correct ($SD = 4.6$), again demonstrating a strong ceiling distribution. To specifically assess the relationship between verbal memory ability and CARB scores, the neurological patients were then stratified into two equal-sized groups based on scoring above or below the mean for total words learned on the CVLT. As expected, these subgroups were quite different from one another on total CVLT words learned ($p < 0.0001$), short-delayed free recall ($p < 0.0001$), and long-delayed free recall ($p < 0.0001$), as well as WMT short-delay ($p < 0.002$) and long delay free recall measures ($p < 0.01$). Nevertheless, the mean total CARB scores differed by less than 0.6% ($p = 0.58$) between these groups. These CARB results in patients with neurological disease are consistent with the findings for patients with moderate to severe TBI.

Taken as a whole, the available research indicates that CARB is not measuring learning or memory; rather, this is a test designed to measure effort. The test is easy for patients with diverse forms of damage to the structure and/or function of their brains.

Analogue Malingering Studies

Conder et al. (1992) compared two groups of eight volunteers asked to malinger on the CARB to eight patients with severe TBI (briefly described earlier) who were asked to perform their best. In the "Gross" exaggeration condition, simulators were told to clearly demonstrate their cognitive impairment on CARB for the examiner. The "Subtle" group of simulators was asked to demonstrate cognitive impairment but to be somewhat subtle in their portrayal since test examiners were likely to be suspicious of patients who performed too badly on this test. The Gross simulation group obtained an average mean CARB score of 35.3% correct (*SD* = 29.1) which was significantly worse than the Subtle simulators' average score of 62.5% correct (*SD* = 15.8). In turn, the performance of Subtle simulators was significantly below that of the patients with severe brain injuries who obtained an average total CARB score of 96.8% correct (*SD* = 3.6).

Iverson, Ropacki, Allen, and Elias (2001) conducted an analogue study in which 44 university students were randomly assigned to two groups, controls ($n = 21$) and experimental-malingerers ($n = 23$). As expected, students instructed to perform their best obtained nearly perfect scores on Blocks 1, 2, 3, and the total score (i.e., 99.2 [*SD* = 1.9], 99.1 [*SD* = 1.3], 99.0 [*SD* = 2.0], and 99.1 [*SD* = 1.1], respectively). The experimental-malingerers obtained very low scores (i.e., 47.0 [*SD* = 27.7], 43.3 [*SD* = 30.6], 47.1 [*SD* = 28.0], and 45.8 [*SD* = 27.6], respectively). The sensitivity of the total score cutoff for detecting malingering was .87, and the specificity was 1.0.

Dunn, Shear, Howe, and Ris (in press) employed a between-group simulation design using CARB and several other neurocognitive measures with 125 undergraduate volunteers to examine the robustness of various symptom validity measures. The use of information concerning the effects of brain injury was assessed in combination with the presence or absence of specific information on how to "defeat" symptom validity measures in a 2 × 2 experimental design in which participants were asked to feign brain damage. A fifth control group was comprised of participants asked to perform their best, but who were otherwise naïve and not provided with additional information. Post-administration self-assessments of motivation for participation, memory for the materials used in the manipulations, and perceived success in following experimental instructions failed to reveal any differences between the groups, indicating that the experimental manipulations were successfully administered. Control participants obtained a mean total CARB score of 99.6% correct (median = 100%; *SD* = 0.71), which was significantly above the median score of 58% obtained from a group comprised of all experimental participants feigning brain injury ($U = 85$; $p < 0.001$). The feigning participants also produced significantly slower ($p < .001$) and more variable ($p < 0.001$) CARB trial response times, confirming the findings of Allen and colleagues (1997) for patients passing and failing CARB. Dunn and his colleagues also found a significant main effect for coaching that elevated coached participants' scores on CARB above those who had not received this information. In spite of this difference, 78% of the coached participants failed CARB. No main effect was found for the provision of information concerning brain injury, and no significant differences were found between any of the four experimental groups in their response times. All control patients passed CARB and the WMT. CARB failure identified 84% of all experimental patients as exaggerating and produced an overall classification rate of 87.2%. Identical classification results were obtained using the combination of WMT-IR and WMT-DR to define WMT failure. Employing the cutoffs from both instruments to identify poor effort improved overall classification to 93% of the entire sample.

Researchers have demonstrated that the majority of subjects instructed to malinger perform very poorly on CARB. The authors are aware of anecdotal evidence of client coaching concerning symptom validity tests by attorneys, disreputable healthcare practitioners, and patient "support groups" (e.g., Youngjohn, 1995). Although the details and incidence of this practice have not been well studied, it is believed that coached patients are taught to identify forced choice digit recognition tests and/or the forced choice method that is common to nearly all SVTs. The first author has received several reports of patients in certain locales who have offered answers to the TOMM *before* the choices were actually presented, and of patients who rapidly obtained flawless performances on CARB but went on to score less than chance on the WMT. A wealth of information about symptom validity tests is publicly available, as well as comprehensive data on the performance of patients with bona fide brain injuries on neuropsychological tests of ability and effort. Given these factors, future analogue malingering studies should investigate more sophisticated issues relating to the effects of internet-based research, attorney coaching, and access to published literature on participants' malingering behavior.

Coaching Patients on CARB

Many clinical neuropsychologists have long sought a special set of instructions that would reliably compel patients involved in compensation-related evaluations to put forth their best effort during the neuropsychological examination in order to obtain valid test results. Gervais, Green, Allen, and Iverson (2001) used information and warnings during patients' actual compensation-related evaluations to virtually eliminate failure on CARB. The authors utilized multiple group comparisons with consecutively referred DSM-IV Pain Disorder patients to assess the effect of warning (providing additional and truthful information) on CARB and WMT performances. During the CARB warning phases of the study, patients were given CARB at the conclusion of the examination and told that failure would cast significant doubt on the validity of their claimed impairment. Prior to implementing these warning procedures, patients with this referral diagnosis were found to be at high risk for suboptimal performance, with 50% failing CARB, 49% failing the WMT, and 53% failing either test. When CARB warning procedures were implemented, the rate of failure dropped significantly to 6%. However, when these warning procedures were reversed and shifted to the WMT, the incidence of CARB failure returned to levels observed when participants were not warned. Group failure rates on the WMT did not differ at any time during the study.

Studies Involving CARB with Other Diagnostic Groups

DSM-IV Pain Disorder. Researchers have demonstrated that patients with DSM-IV Pain Disorder sometimes fail cognitively-oriented symptom validity measures (Allen, Green, & Eimer, 1999; Schmand, Lindeboom, Schagen, Heijt, Koene, & Hamburger, 1998; Vickery, Ranseen, Cooley, & Berry, 1999). The CARB warning procedures employed by Gervais and colleagues with DSM-IV Pain Disorder patients provide support for the use of CARB in detecting suboptimal performance in this population of disability claimants (Gervais, Allen, Green, Cunningham, & Iverson, 1998). The pain patients in this study reported significantly more overall memory complaints on the Memory Complaints Inventory (Green & Allen, 1997; Green, Allen, & Iverson, 1999) compared with a group of 97 patients suffering from severe TBI or neurological disease. The average total CARB score for all of the 118 pain patients studied was also significantly below the patients who evidenced acquired brain impairment ($p < 0.0005$), in spite of the fact that the sample contained 30 pain patients who were successfully coached on CARB.

Fibromyalgia. The performances of 96 patient volunteers with fibromyalgia (FM) and 16 patients with rheumatoid arthritis (RA) on a variety of cognitive measures including CARB and the WMT have also been studied (Gervais, Russell, Green, Allen, Ferrari, & Pieschl, 2001). Fifty of the FM patients were not involved in any kind of disability-related claims for their illness. The remaining 46 FM patients were either receiving disability or were in the process of applying for initial or additional disability benefits. None of the RA patients failed either CARB or the WMT, and none of the FM patients who were not involved in disability claims failed CARB. In contrast, 24% of the FM patients involved in disability claims failed CARB, 30% failed the WMT, and 35% of these patients failed either CARB or the WMT. As in the previous study of pain patients, the FM patients who failed CARB or the WMT evidenced significant elevations on six of the nine scales of the Memory Complaints Inventory, compared with those who passed. However, the 16 FM patients suspected of suboptimal performance scored 6.1 standard deviations below a comparison group of patients with severe TBI and 8.0 standard deviations below a subgroup of these patients selected for impaired verbal memory on the CVLT. The researchers concluded that the performances of the FM patients failing CARB or the WMT were implausible and most likely represented suboptimal performance.

Depression. Depression is a common complaint in outpatients evaluated for various forms of disability. Findings are mixed regarding the relation between depression and cognitive impairment, but no published studies have utilized symptom validity tests to examine the potential confound of exaggeration. Rohling, Green, Allen, and Iverson (2002) addressed this by comparing neuropsychological test performance in two large groups of disability claimants with heterogeneous diagnoses selected for extreme performance on the Beck Depression Inventory (BDI; Beck, 1978). From an initial pool of 719 patients, the authors initially excluded 299 patients (42%) for failing either CARB or the WMT. In a previously studied subgroup of 307 consecutive patients referrals, these SVTs had an 87% rate of overall agreement with regard to poor effort (Allen, Conder, Green, & Cox, 1997). Patients excluded for poor effort scored significantly worse than a sample of 57 patients with severe TBI on the symptom validity measures. The two study groups differed markedly on three measures of self-reported depression (average effect size [g] = −3.89) and symptoms of memory impairment on the MCI ($p < .0001$; $g = -1.01$). Nevertheless, the low depression and high depression groups produced an insignificant mean effect size difference ($g = -0.01$) on 38 measures of cognitive performance assessing executive functioning, immediate and delayed free recall for verbal and nonverbal stimuli, cued recall and recognition memory for words, attention and concentration, and six of eight manual performance measures. The high depression group was worse only on left hand performance on Grooved Pegboard ($p < 0.01$) and Finger Tip Number Writing tests ($p < 0.001$). The third author has replicated the major findings of this study by employing a subsample of the high depression patients who also met the DSM-IV criteria for depression. These two studies provide indirect support for the use of CARB in outpatient disability evaluations, where self-reported depression may be a prominent factor or even the primary complaint. Given the low level of difficulty posed by CARB and the WMT it is very unlikely that the patients excluded from the study for suspicious effort were failing these tests due to depression. More research on CARB is necessary in this population, and there is no evidence to support the use of CARB in disability evaluations of depressed inpatients.

Use of CARB with Children

While the research on CARB with adults is extensive, the use of CARB with children has received far less attention. Flaro, Green, and Allen (2000) studied 69 children between the ages of 8 and 18, referred from "various social service agencies or justice departments for psychological evaluation" (p. 2). The children carried heterogeneous diagnoses, which included Learning Disability (33%), Conduct Disorder (29%), ADHD (17%), Fetal Alcohol Syndrome (17%), and miscellaneous disorders (4%). The average age was 13.3 years (*SD* = 2.6) and measured FSIQ was 92.1 (*SD* = 13.7). Applying the adult cutoff for total CARB score of 89%, 55 out of the 60 children (92%) passed CARB. A total of 13% of the children failed CARB or the WMT effort measures according to the adult norms. The mean age of children who failed CARB averaged 11.0 years (*SD* = 3.9) compared with 13.5 years (*SD* = 2.4) in those who passed. While no statistics were reported for this comparison, the authors acknowledged that CARB might have challenged some of the younger children. They recommended additional research.

Courtney, Dinkins, Allen, and Kuroski (2002) summarized CARB results in 90 children with an average age of 11.2 years (*SD* = 3.1) who were referred for an evaluation related to attention and concentration problems. The children ranged from 6 to 18 years in age, with the years 7 through 10 each having a minimum of 10 individuals. Children 10 years and older almost always exceeded the adult cutoff scores for effort and on average performed much like adults. However, a scatter plot of scores by age fitted with a third order polynomial suggests that CARB performance is sensitive to age effects in children under the age of 10 years. These data from Courtney and his colleagues underscore the need for age-based normative samples in children, especially for those who are 10 years of age or younger.

ON THE ADMISSIBILITY OF CARB EVIDENCE

Trial judges have long had broad discretion regarding the admissibility of expert testimony. Since the 1920s, the *Frye* standard of "general acceptance" was used in most jurisdictions. Quite simply, under this standard expert evidence based upon a scientific technique is inadmissible unless the technique is generally accepted in the scientific community. Arguably, the landmark *Daubert v. Merrell Dow Pharmaceuticals, Inc.* ruling, although replacing *Frye*, also could be conceptualized as *explaining Frye*. The *Frye* test relied heavily on the scientific community's general acceptance of a technique as a proxy for the reliability of the evidence, whereas *Daubert* continues to rely on the scientific community but also elaborates on the method by which the technique should be evaluated (i.e., "The Scientific Method"). The *Daubert* ruling indicated that in Federal Courts the *Frye* test was superseded by the Federal Rules of Evidence. This Supreme Court decision sparked tremendous interest and controversy throughout legal, academic, and professional communities, and scores of articles have been written on the topic.

When evaluating the admissibility of expert evidence, trial judges must make a preliminary determination regarding whether the reasoning or methodology that underlies the testimony is scientifically valid, and, importantly, whether that reasoning or methodology can be applied properly to the facts in the particular case. A fairly conservative interpretation of *Daubert* suggests that the Court has indicated a preference for scientific knowledge being offered as expert testimony, and that scientific knowledge is best derived using scientific methods. Arguably, this poses a problem for a large amount of psychological testimony that is based on clinical experience and clinical judgment. A trial strategy might be to argue that this expert testimony is not being offered as "scientific evidence," and thus the strict *Daubert* criteria should not apply. However, in a 1999 ruling, the Supreme Court has extended *Daubert* to include all forms of expert evidence, not just scientific evidence (*Kumho Tire Company, Ltd. v. Carmichael*).

Four factors were suggested to aid the judges in evaluating admissibility of expert testimony according to the *Daubert* ruling: (a) whether the methods upon which the testimony relies are based on testable hypotheses, (b) the known or potential error rate (e.g., false positives and false negatives) of the method, (c) whether the method has been subjected to peer review, and (d) whether the method is generally accepted in the relevant scientific community. In regards to the CARB, or any other test, we cannot make a sweeping generalization regarding admissibility under *Daubert*. The admissibility of CARB-related evidence depends upon the specific clinical inference (i.e., opinion) that is proffered, and whether that inference can be applied properly to the specific case at hand. In a general sense, the CARB (or any other psychological or neuropsychological test) is not "reliable" and/or "valid." Rather, it is the inferences drawn from the test that possess varying degrees of reliability and validity for specific purposes, with specific populations, under specific circumstances (Franzen, 1989, 2000). Therefore, in regards to the admissibility of CARB evidence, the opinions listed below could be tested using the *Daubert* criteria.

1. The plaintiff, who sustained a very mild traumatic brain injury two years prior to the evaluation, scored 65% correct on the CARB. This score indicates that the plaintiff was malingering.
2. The plaintiff, who sustained a very mild traumatic brain injury two years prior to the evaluation, scored 65% correct on the CARB. This score indicates that the plaintiff was not trying his best on the test. His score was much lower than typical patients with traumatic brain injuries and is very unlikely to be associated with the effects of a traumatic brain injury. His score is very similar to scores obtained by experimental subjects who are given instructions to malinger.
3. The plaintiff obtained a score of 94% correct on the CARB. Therefore, there is no evidence that the plaintiff was exaggerating or malingering during the neuropsychological evaluation.

It is very likely that the opinions presented in points #1 and #3 would not be admissible if they were subjected to a thorough *Daubert* challenge. The first opinion is inadequate because an inference of malingering cannot be based upon a single test. Instead, this inference requires ruling out a number of alternative explanations and differential diagnoses (Iverson & Binder, 2000). The third opinion represents a fundamental error in logic: the absence of evidence is not evidence of absence. Moreover, it would be extraordinarily naïve to believe that all persons who deliberately exaggerate their problems would necessarily do so on the CARB. The second opinion likely would sustain a *Daubert* challenge, as illustrated by the "Validation Research" section of this article. The strength of CARB, in relation to the *Daubert* criteria, is that it is a test designed for a single purpose that has been extensively studied. Moreover, its basic methodology (i.e., the forced choice recognition paradigm) has been applied and validated in dozens of studies.

CONCLUSION

The Computerized Assessment of Response Bias (CARB) is a well-validated forced-choice digit recognition test that can screen for sub-optimal performance and related symptom invalidity. Primary validation for CARB has utilized patients who have suffered significant impairments related to either moderate to severe brain injury or neurological disease. These carefully studied patient groups have a combined average total CARB performance score of 97.8% correct (*SD* = 3.6; Allen & Green, 1999; Green & Allen, 1999). Besides these conditions, CARB has also been validated in analogue malingering studies and in patients with DSM-IV pain disorder. Published research also suggests that CARB is sensitive to suboptimal performance in evaluations with primary complaints of fibromyalgia, depression and a variety of other diagnoses, due to the tendency of many patients to over-generalize symptoms. In an article reviewing symptom validity tests, Iverson and Binder (2000) concluded that CARB was among the best validated of the forced-choice procedures, based on its 1997 test manual. CARB incorporates a number of unique and time saving features that set it clearly apart from other forced choice tests. CARB is expected to hold up under *Daubert* challenges due to its specific focus and purpose, and extensive validation research.

REFERENCES

Allen, L. M., Conder, R. L., Green, P., & Cox, D. R. (1997). *CARB '97: Manual for the Computerized Assessment of Response Bias*. Durham, NC: CogniSyst, Inc.

Allen, L., & Green, P. (1999). Severe TBI sample performance on CARB and the WMT: *Supplement to the CARB '97 and Word Memory Test Manuals*. Durham, NC: CogniSyst, Inc.

Allen, L. M., Green, P., & Eimer, B. N. (1999). The effect of pain on neurocognitive measures in patients demonstrating good effort, Part I: Data on objective and self-reported assessment of memory ability (Abstract). *Archives of Clinical Neuropsychology*, *14*, 742-743.

Allen, L. M., Richards, P. M., Green, W. P., Iverson, G. L., & Condor, R. L. (1998). Performance patterns on the Computerized Assessment of Response Bias in 1752 compensation cases (Abstract). *Archives of Clinical Neuropsychology*, *13*, 15-16.

Beck, A. T. (1978; Beck, A. T., & Steer, R. A., 1993). *Beck Depression Inventory*. Manual. San Antonio, TX: Psychological Corporation.

Binder, L. M. (1993). Assessment of malingering after mild head trauma with the Portland Digit Recognition Test. *Journal of Clinical and Experimental Neuropsychology*, *15*, 170-182.

Binder, L. M., & Kelly, M. P. (1996). Portland Digit Recognition Test performance by brain dysfunction patients without financial incentives. *Assessment*, *3*, 403-409.

Binder, L. M., & Willis, S. C. (1991). Assessment of motivation after financially compensable minor head trauma. *Psychological Assessment*, *3*, 175-181.

Conder, R., Allen, L, & Cox, D. (1992). *Manual for the Computerized Assessment of Response Bias*. Durham, NC: CogniSyst, Inc.

Courtney, J. C., Dinkins, J. P., Allen, L. M., & Kuroski, K. (2002). Age Related Effects in Children Taking the Computerized Assessment of Response Bias and Word Memory Test. Manuscript in preparation.

Daubert v. Merrell Dow Pharmaceuticals, Inc, 509 US 579 (1993).

de Armas, A. (1996). Detection of malingering in forensic psychological evaluations. The *Forensic Examiner*, July-August, 26-28.

Delis, D. C., Kramer, J. H., Kaplan, E., & Ober, B. (1987). The California Verbal Learning Test: Research Edition. New York: The Psychological Corporation.

Dunn, T. M., Shear, P. K., Howe, S. R., & Ris, M. D. (in press). Detecting neuropsychological malingering: Effects of coaching and information. *Archives of Clinical Neuropsychology*.

Flaro, L., Green, P., & Allen, L. M. (2000). Symptom validity test results with children: CARB and WMT (Abstract). *Archives of Clinical Neuropsychology*, *15*, 840.

Franzen, M. D. (1989). *Reliability and Validity in Neuropsychological Assessment*. New York: Plenum Press.

Franzen, M. D. (2000). *Reliability and Validity in Neuropsychological Assessment*. (2nd Edition) New York: Kluwer Academic/Plenum Press.

Frederick, R. I. (2000). A personal floor effect strategy to evaluate the validity of performance on memory tests. *Journal of Clinical and Experimental Neuropsychology*, *22*, 720-730.

Gervais, R., Allen, L. Green, P., Cunningham. S., & Iverson, G. (1998). Exaggeration and malingering in persons with DSM-IV pain disorders. Poster session presented at the 18th annual meeting of the National Academy of Neuropsychology, Washington, DC.

Gervais, R. O., Green, P., & Allen, L. M., & Iverson, G.L. (2001). Effects of coaching on symptom validity testing in chronic pain patients presenting for disability assessments. *Journal of Forensic Neuropsychology* 2, (2) 1-19.

Gervais, R. O., Russell, A. S., Green, P., Allen, L. M., Ferrari, R., & Pieschl, S. D. (2001). Effort testing in fibromyalgia patients with disability incentives. *Journal of Rheumatology 28*, 1892-1899.

Green, P., & Allen, L. M. (1997). Memory Complaints Inventory: A Computerised Test of Memory Complaints. Durham, NC: CogniSyst, Inc.

Green, P., & Allen, L. M. (1999). Performance of Neurological Patients on the Word Memory Test (WMT) and Computerised Assessment of Response Bias (CARB): Supplement to the Word Memory Test and CARB '97 Manuals. Durham, NC: CogniSyst, Inc.

Green, P., & Allen, L. M. (2000). Patterns of memory complaints in 577 consecutive patients passing or failing symptom validity tests. Poster session presented at the 18th annual meeting of the National Academy of Neuropsychology, Washington, DC.

Green, P., Allen, L. M., & Astner, K. (1996). *The Word Memory Test: A User's Guide to the Oral and Computer-Administered Forms, US Version 1.1.* Durham, NC: CogniSyst, Inc.

Green, P., Allen, L. M., & Iverson, G. L. (1999). Utility of the Memory Complaints Inventory for identifying symptom exaggeration in mild to moderate traumatic brain injury (Abstract). *Archives of Neuropsychology*, *14*, 743-744.

Green, P., Gervais, R., Astner, K., Kiss, I. & Allen, L. (1993). CARB malingering test results in 210 accident/compensation cases with and without head injury. Poster session presented at the annual meeting of the National Academy of Neuropsychology, Phoenix, AZ.

Green, P., & Iverson, G. L. (2001). Validation of the Computerized Assessment of Response Bias in litigating patients with head injuries. *The Clinical Neuropsychologist 15*, 492-497.

Green, P., Rohling, M. L., Lees-Haley, P. R., & Allen L. M. (2001). Effort has a greater effect on neuropsychological test scores than severe brain injury. *Brain Injury*, *15*, 1045-1060.

Hiscock, M., & Hiscock, C. (1989). Refining the forced-choice method for the detection of malingering. *Journal of Clinical and Experimental Neuropsychology*, *11*, 967-974.

Iverson, G. L., & Binder, L. M. (2000). Detecting exaggeration and malingering in neuropsychological assessment. *Journal of Head Trauma Rehabilitation*, *15*, 829-858.

Iverson, G. L., & Franzen, M. D. (1996). Using multiple objective memory procedures to detect simulated malingering. *Journal of Clinical and Experimental Neuropsychology*, *18*, 38-51.

Iverson, G. L., Ropacki, M. T., Allen, L. M., & Elias, J. W. (2001). Analog malingering on the Computerized Assessment of Response Bias (Abstract). *Archives of Clinical Neuropsychology*, *16*, 850-851.

Kumho Tire Company, Ltd. v. Carmichael, 119 S Ct 1167 (1999).

Millis, S. R., Putnam, S. H., Adams, K. H., & Ricker, J. H. (1995). The California Verbal Learning Test in the detection of incomplete effort in neuropsychological testing. *Psychological Assessment*, *7*, 463-471.

Rogers, R. Harrell, E., & Liff, C. (1993). Feigning neuropsychological impairment: A critical review of methodological and clinical considerations. *Clinical Psychology Review*, *13*, 255-274.

Rohling, M. L., Green, P., Allen, L. & Iverson, G. L. (2002). Depressive symptoms and neurocognitive test scores in patients passing symptom validity tests. *Archives of Clinical Neuropsychology 17*, 205-222.

Schmand, B., Lindeboom, J., Schagen, S., Heijt, R., Koene, T., & Hamburger, H. L. (1998). Cognitive complaints in patients after whiplash injury: The impact of malingering. *Journal of Neurology, Neurosurgery, and Psychiatry*, *64*, 339-343.

Slick, D., Hopp, G., Strauss, E., Hunter, M., & Pinch, D. (1994). Detecting dissimulation: Profiles of simulated malingerers, traumatic brain-injury patients, and normal controls on a revised version of Hiscock and Hiscock's Forced-Choice Memory Test. *Journal of Clinical and Experimental Neuropsychology*, *16*, 472-481.

Slick, D., Hopp, G., Strauss, E., & Spellacy, F. (1996). Victoria Symptom Validity test: Efficiency for detecting feigned memory impairment and relationship to neuropsychological tests and MMPI-2 validity scales. *Journal of Clinical and Experimental Neuropsychology*, *18*, 911-922.

Slick, D. J., Hopp, G., Strauss, E., & Thompson, G. (1997). *The Victoria Symptom Validity Test*. Odessa, FL: PAR.

Slick, D. J., Iverson, G. L., & Green, P. (2000). California Verbal Learning Test indicators of suboptimal performance in a sample of head-injury litigants. *Journal of Clinical and Experimental Neuropsychology*, *22*, 569-579.

Vickery, C. D., Ranseen, J. D., Cooley, A. T., & Berry, D. T. R. (1999). Use of malingering tests in the forensic evaluation of pain patients (Abstract). *Archives of Clinical Neuropsychology*, *14*, 102.

Warrington, E. K. (1984). *Recognition Memory Test Manual*. Windsor, England: NFER-Nelson Publishing Company.

Wiens, A. N., Tindall, A. G., & Crossen, J. R. (1996). California Verbal Learning Test: A normative data study. *The Clinical Neuropsychologist*, *8*, 75-90.

Youngjohn, J. R. (1995). Confirmed attorney coaching prior to neuropsychological evaluation. *Assessment*, *2*, 279-283.

Neuropsychological Profiling of Symptom Exaggeration and Malingering

Wiley Mittenberg

Nova Southeastern University

Gisela Aguila-Puentes

University of Miami-Jackson Memorial Hospital

Christine Patton

Nova Southeastern University

Elizabeth M. Canyock

Nova Southeastern University

Robert L. Heilbronner

Neurobehavior and` Rehabilitation Network

Wiley Mittenberg, Christine Patton, and Elizabeth M. Canyock are affiliated with the Center for Psychological Studies, Nova Southeastern University, Fort Lauderdale, FL.

Gisela Aguila-Puentes is affiliated with the University of Miami, Jackson Memorial Hospital, Miami, FL.

Robert L. Heilbronner is affiliated with the Neurobehavior and Rehabilitation Network, Chicago, IL.

Address correspondence to: Wiley Mittenberg, PhD, Nova Southeastern University, Center for Psychological Studies, 3301 College Avenue, Fort Lauderdale, FL 33314 (E-mail: wiley@nova.edu).

[Haworth co-indexing entry note]: "Neuropsychological Profiling of Symptom Exaggeration and Malingering." Mittenberg, Wiley et al. Co-published simultaneously in *Journal of Forensic Neuropsychology* (The Haworth Medical Press, an imprint of The Haworth Press, Inc.) Vol. 3, No. 1/2, 2002, pp. 227-240; and: *Detection of Response Bias in Forensic Neuropsychology* (ed: Jim Hom, and Robert L. Denney) The Haworth Medical Press, an imprint of The Haworth Press, Inc., 2002, pp. 227-240. Single or multiple copies of this article are available for a fee from The Haworth Document Delivery Service [1-800-HAWORTH, 9:00 a.m. - 5:00 p.m. (EST). E-mail address: getinfo@haworthpressinc.com].

© 2002 by The Haworth Press, Inc. All rights reserved.

SUMMARY. The theory of profile analysis is generally accepted as a basis for forming expert opinions about symptom exaggeration and malingering. Methods that rely on profile analysis are frequently the only ones that can be applied retrospectively to the interpretation of test results contained in case records. Profile patterns may well be more difficult to coach than external measures, and when combined with other methods offer a convenient source of convergent information about test validity. This paper reviews techniques for the identification of malingered head injury by analysis of the Wechsler Adult Intelligence Scale–3rd edition (Wechsler, 1997a), Halstead-Reitan Battery (Reitan & Wolfson, 1985), or Wechsler Memory Scale-Revised (Wechsler, 1987) profile. These techniques lend themselves to the report of specific statements about the probability of malingering that are easily understood by the court and are likely to meet current standards for evidentiary reliability. *[Article copies available for a fee from The Haworth Document Delivery Service: 1-800-HAWORTH. E-mail address: <getinfo@haworthpressinc.com> Website: <http://www.HaworthPress.com> © 2002 by The Haworth Press, Inc. All rights reserved.]*

KEYWORDS. Daubert, malingering, WAIS-III, Halstead-Reitan Battery, Wechsler Memory Scale

A variety of methods are available to determine if a patient's neuropsychological test performance is a valid indication of his or her actual ability. A recent survey of the American Board of Clinical Neuropsychology (Mittenberg, Patton, Canyock, & Condit, in press) demonstrates that neuropsychologists typically rely upon multiple methods for assessing the probability of malingering or symptom exaggeration. In response to the question, "In what percentage of your probable symptom exaggeration or malingering cases do each of the following support your impression?" the 131 respondents indicated the following: severity of cognitive impairment inconsistent with condition (65%), pattern of cognitive test performance inconsistent with condition (64%), scores below empirical cutoffs on forced choice tests (57%), discrepancies among records, self-report, and observed behavior (56%), implausible self-reported symptoms in interview (46%), implausible changes in test scores across repeated examinations (45%), validity scales on objective personality tests (38%), and scores below chance on forced choice tests (30%). The average respondent considered all methods in forming an opinion. Proposed *Diagnostic Criteria for Malingered Neurocognitive*

Dysfunction (Slick, Sherman, & Iverson, 1999) offer a well informed, probabilistic approach to combining these inferential methods that is similar to National Institute of Neurologic Disorders and American Academy of Neurology diagnostic criteria for other conditions.

The first empirical demonstration that patterns of neuropsychological test performance could discriminate head trauma from malingering was reported by Heaton, Smith, Lehman, and Vogt (1978). They showed that discriminant function analysis using subtest scores from the Wechsler Adult Intelligence Scale and Halstead-Reitan Battery could accurately classify these groups. Actual and simulated head injury could not be distinguished by clinical judgment, severity of impairment in IQ, or Halstead Impairment Index. Larrabee (1990) subsequently proposed a general theory of profile interpretation: patterns of test performance that are inconsistent with the neuropsychological profile known to characterize a disorder can be identified as failing to make "neuropsychological sense," and thus raise the suspicion of intentional distortion.

These observations led to the development of pattern analytic methods by our group and others. One advantage of these methods is that the validity measures are "built in" to standard neuropsychological tests. This makes profile analysis a convenient source of convergent information. The methods are frequently the only ones that can be applied retrospectively to the interpretation of test results contained in case records. Profile patterns may well be more difficult to prepare for or coach than external measures because of their complexity and embedded nature. Profile analysis is disorder-specific to the extent that a test pattern is specific to a particular disorder. For example, test score patterns in chronic head injury differ from those associated with acute head injury, cerebrovascular disorders, or psychosis. Patterns of performance caused by chronic head injury are useful for differentiating this condition from malingering, but may not be appropriate for the differential diagnosis of dissimilar conditions. Other methods of malingering detection do not share the disadvantage of being specific to a particular disorder. Profile analysis procedures are available for the identification of malingered head injury when the examination includes the Wechsler Adult Intelligence Scale-3rd edition (WAIS-3; Wechsler, 1997a), the Halstead-Reitan Battery (HRB; Reitan & Wolfson, 1985), or the Wechsler Memory Scale-Revised (WMS-R; Wechsler, 1987).

IDENTIFICATION OF MALINGERED HEAD INJURY ON THE WMS-R

Memory difficulties are common following head trauma of sufficient severity, and the general public expects symptoms of memory impairment to occur as a consequence of concussion (Mittenberg, DiGiulio, Perrin, & Bass, 1992). Memory impairment can be easily simulated and difficult to distinguish from impairment caused by brain dysfunction. In contrast, attention span is relatively preserved in dementia due to chronic head trauma (Levin, Benton, & Grossman, 1982), as it is in most etiologies of dementia and amnesia (American Psychiatric Association, 1994). The discrimination between malingered and head trauma profiles on the WMS-R rests on the tendency for head injured patients to do better and malingerers to do more poorly on measures of attention relative to their own performance on measures of memory.

Mittenberg, Azrin, Millsaps, and Heilbronner (1993) compared the WMS-R performance of 39 non-litigating head injured outpatients with that of 39 subjects who were instructed to malinger head trauma symptoms without being detected. Patients were an average of 14 months (range 1 to 84 months) post-injuries that ranged from mild to severe. These characteristics are similar to those of patients who are examined in the context of disability insurance or personal injury claims. Simulators were employed in a wide range of occupations, and could be characterized as similar to neurologically normal patients who simulate symptoms on the basis of common sense or the demand characteristics of the test. Protocols were matched on age and General Memory Index scores to permit comparisons between patterns of performance. Simulators successfully produced a number of test findings that are typically observed following head injury. The WMS-R Delayed Recall Index was significantly lower than WAIS-R Full Scale IQ, Performance IQ was significantly lower than Verbal IQ, and Full Scale IQ was significantly lower than premorbid IQ.

Simulators obtained Attention/Concentration Index scores that averaged 14 points lower than General Memory Index scores. In contrast, head trauma patients averaged 11 points higher on Attention/Concentration than General Memory (the opposite pattern). A General Memory-Attention/Concentration difference score of 2 points or more accurately identified 76.9% of simulators and 89.7% of head trauma patients. Crossvalidation using the jackknife technique produced minimal (1.3%) shrinkage in diagnostic accuracy. The Index patterns were consistent with those previously reported in the literature for both head injured and malingering groups (Bernard, 1990; Binder, 1990; Boyer, 1991; Reid & Kelly, 1991; Roth, Conboy, Reeder, & Boll, 1990, Wechsler, 1997). Simulated memory impairment appears to be characterized by a pattern that is inconsistent with the neuropsychological profile known to result from traumatic brain injury. As described by Larrabee (1990), the pattern does not make neuropsychological sense. The average simulator in Mittenberg et al. (1993) earned a General Memory Index that was 1 standard deviation and an Attention/Concentration Index that was 2 standard deviations below normal. It is not likely that an individual with severely impaired attention span could demonstrate low average memory ability, because one cannot remember what is not first attended to. Attentional capacity limits memory function so that severely compromised attention should result in memory impairment that is at least equally severe.

Caveats proposed in the 1993 paper are worth repeating. More extreme scores are associated with more diagnostic confidence using this or any other measure. Questions about the validity of apparent memory impairment do not arise when no memory impairment is apparent. The contrast between attention and memory cannot be used to differentially diagnose normal and impaired performance. Procedures that can be followed in order to make informed diagnoses of this type have been reviewed elsewhere (Hannay, Bieliauskas, Crosson, Hammeke, Hamsher, & Koffler, 1998). Premorbid learning disabilities and attention deficit hyperactivity disorder may adversely influence performance on the Attention/Concentration Index and cause false positive errors. Practice effects over short test-retest intervals artifactually inflate the General Memory Index and may also cause false positives.

Attorneys typically prepare clients for neuropsychological examinations, and may discuss test content, expected symptoms, or test validity measures (Essig, Mittenberg, Petersen, Strauman, & Cooper, 2001). Johnson and Lesniak-Karpiak (1997) examined the effects of coaching on simulated memory impairment using the WMS-R. Three age and IQ matched groups were examined. The malingering group was instructed to simulate impairment due to head injury without being obvious. Coached simulators received similar instructions with the added caution that methods to detect exaggeration on the test existed and would be used. A control group was instructed to devote their best effort to the examination. Both simulating groups demonstrated significant memory and attention/concentration impairment compared to controls, but the coached group earned Memory Index scores that were less grossly exaggerated. In contrast, coaching had no significant effect on the Attention/Concentration Index. General Memory-Attention/Concentration Index differences averaged 11 points in malingerers and 13 points in coached simulators. These results suggest that although coaching may well effect more subtle exaggeration, it may not confound the identification of malingering by neuropsychological profiles.

Iverson and Slick (2001) reported the distribution of General Memory-Attention/Concentration difference scores in a sample of 186 nonlitigating patients who were tested within 4 weeks of head injury. Memory impairment (General Memory < 90) was demonstrated by 101 patients. A cutoff of 3 points or less correctly classified 80.2% of this group, and 97% were accurately characterized with a cutoff of less than 18 points. The specificity of the difference score may have been under-estimated in this sample because transient impairment of attention is frequent following acute head trauma. The authors noted that 10% of the patients were in a state of post-traumatic amnesia when they were tested. No clear evidence of memory impairment was reported in 85 patients. Higher frequencies of "false positive" diagnosis were observed in this group. Questions about the validity of apparent memory impairment do not arise when no memory impairment is evident. The performance of patients with intact cognitive ability is therefore not relevant to validation of malingering measures.

Iverson, Slick, and Franzen (2000) examined the frequency of General Memory-Attention Concentration difference scores in 332 noncompensation seeking inpatients within five days following detoxification for alcohol abuse. Memory impairment (General Memory < 90) was present in 145 patients. Of these, 78.6% were correctly diagnosed with a cutoff of less than 3 points, and 96.5% were correctly categorized with a cutoff of less than 15 points. The authors point out that these data are salient because many head injured patients abuse alcohol. The specificity of the malingering index may have been underestimated in this study because recently detoxified alcoholics frequently display attentional impairment (Ryan & Lewis, 1988). The performance of patients with intact memory in this study is not strictly pertinent to a discussion of malingered memory impairment (see caveats above), but many false positive "errors" occurred in this group.

Rosenfeld, Sands, and Van Gorp (2000) criticized use of the difference score on the basis of low positive predictive accuracy at malingering base rates of 15% or lower. Positive predictive accuracy refers to the percentage of all positive diagnoses that are correct. This percentage is affected by the prevalence of malingering in a given population (the base rate). For example, if a method that was 99% accurate in women (i.e., pregnancy tests) were used to examine 100 men, positive predictive accuracy would be 0% because the 1 positive diagnosis would be incorrect. In clinical practice, the solution to this difficulty is intuitively obvious. More confidence in the diagnosis is associated with more extreme scores on a measure and convergent evidence from multiple measures. Rosenfeld et al. (2000) did not consider the former principle, the effects of which are displayed in Table 1. Rosenfeld et al. also failed to consider the base rate of malingering in compensation seeking or mild head injured populations. Empirical studies using several of the well validated measures described elsewhere in this volume demonstrate malingering base rates between 33% and 59% in compensation seeking mild head injured groups (Binder, 1993; Greiffenstein, Baker, & Gola, 1994; Millis, 1992; Youngjohn, Burrows, & Erdal, 1995). Base rate estimates reported by survey of the membership of the American Board of Clinical Neuropsychology were approximately 30% in compensation seeking patients generally and 40% in patients making claims related to mild head trauma (Mittenberg et al., in press).

The Wechsler Memory Scale-3rd edition (WMS-3; Wechsler, 1997b) differs significantly from the WMS-R. The Working Memory Index (formerly the Attention/Concentration Index) no longer includes the Digit Span or Mental Control subtests. The Immediate Memory Index (formerly the General Memory Index) consists of two new subtests and substantially altered versions of two WMS-R subtests. Forced choice recognition subtests have been added to the scale. The methods described above may or may not generalize to the WMS-3, and it is likely

TABLE 1. Effect of Various Base Rates and Memory-Attention Index Differences on Positive Predictive Accuracy

Malingering Base Rate	Difference Score		
	10	15	20
.5	86.2%	86.4%	93.3%
.4	80.1%	80.8%	90.2%
.3	72.7%	73.1%	85.5%
.2	60.9%	61.3%	77.5%

Note: Percentages in the table indicate the proportion of accurate to total malingering diagnoses (positive predictive accuracy) at hypothetical rates of malingering in the sample (base rate).

that more powerful methods of analysis will be developed. Forensic administrations of the WMS-3 should be supplemented with one or more of the forced choice procedures described in this volume. However measured, patterns of attention span and memory ability that do not make neuropsychological sense may well have diagnostic implications.

IDENTIFICATION OF MALINGERED HEAD INJURY ON THE HALSTEAD-REITAN BATTERY

Replication of Heaton et al.'s (1978) methodology for assessing the validity of HRB profiles resulted in a crossvalidated discriminant function equation that correctly identified 93.8% of non-litigating head injured patients and 83.8% of simulators (Mittenberg, Rotholc, Russell, & Heilbronner, 1996). Patients (n = 80) were an average of 2.9 years (SD = 3 years) post-head injuries that ranged from mild to severe. Simulators solicited from the community were instructed to fake deficits without being obvious. Groups were matched on age, gender, and Impairment Index. Simulators performed more poorly than head trauma patients on attentional, sensory, and motor measures. Head injured patients were more impaired than simulators on the Trail Making and Tactual Performance tests. These results were independent of overall level of deficit. The discriminant function was successful when applied retrospectively to previously published data from Heaton et al. (1978) and three other studies of malingering and head trauma (Cullum, Heaton, & Grant, 1991; Faust, Hart, Guilmette, & Arkes, 1988; Trueblood & Schmidt, 1993).

McKinzey and Russell (1997) cross-validated the discriminant function on a sample of 120 non-compensation seeking head injured patients and found 77.5% accurate diagnosis. This accuracy rate is lower than previously reported, but may be viewed as supporting the utility of the procedure. As is generally the case, a higher rate of confidence (87.5%) was associated with a more extreme score on the measure. Of 158 neurologically normal persons, 96.8% were not impaired on the HRB and obviously therefore could be identified as not malingering impairment on the basis of reason and common sense. Questions about the validity of apparent cognitive impairment do not arise when no cognitive impairment is evident. Misuse of the discriminant function in these cognitively intact patients correctly identified 84% of the group as not malingering cognitive impairment. Patients with diagnoses other than head trauma (particularly schizophrenia and cerebrovascular disease) were misclassified more frequently, consistent with the predictable observation that distinct patterns of HRB performance characterize these disorders. Careful reading of the Mittenberg et al. (1996) study suggests that this diagnostic procedure was designed for the identification of malingered head injury (rather than other conditions) on the Halstead-Reitan battery. Methods that do not rely on profile analysis to detect exaggeration are not disadvantaged by specificity to a given condition.

IDENTIFICATION OF MALINGERED HEAD INJURY ON THE WAIS-3

Mittenberg, Theroux, Zielinski, and Heilbronner (1995) derived two methods to identify malingered head injury on the WAIS-R by comparing the subtest profile of 67 non-litigating head trauma patients to the profile produced by 67 age- and IQ-matched uninjured subjects who were instructed to malinger head trauma symptoms without being detected. Test results were obtained an average of 15 months after head injuries that ranged from mild to severe. Given the normally high correlation between Vocabulary and other abilities, and previous research showing disproportionate malingered reduction of Digit Span, differences between these subtest scores were expected to be diagnostic. Differential diagnoses were also made by discriminant function analysis of the overall subtest profile. The subtest equation accurately classified 79% of profiles, with 82% true negatives and 76% true positives. The Vocabulary-Digit Span difference score correctly identified 79% of head trauma, 63% of simulated, and 71% of total cases. Both methods crossvalidated statistically using the jackknife procedure, and when applied retrospectively to previously published data from six other studies of malingering and head injury (Binder, 1990; Cullum et al., 1991; Faust et al., 1988; Heaton et al., 1978; Thompson & Cullum, 1991; Trueblood, 1994).

Millis, Ross, and Ricker (1998) subsequently reported similar diagnostic accuracy in a crossvalidation on groups of 50 moderate/severe and 50 financially compensable mild head injuries. Nonlitigating head trauma patients were accurately classified by either method in 86% of cases. Compensation seeking head trauma patients had performed in the malingering range on the Recognition Memory Test and in the borderline range of intelligence 2 years after mild injuries. Intellectual impairment was characterized as exaggerated in 88% of this group by the discriminant function, and in 72% of cases by the difference score.

Axlerod and Rawlings (1999) cross-validated the formulas in samples of mild, moderate, and severe head trauma who were tested 2, 4, 8, and 12 months after injury. Diagnostic specificity was 90% for the discriminant function and 81% for the difference score in this series of 238 intellectual assessments. Diagnoses were not significantly influenced by practice effects or recovery of function over time, and were reliable across repeated examinations.

These studies suggested that the WAIS-R formulas were robust and could potentially generalize to the WAIS-3. The WAIS-3 shares pertinent subtests with the WAIS-R; these correlate highly and produce nearly identical scaled scores (Psychological Corporation, 1997). The procedures were applied to the WAIS-3 profiles of 36 non-compensation seeking head trauma cases and 36 adults who were instructed to malinger intellectual impairment without being detected (Mittenberg, Theroux, Aguila-Puentes, Bianchini, Greve, & Rayls, 2001). Patients were examined an average of 1 year (range = 1 month to 8 years) following head injuries that ranged from mild to severe. The discriminant function equation accurately characterized 83.3% of the non-litigating patients and 72.2% of simulators, with an overall classification accuracy rate of 77.8%. The Vocabulary-Digit Span difference score correctly classified 86.1% of patients with head injuries and 55.6% of malingerers, with overall diagnostic accuracy of 70.8%. Positive predictive value was about 80% for both methods and could be maintained at acceptable levels in lower base rate situations. Probability tables are offered that provide higher levels of diagnostic confidence in cases that show more extreme scores.

The formulas were also tested in a sample of 36 compensation seeking patients examined an average of 1.5 years (range = 1 month to 9 years) after mild head injuries. Patients were selected who had obtained WAIS-3 IQs that were at least 15 points lower than estimated premorbid level. It seemed reasonable to characterize such a group as probable malingerers on the basis of this magnitude of purported intellectual impairment, which is unlikely to be caused by chronic mild head trauma (Binder, Rohling, & Larrabee, 1997). Average Full Scale IQ was 73 (SD = 12.5). The subtest equation identified 44.4% of these patients as malingerers; 25% of cases were identified by the difference score. It seems likely that gross exaggeration produces relatively uniform global reductions that may be better identified by methods other than profile analysis.

Questions about the validity of the WAIS-3 IQ logically arise only if intellectual impairment is apparent. It is possible that the validity of a normal profile could be mistakenly questioned in a mild head trauma case. Application of the classification procedures to the WAIS-3 standardization data (Psychological Corporation, 1997) suggests that such a profile would probably be identified as valid. Minimum specificity was 71%, with increased accuracy at higher cutoff scores in this sample of 2,450 normal adults. However, the formulas are intended to provide an indication of the validity of observed intellectual impairment rather than a diagnosis of impairment, and are not useful for this latter purpose. Clinical group standardization data also suggests that false positive classifications may result from premorbid learning disability or attention deficit hyperactivity disorder.

ADMISSIBILITY OF TESTIMONY BASED ON NEUROPSYCHOLOGICAL PROFILING

Standards for the admissibility of scientific evidence set forth in the case of *Daubert v. Merrell Dow Pharmaceuticals* (1993) may often guide trial judges in decisions about the validity of the methodology underlying the expert's opinion. These standards for evidentiary reliability suggest that expert opinions are admissible if they are based upon a theory or technique that has been tested, the subject of peer reviewed publication, has a known or potentially specifiable error rate, and has received general acceptance in the scientific community.

The Wechsler Intelligence Scales, Halstead-Reitan Battery, and Wechsler Memory Scales are among the most widely used and accepted neuropsychological tests. Their reliability and validity are documented by a significant body of peer-reviewed studies. Many of these studies address the accuracy and general acceptance of interpretations based on patterns of performance. It is likely that these considerations alone would be sufficient to establish the admissibility of expert opinions about malingering that rely upon profile interpretation of these tests. The theory of profile analysis is generally accepted by neuropsychologists as a basis for forming expert opinions about symptom exaggeration and malingering (Mittenberg et al., in press). A search of Social Science Citation Index indicates that initial validation studies of the techniques reviewed in this paper have been cited almost 100 times since their original publication. These techniques lend themselves to the report of specific statements about the probability of malingering that are easily understood by the court. The known error rate may be best represented by overall diagnostic accuracy (hit rate), which is not affected by changes in the base rate. The potential error rate may be best represented by the positive predictive accuracy associated with the patient's obtained score and the base rate appropriate to the circumstances of the case. The consensus of expert opinion in litigating or compensation seeking mild head injury cases suggests that a base rate of 40% is generally appropriate (Mittenberg et al., in press).

Subsequent to this testimony being admitted, the expert must determine from review of convergent evidence that includes other valid techniques that any conclusions can be made to a reasonable degree of scientific certainty or probability. Whether these conclusions are credible, more likely than not to be correct, or convincing beyond a reasonable doubt, will usually be determined by a jury.

REFERENCES

American Psychiatric Association (1994). *Diagnostic and statistical manual for mental disorders.* Washington, DC: American Psychiatric Association.

Axelrod, B. N., & Rawlings, D. B. (1999). Clinical utility of incomplete effort WAIS-R formulas: A longitudinal examination of individuals with traumatic brain injuries. *Journal of Forensic Neuropsychology, 1*, 15-27.

Bernard, L. C. (1990). Prospects for faking believable memory deficits on neuropsychological tests and the use of incentives in simulation research. *Journal of Clinical and Experimental Neuropsychology, 12*, 715-728.

Binder, L. M. (1990). Malingering following minor head trauma. *The Clinical Neuropsychologist, 4*, 25-36.

Binder, L. M. (1993). Assessment of malingering after mild head trauma with the Portland Digit Recognition Test. *Journal of Clinical and Experimental Neuropsychology, 15*, 170-182.

Binder, L. M., Rohling, M. L., & Larrabee, G. J. (1997). A review of mild head trauma. Part 1: Meta-analytic review of neuropsychological studies. *Journal of Clinical and Experimental Neuropsychology, 19*, 421-431.

Boyer, C. L. (1991). Wechsler Memory-Scale-Revised: Performance following severe closed head injury. *The Clinical Neuropsychologist, 5*, 262.

Cullum, C. M., Heaton, R. K., & Grant, I. (1991). Psychogenic factors influencing neuropsychological performance: Somatoform disorders, factitious disorders, and malingering. In H. O. Doerr & A. S. Carlin (Eds.), *Forensic Neuropsychology: Legal and Scientific Bases* (pp. 141-171). New York: Guilford Press.

Daubert v. Merrell Dow Pharmaceuticals, 509 U.S. 579 (1993).

Essig, S. M., Mittenberg, W., Petersen, R. S., Strauman, S., & Cooper, J. T. (2001). Practices in forensic neuropsychology: Perspectives of neuropsychologists and trial attorneys. *Archives of Clinical Neuropsychology, 16*, 271-291.

Faust, D., Hart, K., Guilmette, T. J., & Arkes, H. R. (1988). Neuropsychologists' capacity to detect adolescent malingerers. *Professional Psychology: Research and Practice, 19*, 508-515.

Greiffenstein, M. F., Baker, J. W., & Gola, T. (1994). Validation of malingered amnesia measures with a large clinical sample. *Psychological Assessment*, *6*, 218-224.

Hannay, H. J., Bieliauskas, L., Crosson, B. A., Hammeke, T. A., Hamsher, K. deS., & Koffler, S. (1998). Proceedings of the Houston Conference on Specialty Education and Training in Clinical Neuropsychology: Policy statement. *Archives of Clinical Neuropsychology*, *13*, 160-166.

Heaton, R. K., Smith, H. H., Lehman, R. A., & Vogt, A. T. (1978). Prospects for faking believable deficits on neuropsychological testing. *Journal of Consulting and Clinical Psychology*, *46*, 892-900.

Iverson, G. L., Slick, D. J., & Franzen, M. D. (2000). Evaluation of the WMS-R malingering index in a non-litigating clinical sample. *Journal of Clinical and Experimental Neuropsychology*, *22*, 191-197.

Johnson, J. L., & Lesniak-Karpniak, K. (1997). The effect of warning on malingering on memory and motor tasks in college samples. *Archives of Clinical Neuropsychology*, *9*, 437-450.

Larrabee, G. J. (1990). Cautions in the use of neuropsychological evaluation in legal settings. *Neuropsychology*, *4*, 239-247.

Levin, H. S., Benton, A. L., & Grossman, R. G. (1982). *Neurobehavioral Consequences of Closed Head Injury*. New York: Oxford University Press.

McKinzey, R. K., & Russell, E. W. (1997). Detection of malingering on the Halstead-Reitan Battery: A cross-validation. *Archives of Clinical Neuropsychology*, *12*, 585-589.

Millis, S. R. (1992). The Recognition Memory Test in the detection of malingered and exaggerated memory deficits. *The Clinical Neuropsychologist*, *6*, 406-414.

Millis, S. R., Ross, S. R., & Ricker, J. H. (1998). Detection of incomplete effort on the Wechsler Adult Intelligence Scale-Revised: A cross-validation. *Journal of Clinical and Experimental Neuropsychology*, *20*, 167-173.

Mittenberg, W., Azrin, R., Millsaps, C., & Heilbronner, R. (1993). Identification of malingered head injury on the Wechsler Memory Scale-Revised. *Psychological Assessment*, *5*, 34-40.

Mittenberg, W., DiGiulio, D. V., Perrin, S., & Bass, A. E. (1992). Symptoms following mild head injury: Expectation as etiology. *Journal of Neurology, Neurosurgery, and Psychiatry*, *55*, 200-204.

Mittenberg, W., Patton, C., Canyock, E., & Condit, D. (in press). A national survey of symptom exaggeration and malingering base rates. *Journal of Clinical and Experimental Neuropsychology*.

Mittenberg,W., Rotholc, A., Russell, E., & Heilbronner, R. (1996). Identification of malingered head injury on the Halstead-Reitan Battery. *Archives of Clinical Neuropsychology*, *11*, 271-281.

Mittenberg, W., Theroux, S., Aquila-Puentes, G., Bianchini, K., Greve, K., & Rayls, K. (2001). Identification of malingered head injury on the WAIS-3. *The Clinical Neuropsychologist*, *15*, 440-445.

Mittenberg, W., Theroux, S., Zielinski, R. E., & Heilbronner, R. L. (1995). Identification of malingered head injury on the Wechsler Adult Intelligence Scale-Revised. *Professional Psychology: Research and Practice*, *26*, 491-498.

Psychological Corporation (1997). *WAIS-3/WMS-3 Technical Manual.* San Antonio, TX: Harcourt Brace.

Reid, D. P., & Kelly, M. P. (1993). Wechsler Memory Scale-Revised in closed head injury. *Journal of Clinical Psychology, 49*, 245-254.

Reitan, R., & Wolfson, D. (1985). *The Halstead-Reitan Neuropsychological Test Battery.* Tucson, AZ: Neuropsychology Press.

Rosenfeld, B., Sands, S. A., & Van Gorp, W. G. (2000). Have we forgotten the base rate problem? Methodological issues in the detection of distortion. *Archives of Clinical Neuropsychology, 15*, 349-359.

Roth, D. L., Conboy, T. J., Reeder, K. P., & Boll, T. J. (1990). Confirmatory factor analysis of the Wechsler Memory Scale-Revised in a sample of head injured patients. *Journal of Clinical and Experimental Neuropsychology, 12*, 834-842.

Ryan, J. J., & Lewis, C. V. (1988). Comparison of recently detoxified alcoholics on the Wechsler Memory Scale-Revised. *The Clinical Neuropsychologist, 2*, 173-180.

Slick, D. J., Sherman, E. M., & Iverson, G. L. (1999). Diagnostic criteria for malingered neurocognitive dysfunction: Proposed standards for clinical practice and research. *The Clinical Neuropsychologist, 13*, 545-561.

Thompson, L. L., & Cullum, C. M. (1991). Pattern of performance on neuropsychological tests in relation to effort in mild head injury patients. *Archives of Clinical Neuropsychology, 6*, 231.

Trueblood, W. (1994). Quantitative and qualitative characteristics of malingered and other invalid WAIS-R and clinical memory data. *Journal of Clinical and Experimental Neuropsychology, 16*, 597-607.

Trueblood, W., & Schmidt, M. (1993). Malingering and other validity considerations in neuropsychological evaluation of mild head injury. *Journal of Clinical and Experimental Neuropsychology, 15*, 578-590.

Wechsler, D. (1981). *Manual for the Wechsler Adult Intelligence Scale-Revised.* San Antonio, TX: Psychological Corporation.

Wechsler, D. (1997a). *Manual for the Wechsler Adult Intelligence Scale-Third Edition.* San Antonio, TX: Psychological Corporation.

Wechsler, D. (1997b). *Manual for the Wechsler Memory Scale-Third Edition.* San Antonio, TX: Psychological Corporation.

Wechsler, D. (1987). *Manual for the Wechsler Memory Scale-Revised.* San Antonio, TX: Psychological Corporation.

Youngjohn, J.R., Burrows, L., & Erdal, K. (1995). Brain damage or compensation neurosis? The controversial post-concussion syndrome. *The Clinical Neuropsychologist, 9*, 112-123.

Category Test Validity Indicators: Overview and Practice Recommendations

Jerry J. Sweet

Evanston Northwestern Healthcare Medical Group
Northwestern University Medical School

John H. King

Evanston Northwestern Healthcare

SUMMARY. The Category Test (CatT) has been one of the most frequently administered neuropsychological tests for many years, in common usage with traumatic brain injury patients and in forensic cases. Since 1985 there have been a number of attempts to delineate the performances of brain injury simulators and malingerers. The present paper reviews the history of these attempts, with particular attention to the CatT validity indicators developed by Bolter (1985) and by Tenhula and Sweet (1996). Similarities and differences between studies are discussed and clinical practice recommendations and limitations are enumerated. In keeping with the universal recommendations for effort tests and valid-

---

Jerry J. Sweet is affiliated with the Evanston Northwestern Healthcare Medical Group and Northwestern University Medical School.

John H. King is affiliated with Evanston Northwestern Healthcare.

Address correspondence to: Jerry J. Sweet, PhD, ABPP, Psychiatry & Behavioral Sciences, ENH Medical Group, 500 Davis Street, 8th Floor, Evanston, IL 60201 (E-mail: j-sweet@nwu.edu).

The authors wish to thank Dr. Jeffrey Gfeller for comments on an earlier draft of this manuscript.

[Haworth co-indexing entry note]: "Category Test Validity Indicators: Overview and Practice Recommendations." Sweet, Jerry J., and John H. King. Co-published simultaneously in *Journal of Forensic Neuropsychology* (The Haworth Medical Press, an imprint of The Haworth Press, Inc.) Vol. 3, No. 1/2, 2002, pp. 241-274; and: *Detection of Response Bias in Forensic Neuropsychology* (ed: Jim Hom, and Robert L. Denney) The Haworth Medical Press, an imprint of The Haworth Press, Inc., 2002, pp. 241-274. Single or multiple copies of this article are available for a fee from The Haworth Document Delivery Service [1-800-HAWORTH, 9:00 a.m. - 5:00 p.m. (EST). E-mail address: getinfo@haworthpressinc.com].

© 2002 by The Haworth Press, Inc. All rights reserved.

ity indicators from reviews of the neuropsychological malingering literature in the last 12 years, CatT validity indicators should not be viewed in isolation. Rather, they should be considered primarily with regard to validity of CatT results and as one source of relevant information in the detection of insufficient effort and the ultimate complex judgment, among a subset of insufficient effort cases, that the cause is malingering. Implications for meeting *Daubert* evidentiary standards are discussed.
[Article copies available for a fee from The Haworth Document Delivery Service: 1-800-HAWORTH. E-mail address: <getinfo@haworthpressinc.com> Website: <http://www.HaworthPress.com> © 2002 by The Haworth Press, Inc. All rights reserved.]

KEYWORDS. Category test, effort, TBI, malingering, validity indicators

In the 1920s, German researchers (Gelb & Goldstein, 1925; Weigl, 1927) began using concept formation tasks as measures of cognitive functioning. Within the U.S., Halstead (1940) used a concept formation test that required brain-damaged patients to group objects into categories. Halstead and Settlage (1943) modified this procedure and used drawings of geometric designs, rather than actual objects. This version of the Category Test (CatT) had 360 test items divided into nine subtests. Halstead's initial studies (Halstead, 1947) found the CatT to be a sensitive measure of diffuse brain damage. The 360 item version was later revised by Halstead and White (1950); this revision deleted the original Subtests IV and VI. The well known CatT version that resulted involved the projection of seven subtests containing 208 items. The first publication containing data from the seven subtest version of the CatT was apparently Reitan (1955), in which the performances of 50 brain damaged and 50 non-brain damaged subjects were compared. This study found the CatT to be second only to the Impairment Index in differentiating these two groups.

After the initial studies by Halstead and Reitan, numerous other investigators examined the diagnostic utility of the CatT. A preponderance of research evidence has indicated that the CatT is sensitive to cerebral dysfunction (e.g., Bornstein, 1986; Halstead, 1947; Matthews, Shaw, & Kløve, 1966; Reitan & Wolfson, 1992; Vega & Parsons, 1967). Performance on the CatT does not seem to reflect localization or lateralization of conditions (e.g., Anderson, Bigler, & Blatter, 1995; Bornstein, 1986; Chapman & Wolff, 1959; Reitan, 1964; Reitan & Wolfson, 1995; Russell, 1974), nor does duration of cerebral dysfunction (acute vs. chronic) affect CatT performance (Fitzhugh, Fitzhugh, & Reitan, 1961). Used with many neurological conditions (e.g., traumatic brain injury (TBI), multiple sclerosis, alcohol dementia, etc.), but without specific patterns pathognomonic of any particular brain condition, the CatT has been recognized widely as a general measure of brain dysfunction (Choca, Laatsch, Wetzel, & Agresti, 1997).

The skills/constructs assessed by the CatT have been investigated widely. Simmel and Counts (1957) utilized an item analysis to determine the abilities assessed by the CatT. They found the CatT assessed skills including counting, perceptual organization, learning, and maintaining conceptual set. Boll (1981) concluded that the CatT is a test of learning and mental efficiency. Others (Lezak, 1995; Shure & Halstead, 1958) have asserted that the CatT is a test of abstract concept formation, attention, visual concentration, visual memory and conceptual shifts. Studies have found the CatT loads on factors of general intelligence (Barnes & Lucas, 1974; Boyle, 1988) and complex spatial reasoning (Russell, 1974). However, Russell (1974) and Thomas and Trexler (1982) reported that the skills assessed by the CatT may vary by population. Johnstone, Holland, and Hewett (1997) found a three-factor model, with Subtests I and II loading on the first factor (labeled "symbol recogition/ counting"), Subtests III, IV and VII loading on another factor (labeled "spatial positional reasoning"), and Subtests V and VI loading on the last factor (labeled "proportional reasoning"). Allen, Goldstein and Mariano (1999) found the same factor structure of the CatT in patients with schizophrenia, heterogeneous brain dysfunction and controls. When Subtests I and II were eliminated from the analysis, a two-factor model was found, with Subtests III and IV loading on a factor (labeled "spatial positional"), the second factor loading Subtests V and VI (labeled "proportional reasoning"), and Subtest VII loading on both factors.

There are multiple forms of the CatT. In addition to the standard adult version developed by Halstead, White and Reitan, there are at least eight alternate forms of the CatT that have been developed (Mitrushina, Boone, & D'Elia, 1999). These include portable versions (Slay, 1984), paper and pen (Adams & Trenton, 1981; Wood & Strider, 1980), card form (Kimura, 1981), a booklet version (DeFilippis & McCampbell, 1979), and computer versions (Choca, 1987; Choca, Laatsch, Garside, & Arnemann, 1994; DeFilippis, 1992). Due to concerns about the length of the test, several short forms have been developed, including a popular version developed by Wetzel and Boll (1987). Nearly all studies have found the alternate forms of the CatT to be equivalent to the standard version (Boyd, 1980; Boyle 1986; Calsyn et al., 1980; Choca &

Laatsch (1994); DeFilippis & McCampbell, 1979, 1991; Golden, Kuperman, MacInnes, & Moses, 1981; Holz, Gearhard, & Watson, 1996; Mercer et al., 1997; Russell & Levy, 1987; Sherill, 1985, 1987; Wetzel & Boll, 1987). Although Berger, Chibnall, and Gfeller (1994) questioned the equivalence of computerized and standard administrations, the design of this study has been criticized. Considering the Berger et al. study along with many others, Choca, Laatsch, Wetzel, and Agresti (1997) reviewed the literature and concluded that ". . . almost all versions of the Category Test that have been studied have been found to be equivalent to the standard version . . ." (p. 62). Therefore, within the present paper we will *not* focus on differences in study results as possibly being due to different versions of the test being used.

Surveys indicate that the CatT, whether selectively administered or within the Halstead-Reitan Neuropsychological Test Battery (HRNB; Reitan and Wolfson, 1985), continues to be among the most widely utilized measures by neuropsychologists. Seretny, Dean, Gray, and Hartlage (1986) found that 54% of APA Division 40 members and 56% of National Academy of Neuropsychology (NAN) members utilized portions of the HRNB in 1980. By 1985, 65% of APA Division 40 and 59% of NAN members utilized portions of the HRNB. Guilmette, Faust, Hart, and Arkes (1990) found the partial HRNB to be the 7th most popular test and the full HRNB to be the 10th most used test. With specific reference to the CatT, Sellers and Nadler (1992) found that the CatT was one of the two most frequently used tests by neuropsychologists when assessing adults. Lees-Haley, Smith, Williams, and Dunn (1996) found that the CatT was administered 32% of the time by neuropsychologists conducting forensic evaluations, which ranked as the 8th most frequently administered test. A more recent survey by Camara, Nathan, and Puente (2000) found that the CatT ranked 9th in frequency of use by neuropsychologists.

Overall, the impressive popularity and longevity of the CatT has lead to the conclusion, "Few other psychological tests have achieved this same standard" (Reed & Reed, 1997, p. 111). There appears to be no question that the CatT continues to be a widely administered test and, importantly for the present review, is commonly used in forensic evaluations.

HISTORICAL OVERVIEW OF CATEGORY TEST VALIDITY INDICATORS

The notion of developing internal response validity indicators within actual tests of ability, such as the CatT, is straightforward; individuals may demonstrate insufficient effort selectively within or across evaluations. If effort is measured by a specific test of effort or some other means at only one point in the evaluation, there is no means of determining whether that level of effort remained the same throughout the entire evaluation. This notion has resulted in considerable research on effort and response validity with a variety of commonly used tests of ability, such as the Wechsler Adult Intelligence Scale-Revised (WAIS-R; Wechsler, 1981), Wechsler Memory Scale-Revised (WMS-R; Wechsler, 1987), and California Verbal Learning Test (CVLT; Delis, Kramer, Kaplan, & Ober, 1987; see Sweet, 1999 for a listing of 68 such studies). In an ideal forensic neuropsychological evaluation, clinicians would not rely only upon a single effort test, but would be able to examine response validity within and across multiple tests of effort and across and within multiple tests of ability. Although some malingerers perform poorly on all measures administered, more sophisticated malingerers can be expected to be more selective. Moreover, a very brief or isolated indication of insufficient effort may be related to a psychological condition or fatigue, rather than true malingering, and might require numerous validity and effort indicators in order to distinguish. Virtually every serious review of the neuropsychological malingering literature since 1990 has suggested that the diagnosis of malingering is a difficult determination that should be made based upon assessment of multiple dimensions and multiple methods, including measures of effort (Franzen, Iverson, & McCracken, 1990; Haines & Norris, 1995; Miller & Miller, 1992; Millis & Putnam 1996; Rogers, Harrell, & Liff 1993; Nies & Sweet, 1994; Reynolds, 1998; Rogers, 1997; Sweet, 1999; Iverson & Binder, 2000; Vickery et al., 2001). Thus, there is a consensus that response validity indicators within actual tests of ability are not intended to be used in isolation.

With increasing application of clinical neuropsychology to forensic cases, there have been numerous attempts to determine methods of assessing response validity on the CatT, primarily with the purpose of identifying insufficient effort and possible malingering. Consistent with the relevant research on other commonly used neuropsychological ability measures, these efforts primarily have taken several approaches: (1) determination of levels of performance for the specific test that are "too severe" to be realistic for the neurological condition of interest, (2) identification of items or groups of items that constitute relatively rare errors among genuine patients, and (3) evaluation of unrealistic change in performance on retesting. The application of these approaches has typically occurred via decision rules or statistical formulae found to discriminate insufficient effort from performance reflecting adequate effort in patients with genuine brain dysfunction.

Interestingly, the foundation for the above approaches was established many years ago for the CatT within the extensive investigation published by Simmel and Counts (1957). These investigators made several observations relevant to later research on effort and malingering on the CatT, including: (1) normals and brain-damaged make the same erroneous choices and, moreover, "... find the same items 'easy' or 'difficult' ..." (p. 136); (2) "... none of our subjects had any difficulty ..." in Subtest I, and items in Subtest II were "... completed practically without error by all our subjects ..." (p. 137); and (3) upon retesting, both groups showed significant improvement in performance. It is not apparent that *any* of the subsequent malingering researchers credited Simmel and Counts; instead, it appears that each later in the 1980s and 1990s *independently* rediscovered the same types of patterns in their CatT datasets that Simmel and Counts had observed in the 1950s. Separate from research related to detection of insufficient effort and malingering, Laatsch and Choca (1991) reported very similar results to that of Simmel and Counts; among 195 neurological rehabilitation patients, with regard to Subtests I and II "... almost all subjects were able to answer all of the items correctly" (p. 702). Choca and Laatsch concluded that the items of Subtests I and II were too easy to yield useful information regarding brain dysfunction.

Initial Contrary Findings Pertaining to Simulated Malingering

A frequently cited study of malingering by Heaton, Smith, Lehman, and Vogt (1978) employed the HRNB. Within this study a relative difference was reported on the CatT between simulators paid to fake brain damage and moderately to severely (at least 12 hours of loss of consciousness [LOC]) head-injured patients. The performance of the simulators (mean errors = 46.1, *SD* = 20.1) was *better* than that of the genuinely head injured patients (mean errors = 67.4, *SD* = 27.2).

Another early study by Goebel (1983) used the HRNB to investigate malingering and found that simulators produced significantly *fewer* (mean errors = 38.1) CatT errors than heterogeneous brain-damaged patients (mean errors = 86.2). However, a post-experiment debriefing interview found that the vast majority of the simulators were not confident that they had been successful in faking brain damage.

Subsequent to Heaton et al. (1978) and Goebel (1983), numerous studies with more sophisticated design and procedures have reported *opposite* results with the CatT (i.e., simulators and malingerers perform *worse* than genuinely injured patients putting forth good effort), which is consistent with the general literature pertaining to how insufficient effort and simulated or actual malingering are reflected on neuropsychological measures. For example, in two separate validation studies, using samples of age, gender, and Impairment Index matched subjects, Mittenberg, Rotholc, Russell, and Heilbronner (1996) administered the HRNB to non-litigating head injury patients and to simulators. In both the validation and cross-validation samples, the CatT results were significantly worse in the simulated malingering groups (simulator mean errors = 81.2, *SD* = 31.1 in study 1 and 85.2, *SD* = 34.8 in study 2; head injury mean errors = 63.8, *SD* = 31.5 in study 1 and 61.6, *SD* = 30.0 in study 2). Findings with a variety of neuropsychological measures are nearly universal in demonstrating *worse* performance among those feigning brain injury, and have greatly influenced strategies for detecting insufficient effort, including those related to the CatT.

The "Bolter Index" of Performance Validity

The first attempt to assess response validity within the CatT appears to have been that of Bolter, Picano, and Zych (1985). These investigators compared 50 documented heterogeneous brain-damaged patients to 50 patients whose symptoms were believed to be non-neurological in nature. The description of the non-neurological patients appears to suggest a psychiatric etiology to their complaints. None of the participants was described as malingering. All 208 CatT items were scrutinized with regard to the number of patients failing the item. From Subtests III through VII, 15 items were correctly answered by 90% or more of the patients. In order to make the validity index more representative of the entire test, three additional items from Subtests I and II were added (only one of the 28 items from Subtest I and II had been missed by more than 3% of the entire sample). When considered as a whole, 76% of the entire sample made no errors on the 18 validity items, and 97% failed two items or less.

In a later revision of the performance validity index, Bolter (unpublished manuscript) eliminated 4 of the 18 items after attempting to cross-validate his original results. This study involved 55 heterogeneous brain-damaged patients (mean CatT errors = 69.7, *SD* = 24.4) and 50 healthy college students, and employed a more stringent cutoff of 95% success on an item in order for it to be included. Results of individual CatT item analysis revealed that all original 18 validity index items were passed by at least 95% of control subjects. However, among the brain-damaged patients, 4 items were missed by more than 5% of the participants. These items were then eliminated in the revised Bolter index of performance validity. However, most subsequent studies of the CatT that used a "Bolter index" or refer to "Bolter items" are actually referring to the original 18 item index of Bolter, Picano, and Zych (1985).

Trueblood and Schmidt (1993) reported on small samples of mild head injury patients who demonstrated normal effort, questionable validity, or malingering as defined primarily by degree of poor performance on a forced-choice digit recognition procedure based on the Multi-Digit Memory Test (MDMT; Hiscock & Hiscock, 1989; computerized MDMT; Bolter & Niccolls, 1990). The malingerers performed at below chance levels, while the questionable validity group performed at or above chance digit recognition performance and had at least one improbable neuropsychological performance. Among numerous other measures, the CatT was administered. Normal effort on the CatT was associated with significantly fewer errors on Subtest VII, but did not result in a significant difference in scores on the 18 Bolter items. Among the four small samples of 8 patients each, mean numbers of Bolter items failed were 0.0 and 0.1 (range 0-1) in separate groups of good effort, 0.1 (range 0-1) in the questionable validity group and 0.8 (range 0-4) in the malingering group. With such small samples, lack of a statistically significant difference may not be meaningful. Even though results of individual classifications based on a decision rule were not provided, the tabular information provided by the authors indicates that the number of correct classifications of good effort was 100% (i.e., the *range* in the two groups of patients with good effort did not exceed Bolter's cutoff). Further, one or more of the malingerers would have been identified as having produced an invalid result by exceeding Bolter's cutoff.

In a study of litigation and motivation effects on personality and neuropsychological performance among 46 litigating and 30 non-litigating TBI patients, Conder, Guerro, and Conder (1994) administered a variety of measures, including the CatT, and also looked at the Bolter validity index. Motivation was defined as high or low based upon the results of the Computerized Assessment of Response Bias (CARB; Allen, Conder, Green, & Cox, 1997), a forced-choice digit recognition procedure, being in the top or bottom decile with regard to number of correct CARB responses. Among litigants, the total number of CatT errors was found to be significantly greater for the low motivation group comprised entirely of mild TBI (mean = 94.3 errors, *SD* = 22.5) compared to the high motivation group that included 44% of patients with moderate and severe TBI (mean = 59.5 errors, *SD* = 34.5). Among *non-litigants*, most of whom had severe TBI, results of the Bolter validity index showed *no* errors on any item. There were no significant differences in Bolter index scores between the high and low motivation *litigants*.

A recent unpublished study by Ashendorf, O'Bryant, Constantinou, Weber, Palav, and McCaffrey (2001) investigated the 14 item revised Bolter index as it relates to results of the Test of Memory Malingering (TOMM; Tombaugh, 1996) and the Rey Memory for 15 Item Test (Rey-15; Rey, 1964). Using subgroup classifications based upon passing or failing malingering cutoffs on the TOMM or the Rey-15, they found that agreement with the revised Bolter index in regard to *good* effort was high, at .86 with the former and .97 with the latter criteria. Agreement regarding *poor* effort between the revised Bolter index and the two effort measures was low (.14 and .30, respectively). Unfortunately, there are several methodological aspects of this study that limit its relevance to the present discussion, including an unacceptably low number of "malingerers."

Tenhula-Sweet Validity Indices

Tenhula and Sweet (1996) extended the type of approach used by Bolter, Picano, and Zych (1985) and Trueblood and Schmidt (1993) in developing strategies to determine response validity on the Booklet CatT. Two separate sequential investigations were carried out, each comparing samples of normal controls, malingering simulators, and TBI patients who completed the CatT. In the first study, there were 28 simulators, 26 TBI patients, and 34 normal control participants; in the second study, there were 17 simulators, 24 TBI patients, and 24 normal controls. In both studies, mean subtest and total scores were found to be significantly different between the groups, with simulators performing more poorly. For example, TBI patients attained mean total error scores of 49.0 (*SD* = 27.0) and 41.9 (*SD* = 22.5), respectively, in the two studies, while simulators attained mean scores of 79.6 (*SD* = 36.0) and 88.8 (*SD* = 30.9), respectively. Comparisons of mean subtest scores and total scores indicated that Subtests I, II, and VII, and Total errors might differentiate the groups. Additionally, items were analyzed to determine those most commonly passed ("Easy" items), as Bolter had done, and those most commonly failed ("Difficult" items). The latter group of items was of interest because of literature suggesting that malingerers have difficulty identifying degree of difficulty of neuropsychological tasks, and therefore may perform in a manner that is discrepant from that found after legitimate TBI.

A series of discriminant function analyses were performed with the functions from each study then applied to the other study, in a double cross-validation. Because the discriminant functions achieved similar hit rates with minimal reduction on cross-validation, optimal discriminant functions were developed using the samples from both studies. Overall hit rates ranged from a low of 72.5% for the Difficult items to 92.2% for the combination of Subtests I and II. Clinical cutoffs were derived for six indices: total errors, combined errors on Subtests I and II, errors on Subtest VII, Bolter items (18 item version), Easy items, and Difficult items. Not surprisingly, the Difficult items again showed the lowest classification accuracy, in terms of both sensitivity (73.3%) and specificity (72.2%), which is the basis for the authors subsequently having actively discouraged its use when releasing cutoffs to clinicians. The other methods ranged in sensitivity from 68.9% to 77.8% in sensitivity and 86.1% to 100% in specificity. Tenhula and Sweet also reported that of the six validity indicators, the simulators attained a mean of 3.6 (SD = 1.9) invalid indices, whereas combined groups of normals and TBIs attained a mean of 0.5 (SD = 0.8). Using a cutoff of more than one invalidity indicator resulted in 88.9% correct classification of all subjects, with 7.4% false positives and 20% false negatives.

In an unpublished study that followed an early conference presentation by Tenhula and Sweet's study one, Iverson, Myers, and Adams (1994) examined three of the six CatT validity indicators for false positive rates among 108 non-litigating closed head injury patients. The following false positive error rates were found: 12% on Subtest I and II errors, 34% on Subtest VII errors, and 21% on Total errors. Iverson et al. did not evaluate the remaining three indicators and thus could not report on the overall number of indicators exceeded by the patients. Of the CatT validity indicators reported, it appears that the combined number of Subtest I and II errors was substantially more accurate (88%) in classifying closed head injury patients.

Ellwanger, Tenhula, Rosenfeld, and Sweet (1999) evaluated 25 normal controls and 35 malingering simulators in an attempt to determine whether the CatT and event-related potentials (ERPs) offered redundant or unique information in identifying feigned cognitive deficits. In this instance, the ERP data was collected while subjects engaged in a modified MDMT. A series of prior studies by this group (e.g., Rosenfeld, Sweet, & Ellwanger, 1995) had demonstrated potential for ERPs to detect insufficient effort. The Ellwanger et al. study found that, with the exception of the Difficult items, normal controls did not surpass CatT indicators and that 30% to 90% of simulators surpassed an indicator (simulator mean CatT errors = approximately 79). Strongly suggesting the usefulness of the CatT validity indicators as an adjunct to other performances pertaining to effort, Ellwanger et al. found that *all* normals and simulators were correctly classified when the information from the CatT and the ERPs was considered together.

DiCarlo, Gfeller, and Oliveri (2000) used the CatT and five indicators from the Tenhula and Sweet (1996) study, excluding the Bolter items and the Difficult items, to evaluate 122 participants divided into four groups: normal controls, TBI patients, uncoached malingering simulators, and coached malingering simulators. DiCarlo et al. found that all controls passed all of the five indicators. Among TBI patients (mean CatT errors = 55.6, *SD* = 29.4), all passed the Subtest I and II indicator, and 90% each passed the Easy items and the number of criteria exceeded, 70% passed the Subtest VII indicator, and 83.3% passed the total errors indicator. The effect of coaching was pronounced, with the naïve or uncoached simulators (mean CatT errors = 107.4, *SD* = 30.0) detected at rates between 76.7% and 93.3%, whereas sophisticated or coached simulators (mean CatT errors = 77.5, *SD* = 17.9) were detected at rates between 34.4% and 71.9%. DiCarlo et al. concluded that their classification rates with the CatT validity indicators were ". . . consistent with and slightly higher than Tenhula and Sweet . . ." and further noted that the Subtest I and II indicator and the criteria exceeded indicator remained reasonably effective with sophisticated simulators.

In a currently unpublished study, Willamson, Green, Allen, and Rohling administered either the computerized version of the CatT or the Booklet CatT, along with other measures to 244 patients seeking compensation for head injury. The patients were divided by severity of TBI into mild and definite. Results reported from the available CatT validity indicators were limited to total errors on Subtests I and II and the criteria exceeded indicator, referred to as the "tally" approach. Results of the Word Memory Test (WMT; Green, Allen, & Astner, 1996) and a variety of other measures, such as the Minnesota Multiphasic Personality Inventory-2nd Edition (MMPI-2; Hathaway et al., 1989), CARB, and CVLT were also reported. Based on extensive data included in the manuscript, the authors concluded that the CatT indicators should be used only with great caution, as their findings did not show a convergence of findings with measures of effort, personality, or other ability indicators. Perhaps the most striking finding of this study is the data showing little relationship between poor performance on specific effort measures and two of the Tenhula and Sweet CatT validity indicators. In the mild TBI group, the WMT and CatT "tally" approach identified a similar number of patients with poor effort (26% and 30%, respectively), but in the overall sample, the measures disagreed on 36% of individual cases. Further, when limited to the definite TBI group, there were no instances of classification agreement when both the WMT and the two CatT indicators showed invalid performances. Williamson et al. (in press) discussed possible significant effects of variables, such as education and injury severity, on CatT performances in their data, which may affect and detract from the utility of validity indicators within the CatT. The negative influence of including the previously documented ineffective Difficult items in their "tally" classification is not reported in the manuscript. However, the effect likely was negative, as it appears that the "tally" approach was less accurate than errors on Subtests I and II, which was not reported in the DiCarlo et al. study that had excluded the Difficult items from consideration.

Barrett-Putnam "Easy" Items

Using the same approach that defined the Bolter index and the Tenhula-Sweet "easy items," Barrett and Putnam (1998) identified CatT items that 90% of 58 moderate and severe TBI patients had answered successfully. However, unlike the previous investigators, Barrett and Putnam identified a relatively large number (46) of such items, and nearly all of their patients were involved in litigation. By comparison, Bolter originally identified 18 items that 90% of TBI patients answered correctly and on revision reduced the number to 14 answered correctly by 95%, and Tenhula and Sweet identified 19 items that 95% of TBI patients answered correctly. Interestingly, the items identified by Barrett and Putnam included all items from Subtest I and all but one item from Subtest II. A group of 125 mild head injured patients was divided into two groups, depending upon whether they scored above or below the insufficient effort criteria on the Recognition Memory Test (RMT; Warrington, 1984) established by Millis (1992). When compared to the resulting groups of 104 "honest" mild head injured and 21 "suspicious" mild head injured patients, the moderate and severe head injured group did not differ significantly in mean numbers of the 46 easy items that had been identified. The distributions differed somewhat, leading Barrett and Putnam to suggest that level of motivation and effort of any patient be questioned when he/she makes more than three rare errors. This criterion identified 10% of the moderate to severe, 6% of the "honest" mild and 24% of the "suspicious" mild TBI patients. The Bolter index and the Tenhula and Sweet indicators were not investigated by Barrett and Putnam.

Unlike Tenhula and Sweet (1996) and DiCarlo et al. (2000), who had evaluated Subtest I and II errors separately from "easy" items, Barrett and Putnam combined these items. If items from Subtests I and II are excluded, the following item overlap is evident from the three independent attempts to identify CatT items that most brain injured patients answer correctly: Bolter and Tenhula-Sweet share 12 items, Tenhula-Sweet and Barrett-Putnam share 12 items, Bolter and Barrett-Putnam share 15 items. It appears that there is at least some consistency across investigations with regard to items most brain injured patients answer correctly.

Retest Consistency on the CatT

Reitan and Wolfson (1996) used a number of tests with proven sensitivity to cerebral dysfunction to demonstrate the effect of litigation on repeated testing. The CatT was among the measures administered on two occasions to litigants and non-litigants, all having sustained a head injury. Of interest to the present review, the CatT was found to have been performed better initially among *non-litigants* (mean errors = 45.9) than the litigants (mean errors = 65.8) on first administration, and on the second administration non-litigants made approximately 10 fewer errors than on their first testing. Improved performance with the CatT on retesting has been reported consistently for decades (e.g., Dikmen, Heaton, Grant, & Temkin, 1999; Simmel & Counts, 1957). By comparison, errors made by *litigants* increased by approximately 14 on the second administration. Reitan and Wolfson (1996) went on to devise a Dissimulation Index based on these results and similar findings on the other common measures used in their study. Thus, it would appear that comparison of CatT performance on repeat testing can shed light on performance validity, although the Reitan and Wolfson findings await published cross validation.

Variability of Results Across Studies

There are numerous reasons that independent studies of a neuropsychological topic produce different findings. Several variables have been shown unquestionably to affect CatT results significantly: age, education, and IQ. IQ has not been reported consistently across the CatT validity indicator studies, and thus cannot be explored. Among studies that report at least one CatT validity indicator and also report age (Bolter, 1985; DiCarlo et al., 2000; Iverson et al., 1994; Tenhula & Sweet, 1996; Williamson, Green, Allen, & Rohling, in press), it appears that age is not a likely factor in producing different results; all studies consisted of relatively young participants. Education on the other hand varied. Bolter reported a mean of 13.6 years of education; Tenhula and Sweet reported 13.9 years in study 1 and 13.9 years in study 2; Iverson reported 12.0 years; DiCarlo reported 12.7 years; and Williamson et al. reported 12.0 years. The studies that are the most discrepant with regard to reporting false positives (Tenhula & Sweet, Iverson et al., Williamson et al.) are the most discrepant in education. Only two of these studies reported ranges of education, with that information showing that Williamson et al. included participants as low as 5th grade education, while Tenhula and Sweet only went as low as 10th grade in study 1 and 9th grade in study 2. Given that Leckliter and Matarazzo (1989) reported that a combination of five studies showed a −.31 correlation between CatT errors and education, one wonders whether these differences contribute to differences in study outcomes. It appears likely that individuals with very low educational attainment, which can also be associated with low IQ (another variable known to contribute to poor CatT performance) will ordinarily perform more poorly on the CatT and therefore be more prone to make errors even on validity indicators.

Severity of injury has routinely been reported in the studies reviewed within this paper, and was discussed by Williamson et al. (in press) as one possible contributing factor to differences in study results. However, the relationship of brain injury severity to CatT errors in such well-controlled studies as Dikmen, Machamer, Winn, and Temkin (1995) is not as potent as might be imagined. Even severe TBI patients with 7 to 13 days of inability to follow commands produced a median score of 32 errors and a mean score of 49 errors. It seems unlikely that severity differences alone account for variable study results, but in individuals with *very* severe brain injury, this concern may become more important.

CLINICAL EXAMPLES

In this section, we provide several examples regarding how CatT validity indicators may be used by clinicians. Data in Table 1 are from an unsophisticated malingerer who claimed a mild TBI. This litigant is presented because he was later "caught" in real life; there is no question that an accurate conclusion was reached. The plaintiff had undergone numerous prior evaluations after a *possible* trivial blow to the head several years earlier. Results of these prior serial evaluations had declined significantly on each occasion, and were depicted on the last occasion as showing the plaintiff to be "obtunded," "confused," "dementia-like" and so unable to perform even very easy ability tasks that he was virtually untestable. Extensive medical testing was completely normal. At our neuropsychological evaluation, the plaintiff complained bitterly of the difficulty of the tasks presented to him as he produced the data presented in Table 1. Subsequent independent data gathered by a private investigator found the patient to be working effectively under a false name. There was no question that the insufficient effort across evaluations represented malingering.

In Table 2, detailed test data concerning six litigants is presented. We have deliberately juxtaposed three TBI litigants with varying ranges of injury severity who also demonstrated good effort and three litigants who either may have experienced mild TBI or experienced severe TBI and also demonstrated some degree of insufficient effort. As clinicians

TABLE 1. Test Results of an Unsophisticated Malingerer

Test	Raw Score/Metric	Test	Raw Score/Metric
Category Test (errors)		Rey-15	
Subtest 1	4*	Rows	1*
Subtest 2	2*	Items	6*
Subtest 3	32		
Subtest 4	35	Multi-Digit Memory Test	27*/72
Subtest 5	28		
Subtest 6	25	Recognition Memory Test	
Subtest 7	11*	Words	20*, < 1st %ile
Total	137*, T = 9	Faces	25*, < 1st %ile
Easy Items	8*		
Bolter Items	5*	Reliable Digit Span	2*
		WMS-R (Information/Orientation raw score)	8*

Note. T score for Category total errors is from DeFilippis & McCampbell (1979). Percentiles for the Recognition Memory Test are from the test manual (Warrington, 1984).

* These scores are suggestive of insufficient effort in a case of possible mild traumatic brain injury.

Tests and references in alphabetical order:
Category Test (DeFilippis & McCampbell, 1979)
Multi-Digit Memory Test (Bolter & Niccolls, 1990)
Reliable Digit Span (Greiffenstein, Baker, & Gola, 1994)
Rey Memory for 15 Item Test (Rey-15; Rey, 1964)
Recognition Memory Test (Warrington, 1984)
Wechsler Memory Scale-Revised (WMS-R; Wechsler, 1987).

TABLE 2. Neuropsychological Test Results of Three (Mild and Severe) TBI litigants with Good Effort and Three (Questionably Injured and Severe) TBI Litigants with Degrees of Insufficient Effort

Test Raw Score	Case 1 Age = 49 Educ = 13	Case 2 Age = 30 Educ = 15	Case 3 Age = 56 Educ = 14	Case 4 Age = 33 Educ = 12	Case 5 Age = 38 Educ = 12	Case 6 Age = 35 Educ = 14
Category Test (errors)						
Subtest 1	0	0	0	1	2	0
Subtest 2	0	0	0	0	3	4
Subtest 3	3	29	4	29	31	28
Subtest 4	1	2	2	26	30	31
Subtest 5	13	3	3	16	15	22
Subtest 6	5	1	1	16	7	10
Subtest 7	0	3	1	11	7	6
Total	22	38	11	99	95	101
Easy Items	0	0	0	4	2	4
Bolter Items	0	0	0	0	2	3
Rey-15						
Rows	5	4	5	4	1	3
Items	15	15	15	15	11	11
Victoria Symptom Validity Test						
Easy (correct)	24	N/A	N/A	N/A	N/A	N/A
Difficult (correct)	23					
Easy (latency)	1.84					
Difficult (latency)	1.93					
Word Memory Test						
Immediate Recall (% correct)	100	N/A	N/A	N/A	N/A	N/A
Delayed Recall (% correct)	100					
Multi-Digit Memory Test (raw)	N/A	72	72	55	71	38
Reliable Digit Span	10	10	9	10	6	5
MMPI-2 (Fake Bad Scale)	19	17	4	22	42	29
Recognition Memory Test (raw)						
Words	N/A	50	46	27	41	24
Faces		36	41	25	33	28
WAIS-R (age scaled score)						
FSIQ	103	101	112	79	69	78
PIQ	117	104	139	75	72	77
VIQ	110	102	125	76	69	77
Information	12	11	11	4	4	6
Digit Span	10	11	11	10	4	3
Vocabulary	14	10	14	6	4	7
Arithmetic	8	12	9	6	4	6
Comprehension	10	9	13	7	7	6
Similarities	12	10	13	6	4	7
Picture Completion	12	11	15	6	6	5
Picture Arrangement	12	8	13	6	5	5
Block Design	13	13	17	6	6	5
Object Assembly	14	11	17	7	4	5
Digit Symbol	12	12	15	6	5	6
# pairs	7	N/A	7	6	5	4
# symbols	7	N/A	9	6	8	7

Test Raw Score	Case 1 Age = 49 Educ = 13	Case 2 Age = 30 Educ = 15	Case 3 Age = 56 Educ = 14	Case 4 Age = 33 Educ = 12	Case 5 Age = 38 Educ = 12	Case 6 Age = 35 Educ = 14
IQ difference (predicted-actual)	0	7	−13	23	24	33
Shipley						
Vocabulary (raw)	38	34	36	24	N/A	
Abstraction (raw)	26	30	38	12		
AQ (SS)	91	104	117	87		
WCST (raw)						
Categories	6	6	6	2	0	0
Errors	14	29	45	62	97	55
Perseverative Responses	7	11	23	43	118	51
Failure to Maintain Set	0	0	0	3	0	1
"Other" Responses	0	4	3	1	2	1
WRAT-3 (Standard Score)						
Reading	100	93	107	105	45	51
Spelling	104	106	N/A	89	N/A	53
Arithmetic	99	111	N/A	75	N/A	28
PIAT-R (Standard Score)						
Reading Comprehension	111	114	115	97	55	55
PASAT (% correct)						
Trial 1	N/A	90	60	54	NA	68
Trial 2		92	50	38		64
Trial 3		72	48	46		52
Trial 4		52	40	28		50
Gordon Diagnostic System						
Vigilance (correct)	40	44	45	42	N/A	30
Vigilance (commissions)	1	0	0	7		17
Distractibility (correct)	31	42	38	23		17
Distractibility (commissions)	3	3	6	23		28
Stroop (age corrected raw)						
Word	100	91	113	77	79	31
Color	78	71	64	60	49	31
Color-Word	46	59	55	30	20	32
Trail Making Test (seconds)						
Trails A	25	28	27	32	41	79
Trails B	95	104	51	106	344	122
Multilingual Aphasia Exam (raw)						
Naming	60	54	54	48	38	44
COWA (CFL)	43	32	51	31	30	22
Animal Naming Fluency (raw)	13	22	22	11	7	N/A
Ruff Figural Fluency (age corrected)						
Unique	73	88	107	71	46	52
Error Ratio	.04	.10	.05	.16	.99	.06
Finger Tapping (raw)						
Dominant Hand	39	49.4	47.6	49.2	42.6	N/A
Non-Dominant Hand	50	43.4	44.6	N/A	36.8	
Dynamometer (kg)						
Dominant Hand	19	31	27.5	28	44	18
Non-Dominant Hand	22	23	30.5	N/A	41	16.5
Grooved Pegboard (raw)						
Dominant Hand	90	61	74	68	80	99
Non-Dominant Hand	71	70	75	N/A	70	116

TABLE 2 (continued)

Test Raw Score	Case 1 Age = 49 Educ = 13	Case 2 Age = 30 Educ = 15	Case 3 Age = 56 Educ = 14	Case 4 Age = 33 Educ = 12	Case 5 Age = 38 Educ = 12	Case 6 Age = 35 Educ = 14
WMS-R (raw)						
Logical Memory I	26	35	26	16	15	13
Logical Memory II	20	32	26	12	11	8
Logical Memory % Retained	77	91	100	75	73	62
Visual Reproduction I	33	35	36	24	22	23
Visual Reproduction II	28	34	30	16	17	19
Visual Reproduction % Retained	85	97	81	67	77	83
Digit Span Forward	8	8	8	7	4	4
Digit Span Backward	4	9	6	5	3	3
Verbal Paired Associate I	20	22	18	11	18	12
Verbal Paired Associate II	8	8	8	5	5	5
Information/Orientation	14	14	10	11	12	14
Mental Control	5	6	6	6	2	6
CVLT (raw)						
Trial 1	7	7	8	5	5	7
Trial 2	7	10	12	8	8	6
Trial 3	11	8	14	8	9	8
Trial 4	12	11	14	8	9	8
Trial 5	13	11	15	8	10	8
Total 1-5	50	47	63	37	41	37
Interference	8	8	9	4	5	5
Short Free Recall	10	8	12	7	6	6
Short Cued Recall	11	12	16	8	8	7
Long Free Recall	11	10	14	7	7	6
Long Cued Recall	12	11	15	8	7	7
Recognition Hits	15	16	16	8	13	9
Recognition Discriminability (%)	98	98	100	77	82	52
Perseverations (free recall)	5	4	1	7	19	6
Intrusions (free recall)	1	6	8	5	25	1
MMPI-2 (T scores)						
L	43	66	57	71	52[b]	56
F	61	41	41	79	144	61
K	52	70	63	32	37	47
Hs	59	59	49	76	63	79
D	59	53	51	81	62	81
Hy	65	68	47	65	42	91
Pd	53	68	53	73	57	57
Mf	43	57	65	65	54	60
Pa	52	52	37	59	83	72
Pt	55	57	44	77	78	89
Sc	63	53	44	81	94	86
Ma	41	49	47	65	94	62
Si	46	38	41	84	58	54
Beck Depression Inventory-II (raw)	4	4	0	30	16	24
Beck Anxiety Inventory (raw)	1	1	0	18	N/A	12
Beck Hopelessness Scale (raw)	3	0	0	17	N/A	16

Note. The MMPI-2 and FBS for case 5 was from a previous neuropsychological evaluation completed 15 months prior to other results. For most tests, raw scores are provided to enable the reader to refer to preferred norms. With the exception of effort tests, which vary from patient to patient, measures not completed by the majority of the patients have been omitted from the table.

Tests and references in alphabetical order:
Animal Naming Fluency (Goodglass & Kaplan, 1983)
Beck Anxiety Inventory (Beck & Steer, 1990)

Beck Depression Inventory-II (Beck, Steer, & Brown, 1996)
Beck Hopelessness Scale (Beck & Steer, 1988)
California Verbal Learning Test (CVLT; Delis et al., 1987)
Category Test (DeFilippis & McCampbell, 1979)
Finger Tapping Test (Reitan, 1969)
Gordon Diagnostic System (Gordon, McClure, & Post, 1986)
Grooved Pegboard (Klove, 1963)
Hand Dynamometer (Reitan & Davison, 1974)
Minnesota Multiphasic Personality Inventory-2 (MMPI-2; Butcher et al., 1989)
Multi-Digit Memory Test (Bolter & Niccolls, 1990)
Multilingual Aphasia Examination (Benton, Hamsher, & Svian, 1994)
Paced Auditory Serial Addition Test (PASAT; Levin, Mattis, Rugg, & Eisenberg, 1987)
Peabody Individual Achievement Test-Revised (PIAT-R; Markwardt, 1989)
Recognition Memory Test (Warrington, 1984)
Reliable Digit Span (Greiffenstein, Baker, & Gola, 1994)
Rey Memory for 15 Item Test (Rey-15; Rey, 1964)
Ruff Figural Fluency Test (Ruff, 1988)
Shipley Institute of Living Scale-Revised (Shipley; Zachary, 1986)
Stroop Test (Stroop; Golden, 1978)
Trail Making Test (Reitan & Wolfson, 1985)
Victoria Symptom Validity Test (Slick, Hopp, Strauss, & Thompson, 1997)
Wechsler Adult Intelligence Scale-Revised (WAIS-R; Wechsler, 1981)
Wechsler Memory Scale-Revised (WMS-R; Wechsler, 1987)
Wide Range Achievment Test-3rd Edition (WRAT-3; Wilkinson, 1993)
Wisconsin Card Sorting Test (WCST; Berg, 1948; Grant & Berg, 1948)
Word Memory Test (Green, Allen, & Astner, 1996)

can determine for themselves the patterns of reasonable and unrealistic findings within the extensive data presented, we will point out only some of the history and results for each. In each of the six cases below, results of the CatT validity indicators were consistent with the majority of other effort/validity measures.

Case 1 experienced a mild TBI in a car accident, with subsequent documentation of abnormal EEG and brainstem auditory evoked response, as well as cervical injury. Premorbidly, an episode of childhood LOC and adult onset seizures were documented. All effort measures and validity indicators from tests of ability, including the CatT, were consistent with good effort. Neuropsychological performances were generally average, with circumscribed difficulties. The MMPI-2 did not suggest overreporting of symptoms. Self report suggested improvement across time, with successful return to previous occupation.

Case 2 experienced a serious TBI and other bodily injuries in a car accident. Retrograde amnesia of two days and posttraumatic amnesia (PTA) of six weeks were documented in medical records, although intervening surgeries may have obscured actual PTA. LOC, depressed right frontal parietal skull fracture, shift of midline structures, epidural hematoma, and multiple areas of parenchymal hemorrhage were documented, along with a ten day acute care hospitalization, ten week rehabilitation hospitalization, and subsequent outpatient rehabilitation treatment. Effort and validity indicators, including those of the CatT, were consistent with good effort. Evaluation results were relatively limited and consistent with executive dysfunction. Despite significant frontal brain injury, CatT results were not impaired.

Case 3 experienced a serious TBI and other bodily injuries in a car accident. In addition to external signs of head injury, such as contusions and Battle's sign, the plaintiff suffered cardiac arrest and required cardiopulmonary resuscitation at the scene. Retrograde amnesia of less than one hour and PTA of more than six days was present, with the portion attributable to the TBI complicated by the possible anoxia associated with the cardiac arrest. Pre-accident history of epilepsy had been well documented for decades. CatT validity indicators and other measures were consistent with good effort; neuropsychological impairments were relatively limited despite pre-injury epilepsy, unquestionable TBI, and documented cardiac arrest.

Case 4 experienced a very severe TBI and other bodily injuries in a car accident. A protracted period of coma followed by significant behavioral and cognitive changes were well documented in medical records. A mild hemiparesis was present, as was affective lability, at the time of the evaluation. Results were complex and were interpreted as showing personality and cognitive effects of the TBI, with the specific effects of the latter at times obscured by evidence of possible insufficient effort (i.e., MDMT [administered twice], CVLT, RMT) which was at least suggestive of *variability* of effort. The patient's score from the Fake Bad Scale (FBS; Lees-Haley, English, & Glenn, 1991) from the MMPI-2 approached the recommended cutoff. The discrepancy between predicted and measured IQ was more similar to insufficient effort than TBI (Demakis, Sweet, Sawyer, Moulthrop, Nies, & Clingerman, 2001). Regarding the CatT, four validity indicators were surpassed (Subtest VII errors, total errors, "easy item" errors, number of criteria exceeded), which is in keeping with the majority of other effort measures. Nevertheless, obvious gross effects of the injury were clearly devastating and well connected through extensive documentation to the accident. Therefore, although test interpretation limitations due to insufficient effort were noted, an inference of malingering was *not* made.

Case 5 represents an alleged mild TBI from being struck in the head by an outdoor restaurant umbrella that was blown out of its holder at the plaintiff's table by strong winds. Although an extended period of LOC was claimed by the plaintiff, statements of witnesses did not support this. A variety of physical and cognitive complaints were attributed to this incident and ostensibly had been supported by a previous neuropsychological evaluation. Of interest, the MDMT, which has been shown in meta-analytic review (Vickery et al., 2001) to have greater sensitivity to insufficient effort than the Portland Digit Recognition Test (PDRT; Binder, 1993), Rey-15, and Dot Counting Test (Rey, 1941), suggested good effort. However, results of other effort indicators (Rey-15, Reliable Digit Span, CVLT) and unrealistic performances on tests of ability (Trail Making Test, WAIS-R, Wisconsin Card Sorting Test, Wide Range Achievement Test-Revised Reading subtest; Peabody Individual Achievement Test-Revised Reading Comprehension subtest) indicated otherwise. Because of low reading performances, a number of measures were not administered; the Beck Depression Inventory was read to the plaintiff, whereas the FBS and other MMPI-2 data (suggestive of overreporting) were administered elsewhere in a prior evaluation. Four CatT validity indicators were surpassed (errors on Subtests I and II, Subtest VII errors, total errors, number of criteria exceeded). Although low premorbid intelligence was considered, a history of high school graduation without any grade retention or special assistance and having passed a state licensing exam for his profession and a written driver's examination did not support this hypothesis. In this instance, CatT and other effort measures, along with history information, strongly suggested that the plaintiff was malingering.

Case 6 experienced a *possible* mild TBI in a car accident. There was no indication of altered consciousness. No medical treatment was deemed necessary. Despite an Associate's Degree and prior success in two white collar professions, previous post-accident testing (FSIQ of 76 and *very* abnormal performances on a variety of other measures, such as the Connors Continuous Performance Test [CPT; Conners and Multi-Health Systems Staff, 1995], WMS-R, and MMPI-2) had been interpreted as indicative of brain injury. Results of the second evaluation, presented in Table 2, reveal chance level performances on the MDMT and RMT, a variety of positive invalidity indicators, such as CVLT, MMPI-2 (FBS), and Reliable Digit Span, and a number of unrealistically poor performances (e.g., WRAT-R, PIAT-R, hand dynamometer) that are *inconsistent* with possible mild TBI. All six of the CatT validity indicators were surpassed. There seemed little question that the prior and present testing could not be viewed as valid.

In summary, these cases illustrate numerous points. First, the presence or absence of insufficient effort can be independent of injury severity. Case 1 represents an individual with a mild injury and discrete abnormal neuropsychological findings, who does not show any effort or psychological difficulties. Even with very serious injury, CatT performance may not be impaired. In this regard, the results of Cases 2 and 3 are not unusual; severe injuries did not result in impaired CatT scores. In fact, Dikmen et al. (1995) demonstrated that only in cases of TBI associated with 14 to 28 days of inability to follow commands does the mean of CatT errors appear to be near that found in the simulators and malingerers investigated within the studies cited in the present review paper. Moreover, as represented in Case 4, serious injury can also be accompanied by insufficient effort. In the instance of Case 4, the insufficient effort was apparent on CatT validity indicators and other effort measures. Further, as demonstrated by Case 5, effort measures, validity indicators, and other methods of analyzing effort will not always be in complete agreement in an individual case. Although the MDMT has been shown to be among the most sensitive of well known effort measures studied in a meta-analytic review (Vickery et al., 2001), in the instance of Case 5, the MDMT produced a result that was very inconsistent with the overall presentation of this individual. In this same vein, the CatT validity indicators may not always match other effort tests or validity indicators, both because of sensitivity and specificity differences between measures and because an examinee's effort may vary within an evaluation. For example, individuals attempting to feign memory impairment may not view the CatT as relevant to that goal and therefore may not demonstrate deliberately poor performance. On the other hand, individuals such as Case 6 appear to show indifference to test domain and perform poorly on a wide range of types of measures (i.e., memory, reasoning, intellectual, etc.).

PRACTICE RECOMMENDATIONS

1. Use multiple measures of effort in all cases that are, or are likely to become, adversarial. Classification rates have been shown to be higher when multiple measures are used (e.g., Ellwanger et al., 2000; Iverson & Franzen, 1996).
2. Beyond the use of multiple effort measures, virtually all serious reviews of the neuropsychological malingering literature in recent years have recommended that multiple sources of information be considered, rather than just effort measures (Franzen, Iverson, & McCracken, 1990; Haines & Norris, 1995; Iverson & Binder, 2000; Miller & Miller, 1992; Millis & Putnam, 1996; Nies & Sweet, 1994; Reynolds, 1998; Rogers, 1997; Rogers, Harrell, & Liff 1993; Sweet, 1999; Vickery et al., 2001).

3. Effort measures and validity indicators need not be used only in adversarial cases. In fact, use in clinical cases can be helpful and should be considered in any clinical case in which motivation may be problematic. Examples of non-adversarial clinical cases in which effort measures should at least be considered include individuals who on clinical interview report any of the following: prior suspicion by family or health care professionals of the validity of his or her symptoms; unusual, incredible or rare symptoms that appear to have garnered sympathy or attention of family or significant others; significant history of frequent health care usage with little or no documentation of medical necessity.
4. In addition to effort measures, when available, use validity indicators contained within neuropsychological measures. For each such indicator, consider the intended clinical population and the known effectiveness with that population.
5. The CatT validity indicators to date have only been developed for use with TBI. They should not be used with other neurological conditions, unless future research supports such use. Current specific usage recommendations and limitations are as follows:

    a. With TBI cases, within the CatT, consider whether more than one criteria of the following are met: Subtest I and II errors, Bolter items, "easy" items, Subtest VII errors, total errors.
    b. Do *not* consider errors on the "difficult" items, as these were shown to have inadequate specificity (Tenhula & Sweet, 1996). Inclusion of "difficult" items in the determination of whether more than one criterion has been exceeded appears to be associated with *decreased* convergence with other measures (Williamson et al., in press).
    c. With the CatT validity indicators, place a greater degree of confidence in the results of Subtests I and II, as this indicator appears to be the least affected by genuine brain dysfunction across studies (e.g., DiCarlo et al., 2000; Iverson et al., 1994; Laatsch & Choca, 1991; Simmel & Counts, 1957; Tenhula & Sweet, 1996), and in some studies has shown adequate sensitivity to insufficient effort (DiCarlo et al., 2000; Tenhula & Sweet, 1996).
    d. Reduce the risk of false positives by considering the significant effects that age and education are known to have on the CatT (cf. Garb & Lutz, 2001). With an individual who is older or less educated than the subjects of the Tenhula and Sweet (1996)

and DiCarlo et al. (2000) studies, apply these criteria very cautiously. Do not apply the indicators at all in patients with very discrepant age and education or with *very* severe TBI.

e. With the CatT indicators, as with any other measures that may detect insufficient effort, do not expect that all individuals who are motivated to perform poorly will necessarily do so on this particular test. In fact, more sophisticated malingerers are known to be able to apply their insufficient effort selectively (Youngjohn, Lees-Haley, & Binder, 1999). We have seen litigants we felt confident were malingering perform poorly on the CatT Test indicators, while other malingerers performed well not only on the validity indicators, but on the CatT overall. This is not surprising and parallels our experience with validity indicators of other neuropsychological measures (e.g., Digit Span, CVLT, RMT) and actual effort measures in malingering patients. Stated differently, there may not be a complete convergence of all validity indicators (see Case 5). For example, the MMPI-2 validity indicators may or may not agree with cognitive validity indicators (Boone & Lu, 1999; Greiffenstein, Gola, & Baker, 1995; Slick, Hopp, Strauss, & Spellacy, 1996).
f. Do *not* interpret the CatT indicators in isolation. These indicators *suggest* possible insufficient effort; alone, they do not confirm insufficient effort. If insufficient effort is suspected on the basis of the CatT indicators, examine other neuropsychological tests and personality and effort tests as well for additional indications. Moreover, when available, compare evaluation results across time. Worsening performances across evaluations *may* indicate malingering. In instances of stable neurological status, such changes indicate the presence of some non-neurological factor (e.g., fatigue, medications, deteriorating emotional state, insufficient effort) that should be distinguished from effects of brain dysfunction. Also, compare evaluation results against real life functioning.

As one should not conclude that an individual is malingering based only on an isolated indicator of invalidity or insufficient effort, conversely, it is not necessary to have complete agreement of measures in order to conclude that malingering is present. This differential diagnostic decision ultimately is a *clinical* judgment, which, as is almost always the case for any important clinical decision, often requires integration of test data, patient behavior, and historical information. Similar to many clinical decisions (cf. Kleinmuntz, 1990), the determination that someone is malingering is not solely actuarial, even though strongly aided by data-based decision rules. Malingering is not likely to be diagnosed accurately by neuropsychologists who choose not to be informed by current relevant literature or who do not use multiple available methods to examine proactively for this possibility.

DAUBERT THRESHOLDS

In some jurisdictions, though certainly not all, forensic neuropsychologists who address issues of acquired brain injury and related matters, such as malingering, must satisfy the evidentiary admissibility standards posited within the US Supreme Court's decision known as *Daubert v. Merrell Dow Pharmaceuticals* (1993). The editors of this special issue have asked that these standards be addressed.

Falsifiability

Basically, this standard requires that the technique or theory be investigated using scientific methodology, in part to identify conditions under which the ability to identify an erroneous conclusion is compromised. As evident within our review, the use of the CatT to identify brain injury and malingering has been subjected to scientific investigation; variables have been identified that will reduce the diagnostic accuracy of the CatT and its validity indicators. When such variables are present in an individual forensic case, an expert witness should insure that these variables have been examined and their impact considered. For example, variables other than brain dysfunction, such as limited education or limited IQ, can affect overall CatT performance and will also affect CatT validity indicators. Thus, as explained earlier in this review, using the CatT and relying upon the CatT validity indicators in an individual whose education or IQ is known to be limited would unreasonably reduce the validity of CatT results, independent of an individual's brain integrity and effort. When the opportunity to prove that the diagnostic impression of brain injury *or* insufficient effort is erroneous has been reduced, then *Daubert* criteria (and common sense) dictate that the CatT and its indicators should not be relied upon.

Peer Review and Publication

The intent of this standard is self-evident and, by virtue of multiple presentations and publications regarding the use of the CatT to differentiate brain injury from malingering, certainly has been met based on present literature. *Daubert* criteria do not set a specific threshold for acceptance or rejection of peer review conclusions. That is, not all studies must find the same exact results in order for this criterion to be satisfied. Thus, when studies demonstrate a range of effectiveness, due to use of different samples or for other methodological reasons, the resulting information regarding important moderator variables should be integrated and considered by expert witnesses as they determine the limitations of relevant opinions.

Known Rate of Error

Associated with the scientific investigation of a technique or theory is the need to address rates of error that could result. The present review has demonstrated in multiple studies that the rates of false positives (identifying malingering among brain-injured patients who show good effort) are typically quite low. The exception to these studies is that of Williamson et al. (in press), which may, in part, relate to inclusion of patients with lower education and to their inclusion of the "Difficult Items" scale. As discussed earlier within the present review, we do not recommend that clinicians use the "Difficult Items" scale.

Although in some CatT studies, sensitivity to the presence of malingering as determined by external measures may at times be low, we do not view this as any different than other indicators of invalidity that are housed within tests of ability, rather than tests specifically of effort. As with other such indicators within tests of ability, and related to known error rates, we believe the CatT validity indicators should *not* be used in isolation. As such, presently known error rates support its use only as one of a number of other invalidity indicators and effort tests.

General Acceptance

This standard addresses the degree to which a technique or theory is widely used or adhered to in the relevant field. The *Daubert* ruling did not specify a means of determining acceptance nor a necessary threshold (e.g., greater than 50%) that must be satisfied. Clearly, the CatT is among the most widely used of neuropsychological tests. We do not know, but expect that the use of the invalidity indicators reviewed in this paper is not nearly as common among clinical psychologists in general. However, the fact that the present topical review concerning CatT validity indicators was thought to be worthy enough to be invited for this special issue likely implies general acceptance among forensic experts in clinical neuropsychology.

REFERENCES

Adams, R. L., & Trenton, S. L. (1981). Development of a paper-and-pen form of the Halstead Category Test. *Journal of Consulting and Clinical Psychology, 49*, 298-299.

Allen, D. N., Goldstein, G., & Mariano, E. (1999). Is the Halstead Category Test a multidimensional instrument? *Journal of Clinical and Experimental Neuropsychology, 21*, 237-244.

Allen, L. M., Conder, R. L. Jr., Green, P., & Cox, D. R. (1997). *Computerized Assessment of Response Bias*. Durham, NC: CogniSyst.

Anderson, C. V., Bigler, E. D., & Blatter, D. D. (1995). Frontal lobe lesions, diffuse damage, and neuropsychological functioning in traumatic brain-injured patients. *Journal of Clinical and Experimental Neuropsychology, 17*, 900-908.

Ashendorf, L., O'Bryant, S., Constantinou, M., Weber, M., Palav, A., & McCaffrey, R. (2001). *An empirical examination of Bolter's validity index for the Halstead Category Test*. Presented at the annual meeting of the National Academy of Neuropsychology, San Francisco, CA.

Barnes, G., & Lucas, G. J. (1974). Cerebral dysfunction vs. psychogenesis in the Halstead-Reitan tests. *Journal of Nervous and Mental Disease, 158*, 50-60.

Barrett, P., & Putnam, S. (1998). *Empirical data as an aide for assessing performance validity on the Halstead Category Test for mild head injury patients*. Presented at the annual meeting of the National Academy of Neuropsychology, Washington, DC.

Beck, A. T. (1978). *Beck Depression Inventory Manual*. San Antonio, TX: Psychological Corporation.

Beck, A. T., & Steer, R. A. (1990). *Beck Anxiety Inventory Manual*. San Antonio, TX: Psychological Corporation.

Beck, A. T., & Steer, R. A. (1988). *Beck Hopelessness Scale Manual*. San Antonio, TX: Psychological Corporation.

Beck, A. T., Steer, R. A., & Brown, G. K. (1996). *Beck Depression Inventory II Manual*. San Antonio, TX: Psychological Corporation.

Benton, A. L., Hamsher, K. de S., & Sivan, A. B. (1994). *Multilingual Aphasia Examination* (3rd ed.). Iowa City; IA: AJA Associates.

Berg, E. A. (1948). A simple objective technique for measuring flexibility in thinking. *Journal of General Psychology, 39*, 15-22.

Berger, S. G., Chibnall, J. T., & Gfeller, J. D. (1994). The Category Test: A comparison of computerized and standard versions. *Assessment, 1*, 255-258.

Binder, L. M. (1993). Assessment of malingering after mild head trauma with the Portland Digit Recognition Test. *Journal of Clinical and Experimental Neuropsychology, 15*, 170-182.

Boll, T. J. (1981). The Halstead-Reitan neuropsychology battery. In S. B. Filskov & T. J. Boll (Eds.), *Handbook of Clinical Neuropsychology* (pp. 577-607). New York: John Wiley & Sons.

Bolter, J. F. (1985). Item error frequencies for the Halstead Category Test: A cross validation study on a performance validity check. (unpublished manuscript).

Bolter, J. F., & Niccolls, R. (1990). *The Multi-Digit Memory Test Manual.* San Luis Obispo, CA: Wang Neuropsychology Laboratory.

Bolter, J. F., Picano, J. J., & Zych, K. (1985). Item error frequencies on the Halstead Category Test: An index of performance validity. Paper presented at the annual meeting of the National Academy of Neuropsychology, Philadelphia, PA.

Boone, K., & Lu, P. (1999). Impact of somatoform symptomatology on credibility of cognitive performance. *The Clinical Neuropsychologist, 13*, 414-419.

Bornstein, R. (1986). Contribution of various neuropsychological measures to detection of frontal lobe impairment. *International Journal of Clinical Neuropsychology, 8*, 18-22.

Boyd, J. L. (1980). Validity of a shortened booklet form of the Halstead Category Test (Doctoral dissertation, Florida State University, 1979). *Dissertation Abstracts International, 40*, 4472B.

Boyle, G. J. (1988). What does the neuropsychological Category Test measure? *Archives of Clinical Neuropsychology, 3*, 69-76.

Boyle, G. J. (1986). Clinical neuropsychological assessment: Abbreviating the Halstead Category Test of brain dysfunction. *Journal of Clinical Psychology, 42*, 615-625.

Butcher, J. N., Dahlstrom, W. G., Graham, J. R., Tellegen, A., & Kramer, B. (1989). *Minnesota Multiphasic Personality Inventory 2: Manual for Administration and Scoring.* Minneapolis, MN: University of Minnesota Press.

Calsyn, D. A., O'Leary, M. R., & Chaney, E. F. (1980). Shortening the Category Test. *Journal of Consulting and Clinical Psychology, 48*, 788-789.

Camara, W., Nathan, J., & Puente, A. (2000). Psychological test usage: Implications in professional psychology. *Professional Psychology: Research and Practice, 31*, 141-154.

Chapman, L., & Wolff, H. (1959). The cerebral hemispheres and the highest integrative functions of man. *Archives of Neurology, 1*, 357-424.

Choca, J. (1987). *Category Test Computer Program.* Ontario, Canada: Multi-Health Systems.

Choca, J., & Laatsch, L. (1994). *Equivalence of the Adaptive Category Test and the Full Halstead Version.* Paper presented at the 102nd Annual Convention of the American Psychological Association: Los Angeles, CA.

Choca, J., Laatsch, L., Garside, D., & Arnemann, C. (1994). *Computer Category Test.* Ontario, Canada: Multi-Health Systems.

Choca, J., Laatsch, L., Wetzel, L., & Agresti, A. (1997). The Halstead Category Test: A fifty year perspective. *Neuropsychology Review, 7*, 62-75.

Conder, R., Guerro, D., & Conder, A. (1994). Relationship between neuropsychological and psychological measures of validity: Associative or dissociative? Paper presented at the annual meeting of the National Academy of Neuropsychology, Orlando, FL.

Connors, C. K., & Multi-Health Systems Staff (1995). *Conner's' Continuous Performance Test.* Toronto, Canada: MHS.

Daubert v. Merrill Dow Pharmaceuticals, Inc. 113 S. Ct. 2786 (1993).

DeFilippis, N. A. (1992). *Category Test: Computer Version, Research Edition.* Odessa, FL: Psychological Assessment Resources.

DeFilippis, N. A., & McCampbell, E. (1979, 1991). *Manual for the Booklet Category Test.* Odessa, FL: Psychological Assessment Resources.

Delis, D. C., Kramer, J. H., Kaplan, E., & Ober, B. A. (1987). *California Verbal Learning Test: Adult Version Manual.* San Antonio, TX: The Psychological Corporation.

Demakis, G., Sweet, G., Sawyer, T., Moulthrop, M., Nies, K., & Clingerman, S. (2001). Discrepancy between predicted and obtained WAIS-R IQ scores discriminates between traumatic brain injury and insufficient effort. *Psychological Assessment, 13*, 240-248.

DiCarlo, M. A., Gfeller, J. D., & Oliveri, M. V. (2000). Effects of coaching on detecting feigned cognitive impairment with the Category Test. *Archives of Clinical Neuropsychology, 15*, 399-413.

Dikmen, S., Heaton, R. K., Grant, I., & Temkin, N. R. (1999). Test-retest reliability and practice effects of Expanded Halstead-Reitan Neuropsychological Test Battery. *Journal of the International Neuropsychological Society, 5*, 346-356.

Dikmen, S., Machmamer, J., Winn, R., & Temkin, N. (1995). Neuropsychological outcome at 1-year post head injury. *Neuropsychology, 9*, 80-90.

Ellwanger, J., Tenhula, W. N., Rosenfeld, J. P., & Sweet, J. J. (1999). Identifying simulators of cognitive deficit through combined use of neuropsychological test performance and event-related potentials. *Journal of Clinical and Experimental Neuropsychology, 21*, 866-879.

Fitzhugh, K. B., Fitzhugh, L. C., & Reitan, R. M. (1961). Psychological deficits in relation to acuteness of brain dysfunction. *Journal of Consulting Psychology, 25*, 61-66.

Franzen, M., Iverson, G., & McCracken, L. (1990). The detection of malingering in neuropsychological assessment. *Neuropsychology Review, 1*, 247-279.

Garb, H., & Lutz, C. (2001). Cognitive complexity and the validity of clinicians' judgments. *Assessment, 8*, 111-115.

Gelb, A., & Goldstein, K. (1925). Ueber farbennamenamnesie [On color-perception amnesia]. *Psychologische Forschungin, 6*, 127-186.

Goebel, R. (1982). Detection of faking of the Halstead-Reitan Neuropsychological Test Battery. *Journal of Clinical Psychology, 39*, 731-742.

Golden, C. J. (1978). *The Stroop Color and Word Test: A Manual for Clinical and Experimental Uses.* Stoelting: Chicago, IL.

Golden, C. J., Kuperman, S. K., MacInnes, W. D., & Moses, J. A. (1981). Cross-validation of an abbreviated form of the Halstead Category Test. *Journal of Consulting and Clinical Psychology, 49*, 606-607.

Goodglass, H., & Kaplan, E. (1983). *Boston Diagnostic Aphasia Examination.* Philadelphia: Lea & Febiger.

Gordon, M., McClure, F. D., & Post, E. M. (1986). Interpretive guide to the Gordon Diagnostic System. DeWitt: Gordon Systems, Inc.

Grant, D. A., & Berg, E. A. (1948). A behavioral analysis of degree of impairment and ease of shifting new responses in a Weigl-type card sorting problem. *Journal of Experimental Psychology, 39*, 404-411.

Gregory, R. J., Paul, J. J., & Morrison, M. W. (1979). A short form of the Category Test for adults. *Journal of Clinical Psychology, 35*, 795-798.

Green, P., Allen, L. M., & Astner, K. (1996). The Word Memory Test: A user's guide to the oral and computer-administered forms, US version 1.1. Durham, NC: CognitSyst, Inc.

Greiffenstein, M., Baker, W.J., & Gola, T. (1994). Validation of malingered amnesia measures with a large clinical sample. *Psychological Assessment, 6*, 218-224.

Greiffenstein, M., Gola, T., & Baker, W. J. (1995). MMPI-2 validity scales versus domain specific measures in detection of factitious traumatic brain injury. *The Clinical Neuropsychologist, 9*, 230-240.

Guilmette, T. J., Faust, D., Hart, K., & Arkes, H. R. (1990). A national survey of psychologists who offer neuropsychological services. *Journal of Clinical Neuropsychology, 2*, 200-202.

Haines, M., & Norris, M. (1995). Detecting the malingering of cognitive deficits: An update. *Neuropsychology Review, 5*, 125-148.

Halstead, W. C. (1940). Preliminary analysis of grouping behavior in patients with cerebral injury by the method of equivalent and non-equivalent stimuli. *American Journal of Psychiatry, 96*, 1263-1294.

Halstead, W.C. (1947). *Brain and Intelligence. A Quantitative Study of the Frontal Lobes.* Chicago: University of Chicago Press.

Halstead, W. C., & Settlage, P. H. (1943). Grouping behavior of normal persons and of persons with lesions of the brain. *Archives of Neurology and Psychiatry, 49*, 489-503.

Halstead, W., & White, J. (1950). *Manual for the Halstead Battery of Neuropsychological Tests.* (Mimeographed manual.) Chicago: University of Chicago Press.

Heaton, R. K., Smith, H. H., Jr., Lehman, R. A. W., & Vogt, A. T. (1978). Prospects for faking believable deficits on neuropsychological testing. *Journal of Consulting and Clinical Psychology, 46*, 892-900.

Hiscock, M., & Hiscock, C. K. (1989). Refining the forced-choice method for the detection of malingering. *Journal of Clinical and Experimental Neuropsychology, 11*, 967-974.

Holz, J. L., Gearhart, L. P., & Watson, C. G. (1996). Comparability of scores on projector and booklet administration of the Category Test in brain-impaired veterans and controls. *Neuropsychology, 10*, 194-196.

Iverson, G. I., & Binder, L. M. (2000). Detecting exaggeration and malingering in neuropsychological assessment. *Journal of Head Trauma Rehabilitation, 15*, 829-858.

Iverson, G. I., Myers, B., & Adams, R. (1994). Specificity of the Category Test for detecting malingering. Paper presented at the annual meeting of the National Academy of Neuropsychology, Orlando, FL.

Johnstone, B., Holland, D., & Hewett, J. E. (1997). The construct validity of the Category Test: Is it a measure of reasoning or intelligence? *Psychological Assessment, 9*, 28-33.

Kimura, S. D. (1981). A card form of the Reitan modified Halstead Category Test. *Journal of Consulting and Clinical Psychology, 49*, 145-146.

Kleinmuntz, B. (1990). Why we still use our heads instead of formulas: Toward an integrative approach. *Psychological Bulletin, 107*, 296-310.

Klove, H. (1963). Clinical neuropsychology. In F. M. Forster (Ed.), *The Medical Clinics of North America*. New York: Saunders.

Laatsch, L., & Choca, J. (1991). Understanding the Category Test by using item analysis. *Psychological Assessment: A Journal of Consulting and Clinical Psychology, 3*, 701-704.

Lees-Haley, P. R., English, L. T., & Glenn, W. J. (1991). A fake bad scale on the MMPI-2 for personal injury claimants. *Psychological Reports, 68*, 203-210.

Lees-Haley, P. R., Smith, H. H., Williams, C. W., & Dunn, J. T. (1996). Forensic neuropsychological test usage: An empirical survey. *Archives of Clinical Neuropsychology, 11*, 45-51.

Levin, H. S., Mattis, S., Ruff, R. M., Eisenberg, H. M., et al. (1987). Neurobehavioral outcome following minor head injury: A three-center study. *Journal of Neurosurgery, 66*, 234-243.

Lezak, M. D. (1995). *Neuropsychological Assessment* (3d ed.). New York: Oxford University Press.

Markwardt, F. C. (1989). *Peabody Individual Achievement Test-Revised*. Circle Pines, MN: American Guidance Service.

Matthews, C. G., Shaw, D. J., & Kløve, H. (1966). Psychological test performance in neurologic and pseudoneurologic subjects. *Cortex, 2*, 244-253.

Mercer, W. N., Harrell, E. H., Miller, D. C., Childs, H. W., & Rockers, D. M. (1997). Performance of brain-injured versus healthy adults on three versions of the Category Test. *The Clinical Neuropsychologist, 11*, 174-179.

Miller, W., & Miller, E. S. (1992). Malingering and neuropsychological assessment. *Physical Medicine and Rehabilation: State of the Art Reviews, 6*, 547-563.

Millis, S. R. (1992). The Recognition Memory Test in the detection of malingered and exaggerated memory deficits. *The Clinical Neuropsychologist, 6*, 406-414.

Millis, S., & Putnam, S. (1996). Detection of malingering in postconcussive syndrome. In M. Rizzo & D. Tranel (Eds.) *Head Injury and Postconcussive Disorder* (pp. 481-498). New York: Churchill Livingstone.

Mitrushina, M. N., Boone, K. B., & D'Elia, L. F. (1999). *Handbook of Normative Data for Neuropsychological Assessment*. New York: Oxford University Press.

Mittenberg, W., Rotholc, A., Russell, E., & Heilbronner, R. (1996). Identification of malingered head injury on the Halstead-Reitan Battery. *Archives of Clinical Neuropsychology, 11*, 271-281.

Nies, K. J., & Sweet, J. J. (1994). Neuropsychological assessment and malingering: A critical review of past and present strategies. *Archives of Clinical Neuropsychology, 9*, 501-552.

Reed, J. C., & Reed, H. B. (1997). The Halstead-Reitan Neuropsychological Battery. In G. Goldstein & T. Incagnoli (Eds.) *Contemporary Approaches to Neuropsychological Assessment* (pp. 93-129). New York: Plenum Press.

Reitan, R. M. (1955). Investigation of the validity of Halstead's measures of biological intelligence. *Archives of Neurology and Psychiatry, 73*, 28-35.

Reitan, R. M. (1964). Psychological deficits resulting from cerebral lesions in man. In Warren, J. M., and Akert, K. A. (Eds.), *The Frontal Granular Cortex and Behavior* (pp. 295-312). New York: McGraw-Hill.

Reitan, R. M. (1969). *Manual for Administration of Neuropsychological Test Batteries for Adults and Children*. Indianapolis, IN.

Reitan, R. M., & Davison, L. A. (1974). *Clinical Neuropsychology: Current Status and Applications*. Washington, DC: V. H. Winston.

Reitan, R. M., & Wolfson, D. (1985). *The Halstead-Reitan Neuropsychological Test Battery*. Tucson, AZ: Neuropsychology Press.

Reitan, R. M., & Wolfson, D. (1992). Conventional intelligence measures and neuropsychological concepts of adaptive abilities. *Journal of Clinical Psychology, 48*, 521-529.

Reitan, R. M., & Wolfson, D. (1995). Category Test and Trail Making Test as measures of frontal lobe functions. *Journal of Clinical Neuropsychology, 9*, 50-56.

Reitan, R. M., & Wolfson, D. (1996). The question of validity of neuropsychological test scores among head-injured litigants: Development of a Dissimulation Index. *Archives of Clinical Neuropsychology, 11*, 573-580.

Rey, A. (1941). L'examen psychologique dans les cas d'encephalopathie traumatique. *Archives de Psychologie, 28*, 286-340.

Rey, A. (1964). *L'examen clinique en psychologie*. Paris: University of France Press.

Reynolds, C. R. (1998). *Detection of Malingering During Head Injury Litigation*. New York: Plenum Press.

Rogers, R. (1997). *Clinical Assessment of Malingering and Deception* (2nd ed.). New York: Guilford.

Rogers, R., Harrell, E., & Liff, C. (1993). Feigning neuropsychological impairment: A critical review of methodological and clinical considerations. *Clinical Psychology Review, 13*, 255-275.

Rosenfeld, J. P., Ellwanger, J., & Sweet, J. J. (1995). Detecting simulated amnesia with event-related brain potentials. *International Journal of Psychophysiology, 19*, 1-11.

Ruff, R. (1988). *Ruff Figural Fluency Test*. San Diego, CA: Neuropsychological Resources.

Russell, E. W. (1974). The effect of acute lateralized brain damage on Halstead's biological intelligence factors. *Journal of General Psychology, 90*, 101-107.

Russell, E. W., & Levy, M. (1987). Revision of the Halstead Category Test. *Journal of Consulting and Clinical Psychology, 55*, 898-901.

Sellers, A. H., & Nadler, J. D. (1992). A survey of current neuropsychological assessment procedures used for different age groups. *Psychotherapy in Private Practice, 11*, 47-57.

Seretny, M. L., Dean, R. S., Gray, J. W., & Hartlage, L. C. (1986). The practice of clinical neuropsychology in the United States. *Archives of Clinical Neuropsychology, 1*, 5-12.

Sherrill, R. E. (1985). Comparison of three short forms of the Category Test. *Journal of Clinical and Experimental Neuropsychology, 7*, 231-238.

Sherrill, R. E. (1987). Options for shortening Halstead's Category Test for adults. *Archives of Clinical Neuropsychology, 2*, 343-352.

Shure, G., & Halstead, W. C. (1958). Developmental variability in frontal lobe functioning. *Psychological Monographs, 72* (No. 465).

Simmel, M. S., & Counts, S. (1957). Some stable determinants of perception, thinking, and learning: A study based on the analysis of a single test. *Genetic Psychology Monographs, 56*, 3-157.

Slay, D. K. (1984). A portable Halstead-Reitan Category Test. *Journal of Clinical Psychology, 40*, 1023-1027.

Slick, D., Hopp, G., Strauss, E., & Thompson, G. (1997). *The Victoria Symptom Validity Test.* Odessa, FL: Psychological Assessment Resources.

Slick, D., Hopp, G., Strauss, E., & Spellacy, F. (1996). Victoria Symptom Validity Test: Efficiency for detecting feigned memory impairment and relationship to neuropsychological tests and MMPI-2 validity scales. *Journal of Clinical and Experimental Neuropsychology, 18*, 911-922.

Suchy, Y., & Sweet, J. J. (2000). Information/orientation subtest of the Wechsler Memory Scale-Revised as an indicator of suspicion of insufficient effort. *The Clinical Neuropsychologist, 14*, 56-66.

Sweet, J. (1999). Malingering: Differential diagnosis. In J. Sweet (Ed.) *Forensic Neuropsychology: Fundamentals and Practice* (pp. 255-286). Lisse, Netherlands: Swets & Zeitlinger.

Tenhula, W. N., & Sweet, J. J. (1996). Double cross-validation of the Booklet Category Test in detecting malingered traumatic brain injury. *The Clinical Neuropsychologist, 10*, 104-116.

Thomas, J. D., & Trexler, L. E. (1982). Behavioral and cognitive deficits in cerebrovascular accidents and closed head injury: Implications for cognitive rehabilitation. In Trexler, L. E. (Ed.), *Cognitive Rehabilitation: Conceptualization and Intervention* (pp. 27-61). New York: Plenum Press.

Tombaugh, T. N. (1996). *Test of Memory Malingering (TOMM).* New York: Multi Health Systems.

Trueblood, W., & Schmidt, M. (1993). Malingering and other validity considerations in the neuropsychological evaluation of mild head injury. *Journal of Clinical and Experimental Neuropsychology, 15*, 578-590.

Vega, A., & Parsons, O. A. (1967). Cross-validation of the Halstead-Reitan tests for brain damage. *Journal of Consulting and Clinical Psychology, 31*, 619-625.

Vickery, C., Berry, D., Inman, T., Harris, M., & Orey, S. (2001). Detection of inadequate effort on neuropsychological testing: A meta-analytic review of selected procedures. *Archives of Clinical Neuropsychology, 16*, 45-73.

Warrington, E. K. (1984). *Recognition Memory Test Manual.* Windsor, England: NFER-Nelson.

Wechsler, D. (1987). *Wechsler Memory Scale-Revised.* San Antonio, TX: The Psychological Corporation.

Wechsler, D. (1981). *Manual for the Wechsler Adult Intelligence Test-Revised.* San Antonio, TX: The Psychological Corporation.

Weigl, E. (1927). Zur psychologie sogenannter abstraktionsprozesse [On the psychology of the so-called abstraction process]. *Zeitschrift fur Psychologie, 103*, 1-45.

Wetzel, L., & Boll, T. J. (1987). *Short Category Test, Booklet Format.* Los Angeles: Western Psychological Services.

Wilkinson, G. S. (1993). *WRAT3 Administration Manual.* Wilmington: DE: Wide Range.

Williamson, D. J., Green, P., Allen, L., & Rohling, M. (in press). Evaluating effort with the Word Memory Test and Category Test–or not: Inconsistencies in a forensic sample. *Journal of Forensic Neuropsychology.*

Wood, W., & Strider, M. (1980). Comparison of two methods of administering the Halstead Category Test. *Journal of Clinical Psychology, 36,* 476-479.

Youngjohn, J., Lees-Haley, P., & Binder, L. (1999). Comment: Warning malingerers produces more sophisticated malingering. *Archives of Clinical Neuropsychology, 14,* 511-516.

Zachary, R. A. (1986). *Shipley Institute of Living Scale-Revised Manual.* Los Angeles, CA: Western Psychological Services.

Detection of Malingering and Invalid Test Results Using the Halstead-Reitan Battery

Ralph M. Reitan

Reitan Neuropsychology Laboratory

Deborah Wolfson

Reitan Neuropsychology Laboratory

SUMMARY. This paper describes procedures that are strikingly effective in demonstrating invalid test results among plaintiffs claiming losses from traumatic head injuries, raises serious questions about the invalidity of test results due to the influence and procedures of different examiners, and presents a description of procedures for evaluating the validity of test results for individual persons. Finally, this paper considers the adequacy of neuropsychological procedures in meeting the four *Daubert* criteria, and finds them generally lacking with respect to identifying the error rate in evaluating individual clients. It is apparent that expert witnesses in clinical neuropsychology must produce evidence that their testing procedures validly differentiate between brain-damaged and non-brain-damaged subjects, together with empirical determination of error-rates, if they are to meet the criteria defined by the Supreme Court. *[Article copies available for a fee from The Haworth Document Delivery Service: 1-800-HAWORTH. E-mail address: <getinfo@haworthpressinc.com> Website: <http://www.HaworthPress.com> © 2002 by The Haworth Press, Inc. All rights reserved.]*

Ralph M. Reitan and Deborah Wolfson are affiliated with Reitan Neuropsychology Laboratory, Tucson, AZ.

Address correspondence to: Ralph M. Reitan, PhD, Reitan Neuropsychology Laboratory, P.O. Box 66080, Tucson, AZ 85728.

[Haworth co-indexing entry note]: "Detection of Malingering and Invalid Test Results Using the Halstead-Reitan Battery." Reitan, Ralph M., and Deborah Wolfson. Co-published simultaneously in *Journal of Forensic Neuropsychology* (The Haworth Medical Press, an imprint of The Haworth Press, Inc.) Vol. 3, No. 1/2, 2002, pp. 275-314; and: *Detection of Response Bias in Forensic Neuropsychology* (ed: Jim Hom, and Robert L. Denney) The Haworth Medical Press, an imprint of The Haworth Press, Inc., 2002, pp. 275-314. Single or multiple copies of this article are available for a fee from The Haworth Document Delivery Service [1-800-HAWORTH, 9:00 a.m. - 5:00 p.m. (EST). E-mail address: getinfo@haworthpressinc.com].

© 2002 by The Haworth Press, Inc. All rights reserved.

KEYWORDS. Malingering, Halstead-Reitan Battery, Daubert, dissimulation

The problem of malingering, dissimulation, or even the non-deliberate production of invalid performances cuts at the core of the scientific basis of clinical practice in neuropsychology. The *Diagnostic and Statistical Manual of Mental Disorders* (DSM-IV; American Psychiatric Association, 1994) cautions that malingering should be strongly suspected if an examination is done in a medicolegal context (e.g., the client was referred by an attorney for an evaluation). Binder (1990), in his review of forensic cases, stated that malingering should be considered a possibility whenever the test results may be related to an opportunity for financial gain.

The obvious need for a valid index of malingering or dissimulation has led to many studies, most of which used normal subjects instructed to pretend that they were brain-injured while taking neuropsychological tests (for a review of this literature, see Franzen, Iverson, & McCracken, 1990; Nies & Sweet, 1994; Reynolds, 1998). Although a number of investigations reported statistically significant differences between feigned malingerers and groups not suspected of malingering, there are two major problems plaguing these research efforts.

First, it is naive to assume that normal subjects instructed to fake the type of deficits that would result from a head injury would actually be able to simulate the neuropsychological impairment caused by brain damage. The subjects–who are usually normal, unimpaired, and relatively young–typically know very little about the behaviors they are instructed to simulate (viz., neuropsychological deficits). In addition, normal subjects pretending to be brain-damaged share none of the stresses, anxieties, guilt, depression, and desperation experienced by many litigants whose future financial stability may depend on the outcome of the neuropsychological examination.

Many plaintiffs may not even realize that they are not putting forth their best possible effort when taking the tests. In such cases, the real-life situation is far different from the laboratory, and laboratory results are open to serious question. Since few subjects ever reveal that they have malingered, no one has been able to assemble a representative group large enough to perform even the first valid comparison of malingerers and non-malingerers. How can the unique characteristics of malingerers be identified if we cannot compose an appropriate group to study?

Second, the conceptual bases underlying the approaches used is open to question. Some approaches presume that a constant presentation of misinformation (for example, telling the client, "This test is difficult" when, in fact, it is quite easy) will be both accepted and dealt with in an invariable manner by each potential subject. We must recognize that variability is the essence of measurement! Some subjects will believe anything they are told, and others will believe little of what they are told, with the majority of subjects falling somewhere in-between.

The degree of impairment represents another potentially confounding variable. Some subjects are so impaired that "easy" tasks are for them quite difficult, and their performances earn scores that fall in the "malingering" range. We learned long ago, in studying neuropsychological test data among normals and brain-injured persons, that use of a cutoff point on a single test, which divides the population into two categories (brain-injured and non-brain-injured), was a conceptually naive undertaking that could hardly produce accurate results for individual subjects. We contend that malingering (and the production of invalid test results, for whatever reason) constitutes a behavior that is complex and has multi-faceted roots; that a "level of performance" approach, implemented by a predetermined cutoff score, can hardly be sufficiently accurate for general use in identifying and separating any sub-population from the population as a whole; and that approaches based on this concept cannot hope to yield anything more than suggestive information while the problem requires definitive information.

A second general approach has used statistical distributions and the probability that any single performance (score) fits under the Gaussian distribution. Although this approach will produce information that quantifies the unlikelihood of a performance with relation to expectation, the very concept on which it is based tends to defeat its purpose. Every response, regardless of its deviation, fits under the normal probability curve, and a finding that it would occur 5% or less of the time among normals (for example) still includes the score within the range of normal responses. A method that represents scores as "very normal," "somewhat normal," and "deviantly normal" does not classify subjects into discrete categories. The problem of identifying malingerers (or producers of invalid test results) requires accurate assignment of individual persons into appropriate categories rather than assignment into positions on a scale of normal variation.

We do not wish to imply that approaches based on the above-stated conceptual models are entirely without merit. We have all seen instances in which the obtained results complement other sources of information in a useful manner to facilitate conclusions about individual persons. In some such instances, test results have served to recommend personal observation of daily activities which, in turn, have produced unequivocal, recorded evidence that the subject can perform activities which controvert the subject's claimed disabilities. In other instances, such testing has led to readministration of previously given tests, which in turn have produced disparities in the results of the two examinations that have inescapable face-validity as indicators of inadequate or essentially invalid performances. However, labeling someone as a malingerer is a serious charge, and we cannot base our diagnoses on evidence prefaced by "the chances are," just as a neurosurgeon can hardly be satisfied with concluding that a patient has a malignant brain tumor, an arteriovenous malformation, or other serious condition based on equivocal findings.

COMMENTS ON RESEARCH REPORTS

Research studies of malingering, dissimulation, and production of invalid test results (knowingly or unknowingly, deliberately or as a result of complex, interacting, and essentially unidentified forces) have only occasionally utilized test batteries designed to evaluate an individual's broad range of adaptive abilities. The approach has customarily been to administer a single test or to examine a single set of performances based on a presumption that the distributions of malingerers and non-malingerers would be essentially non-overlapping, or at most, minimally overlapping. Use of a battery of tests, however, permits evaluation of intraindividual test scores in addition to comparisons of the subject's scores on individual tests with a population sample.

If malingering is viewed in the broader context of invalid test results, the nature of the problem as it relates to cerebral damage or dysfunction can be clarified. The psychologist's task may then be to differentiate between valid and invalid indications of brain impairment rather than to evaluate the sincerity of the subject's motivation or effort when taking the tests. Presumably, malingerers (or subjects instructed to malinger) would not produce test results that reflected the genuine effects of brain damage, and this would reveal the invalidity of the malingerer's test results.

Individual tests are usually interpreted in terms of how well they are performed, and the method generally used to detect malingering is to identify scores that are lower than expected. Considering the range of performances on individual tests among non-malingerers, this simplistic model would be difficult to apply with any degree of accuracy. A battery of tests, however, would produce scores that allow comparisons of the individual's performances across a range of tests. Thus, a subject's scores could be compared to each other (an intraindividual approach) as well as to normative data (an interindividual approach). If the test battery was both sensitive and specific for brain injury, there might be a useful and valid basis for separating legitimate indications of brain damage from simulated scores. A fundamental problem with this approach, however, is that it depends upon the ability of the neuropsychologist to recognize valid manifestations of brain damage, to identify patterns and relationships that are valid indications of brain disorders, and to differentially identify normal inter-test variations, inter-test variations that reflect brain disease or damage, and inter-test variations that do not fall in either of these two categories. This type of insight may well be beyond the clinical skill of many neuropsychologists, and in any case, is difficult to verify with respect to accuracy.

In one sense, these considerations are reminiscent of the history and background from which current clinical procedures for neuropsychological assessment developed. Many neuropsychologists can remember the search to find a test of "brain damage" and the debates (and arguments) concerning which test was most effective. It appears that the approach to identifying malingerers is currently at a similar primitive stage. The field of neuropsychology now views the prior attempts to develop the "ultimate test" for brain damage as simplistic and misguided, and recognizes that such a unidimensional approach would never have led to a scientific understanding of the complexity of the behaviors subserved by the brain.

An example that used a battery rather than one or more tests individually was provided by a study done by Goebel (1983). Goebel used the Halstead-Reitan Battery to identify protocols that genuinely reflected brain damage and to differentiate the legitimate protocols from the test results produced by normal subjects instructed to fake the effects of brain damage. He composed three groups: (1) 52 subjects with documented cerebral disease or damage, (2) 50 volunteer subjects presumed to not have brain damage, and (3) 152 volunteer college students also believed to be non-impaired. The non-brain-damaged subjects were divided into four subgroups: one group of controls and three groups instructed to pretend that they had either right, left, or diffuse cerebral damage. The non-brain-damaged subjects were not given any specific information about the known effects of brain damage; instead, they were instructed only to alter their normal performances as if they had actually sustained brain damage and to attempt to produce believable and realistic test results.

The Halstead-Reitan Battery was individually administered by two technicians trained and supervised by Goebel. Although the technicians were not informed of any subject's classification, they felt that it was "fairly easy" to detect fakers on the basis of the behavioral observations they made during the testing.

Goebel analyzed the results both statistically and through clinical evaluation of protocols. In each case, the brain-damaged subjects were differentiated at a highly significant level from the volunteers pretending to be brain-damaged. Each analysis showed that 97% or 98% of the "pretenders" were unable to successfully simulate the effects of brain damage. The brain-damaged subjects were classified with a somewhat lower accuracy rate; about 79% were identified correctly on the basis of clinical evaluation, and a slightly higher percentage was correctly classified using discriminant functions as a basis for predicting group membership.

Considering the practical problems inherent in this type of research, it is not surprising that several aspects of Goebel's study have been criticized (Faust, Ziskin, & Hiers, 1991). In Goebel's study the majority of the brain-damaged patients were male, and gender distributions were not perfectly equivalent in the subgroups of non-brain-damaged subjects. Goebel cautioned against uncritical generalizations based on the findings, pointing out that normal subjects instructed to fake brain damage do not necessarily perform the same as true malingerers. During the post-experiment debriefing, many subjects reported feeling that they did not know enough about brain damage to be able to simulate the behavioral correlates effectively, and were uncomfortable in attempting to do so.

Finally, in terms of the results based on clinical interpretations, Goebel's study must be viewed as having an *N* of 1. The judgments were made only by the author, and it is unknown whether comparable classifications would have been made by other judges. Despite these possible problems, the results strongly suggest that the data produced by the subjects provided a basis for a rather striking differentiation between brain-damaged subjects and volunteers pretending to be brain-damaged. It should be recognized that this study was based on a major conceptual difference from most studies in this area–it was designed to permit evaluations of *intraindividual* differences in test scores as well as *interindividual* differences (differences in test performances of the individual subject from test scores produced by the population on a single test). However, Goebel's results, which were based on an approach using intraindividual differences among tests as well as normative evaluations (as is routinely done in clinical evaluation of a battery of test scores), deserves further study and exploration in a systematic context.

USE OF INTRAINDIVIDUAL TEST SCORES TO IDENTIFY INVALID TEST RESULTS

The task of identifying individual malingerers or dissimulators on the basis of psychological testing appears to be no different in principle from diagnostic testing that evaluates the full range of psychiatric and neurological conditions. Psychologists have depended principally upon level of performance to draw conclusions about a subject's neuropsychological functioning, and use of this model alone is hardly adequate. Some psychiatric and neurological conditions, for example, are presumed to be associated with impaired performances, but in many cases psychiatric and neurological subjects perform within the normal range. Considering the broad range of performances found in the general population, it is unlikely that valid diagnostic conclusions can consistently be inferred in individual cases using a method based only on interindividual comparisons.

Many years ago, Reitan (1967) published a description of the systematic use of different approaches to interpret neuropsychological test data, and demonstrated with individual case illustrations how to use these various approaches in a complementary manner to draw inferences about neuropsychological diagnoses. The subject's level of performance was useful, but not uncommonly some test scores were in the normal range and some scores were impaired. This fact by itself represented the basis for a second approach to evaluation of test scores.

For example, if a subject performed poorly on tests that were sensitive to brain damage and performed relatively well on tests that were not sensitive, a comparison of these performances might have diagnostic significance. This method, probably used first by Babcock (1930), was utilized by a number of other psychologists, including Wechsler (1955) and Hunt (1943). This approach to interpretation used intraindividual test scores (comparing the subject with himself or herself on various tests) as contrasted with evaluating interindividual test scores (comparing the subject's scores with the rest of the population). Modifications of this procedure, especially in clinical neuropsychology, compared a subject's performance on the same test on each side of the body to make inferences about the status of the two cerebral hemispheres. An intra-individual approach to test interpretation uses the subject as his or her own control, and the wide range of variability, commonly seen in the general population, is thereby largely controlled.

The case of Albert Johnson, presented below, illustrates the critical importance of considering disparities among tests as an additional approach to detection of invalid scores.

THE CASE OF ALBERT JOHNSON

This approach to interpretation is illustrated by the case of Albert Johnson, a 54-year-old man who was involved in a moving vehicle accident and sustained multiple injuries, particularly to his face, chest, and abdomen. The testing was done by a technician under the direction of an experienced clinical neuropsychologist hired by Mr. Johnson's attorney. The purpose of the examination was to determine whether Mr. Johnson demonstrated any impairment that might be attributed to the head injury. Before the testing began, Mr. Johnson was advised to perform as well as he could on every test and to ask for more information if any procedure was not clear to him. The examiner believed that Mr. Johnson put forth his best effort during the examination and that a valid set of test results had been obtained.

At this point it may be instructive for readers who are familiar with the Halstead-Reitan Battery (HRB) to review Mr. Johnson's test results (Figure 1) to determine whether there are any significant indications of impairment. Also, analyze the findings for any inconsistencies in adequacy of performance that might imply that Mr. Johnson was malingering or not putting forth adequate effort when performing a task.

Mr. Johnson earned a Verbal IQ of 104, a score slightly above the Average level. His Performance IQ of 85 was 19 points lower, falling in the Low Average range. His lowest scaled score on the Verbal subtests was 9; his highest scaled score on the Performance subtests was only 7. These results suggest that Mr. Johnson was consistently less able on the Performance subtests than the Verbal subtests. Results of this kind have been associated with right cerebral damage, but before any such conclusions can be drawn it would be necessary, at least, to have determined whether any evidence of cerebral damage was present.

Mr. Johnson's General Neuropsychological Deficit Scale (GNDS) score of 26 was a borderline value, falling just above the cutoff point of

FIGURE 1. Test results for Albert Johnson.

The Halstead–Reitan Neuropsychological Test Battery for Adults

Name: Albert Johnson — Age: 54
Gender: M — Education: 11 — Handedness: (RH) 7 LH 0

Neuropsychological Deficit Scale (NDS) Summary

General NDS	
Level of Performance	15
Pathognomonic Signs	2
Patterns	3
Right/Left Differences	8
Total GNDS Score	28
Left NDS	4
Right NDS	10

WAIS–R

VIQ	104
PIQ	85
FSIQ	95

Verbal Subtests		Performance Subtests	
Information	9	Digit Symbol	6
Comprehension	9	Picture Completion	6
Arithmetic	12	Block Design	7
Similarities	9	Picture Arrangement	6
Digit Span	12	Object Assembly	6
Vocabulary	12		

Minnesota Multiphasic Personality Inventory (MMPI)

		Hs	72
		D	80
		Hy	62
L	73	PD	55
F	55	MF	43
K	55	Pa	44
		Pt	52
		Sc	56
		Ma	43
		SI	62

Strength of Grip

Dominant hand (R) 50.5 kg
Non–dominant hand (L) 49.0 kg

Name Writing

Dominant hand (R) 4 sec
Non–dominant hand (L) 16 sec

Aphasia Screening Test: No dysphasia, but note drawing of the key.

Category Test

Number of errors: 90

Tactual Performance Test

Dominant hand (R)	8.8	Total Time	23.0
Non–dominant hand (L)	9.0	Memory	8
Both hands	5.2	Localization	3

Seashore Rhythm Test

Number correct: 23 — 9

Speech–sounds Perception Test

Number of errors: 14

Finger Tapping Test

Dominant hand (R) 56 — 56
Non–dominant hand (L) 55

Impairment Index

0.7

Trail Making Test

Part A	26 sec	0 error(s)
Part B	36 sec	0 error(s)

Bilateral Simultaneous Sensory Stimulation

RH	0	LH	0	Both: RH	0	LH	0
RH	0	LF	0	Both: RH	0	LF	0
LH	0	RF	0	Both: LH	0	RF	0
RE	0	LE	0	Both: RE	0	LE	0
RV	0	LV	0	Both: RV	0	LV	0
	0		0		0		0
	0		0		0		0

Tactile Finger Recognition

RH 1 ___ 2 ___ 3 ___ 4 ___ 5 ___ RH 0 / 20
LH 1 ___ 2 ___ 3 ___ 4 ___ 5 ___ LH 0 / 20

Finger–Tip Number Writing

RH 1 ___ 2 ___ 3 ___ 4 ___ 5 ___ RH 0 / 20
LH 1 ___ 2 ___ 3 ___ 4 ___ 5 ___ LH 0 / 20

Tactile Form Recognition Test

Dominant hand (R)	12 sec	0 error(s)
Non–dominant hand (L)	9 sec	0 error(s)

©1991, Ralph M. Reitan, Ph.D. Reitan Neuropsychology Laboratory Tucson, Arizona

25/26. The Left Neuropsychological Deficit Scale (LNDS) score of 4 was significantly less than the Right Neuropsychological Deficit Scale (RNDS) score of 10, indicating that Mr. Johnson might have very mild impairment of brain functions, with the right hemisphere more dysfunctional than the left hemisphere.

Three of the other four HRB measures that are most sensitive to brain damage had scores in the impaired range: Impairment Index, 0.7; Category Test, 90 errors; and Tactual Performance Test (TPT)-Localization component, 3. Note, though, that Mr. Johnson performed extremely well on Part B of the Trail Making Test, completing the task in just 36 sec.

Mr. Johnson also tended to perform somewhat poorly on other measures of central processing. Although he did relatively well on the Memory component of the TPT (8), his Total Time score of 23.0 min was clearly in the impaired range. His scores on the Rhythm Test (23 correct) and the Speech-sounds Perception Test (14 errors) were also in the impaired range.

Mr. Johnson's finger tapping speed and grip strength were adequate bilaterally, and there were no significant sensory-perceptual deficits. These scores provide a basis for presuming that the relatively long TPT trials were due to higher-level rather than lower-level deficits. The test results up to this point reveal that Mr. Johnson performed poorly on a number of tests, with the overall findings indicating mild generalized neuropsychological impairment.

Although the RNDS score (10) was considerably higher than the LNDS score (4), clinical evaluation of the lateralized findings suggested that the cerebral dysfunction was approximately equivalent for each hemisphere. Right cerebral indicators included the finding that on the TPT Mr. Johnson was slow with his left hand as compared with his right hand. Although most of the Aphasia Screening Test figures (Figure 2) were drawn quite well, the mistakes he made reproducing the key are characteristic of persons with right hemisphere dysfunction.

There were several indications of left hemisphere impairment: somewhat slow finger tapping speed and grip strength with the right upper extremity as compared with the left upper extremity (even though the level of performance was adequate on both sides) and a somewhat slower response time with the right hand than the left on the Tactile Form Recognition Test. Thus, in terms of overall assessment, the lateralizing indicators were not particularly strong or entirely convincing, but they were fairly characteristic of the type of impairment demon-

FIGURE 2. Aphasia Screening Test drawings for Albert Johnson.

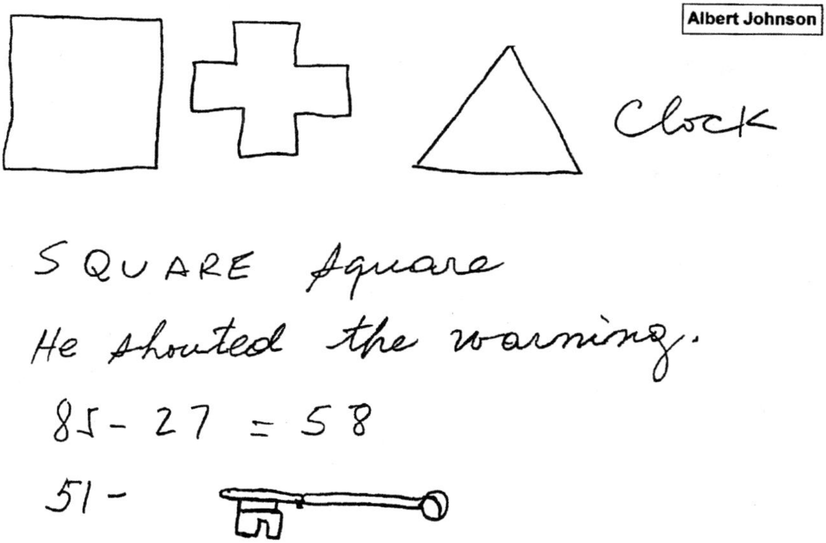

strated by persons with a closed head injury. The rest of the test results were also consistent with this interpretation.

Mr. Johnson's MMPI profile revealed various types of emotional complaints with elements of depression. Although elevated scores on the neurotic triad are not diagnostic of a brain injury, such configurations are not uncommon among head-injured subjects (Reitan, 1955).

These findings led the neuropsychologist hired by the plaintiff's attorney to conclude that Mr. Johnson exhibited mild to moderate brain damage, manifested by impairment of frontal reasoning processes (based particularly on the Category Test score of 90 errors). This conclusion was in turn based on a presumption that the Category Test is a "frontal lobe" test; the neuropsychologist was not aware of the scientific study demonstrating that the Category Test has essentially no specificity for frontal damage (Reitan & Wolfson, 1995a).

This neuropsychologist also concluded that Mr. Johnson had motoric and auditory processing deficits implicating the parietal and temporal areas. (It is somewhat difficult to infer the psychologist's basis for this conclusion. He perhaps incorrectly presumed that the Rhythm Test score of 23 implicated the right temporal area [see Reitan & Wolfson, 1989], and with regard to motor deficits, had noted that finger tapping and grip strength were only slightly better with the right hand than the left hand, whereas TPT performance was comparatively poor with the left hand.) (See the summary sheet for details.)

The neuropsychologist judged that the right hemisphere dysfunction was greater than the left hemisphere impairment, and attributed this to a possible contra-coup effect because the patient was reportedly struck on the left side of the head. The depression and anxiety demonstrated on the MMPI were attributed to Mr. Johnson's physical injury as well as his cognitive deficits. Finally, since the injury occurred 14 months prior to the neuropsychological examination, the neuropsychologist concluded that Mr. Johnson's cognitive impairment was most likely to be permanent.

While it is understandable how a conclusion of brain damage might be inferred from these test results, experienced neuropsychologists would note one particular finding that would cast significant doubt on this interpretation. Mr. Johnson completed Part B of the Trail Making Test in only 36 sec–an extremely good score even for persons of high intelligence and excellent neuropsychological abilities. The neuropsychologist who interpreted the test results observed that the client had performed relatively well on certain tests, and remarked that this was to be expected even in cases of mild to moderate brain injury. In fact, the neuropsychologist claimed that Mr. Johnson's good performances supported his contention that the client was making his best effort to do well on the tests.

If the neuropsychologist had referred to the Manual for Administration of the Trail Making Test, it would have been clear that not a single subject out of a sample of 200 brain-damaged subjects was able to complete Part B in less than 46 sec, and only 4 of these 200 subjects had scores of 69 sec or less. Only 2 of the 84 non-brain-damaged control subjects were able to complete Trails B in 36 sec or less.

If Mr. Johnson could complete Trails B in 36 sec, it is reasonable to conclude that his poor performances, particularly on the Category Test, were unlikely to represent his best effort. Even if a subject decides to do poorly on an examination to support a claim of brain injury, he or she must still expend some effort to perform reasonably well on at least some of the tests in order to make the overall performance appear credible. The malingerer's challenge is to produce a credible performance while still performing more poorly, at least on some tests, than represents his actual ability level–all without benefit of knowledge of normative data. When the subject has no knowledge of normative data, his or her ability to produce a set of test results that credibly reflect brain impairment is naturally limited. As in Mr. Johnson's case, it is likely that a malingerer will have one or more test scores that are entirely incongruous with the other test results and previous examinations.

It must also be recognized that even though internal inconsistencies in a set of test results may cast doubt on the validity of the subject's performances, there is no guarantee that the inconsistencies will reach the level of detection in every case. One of the basic limitations of using a method that identifies inconsistencies among test results on a single examination is that the only way to evaluate a subject's performance on each test is to compare the subject's score to normative standards (performances by the rest of the population). Most subjects demonstrate some variability in performance on a battery of tests, and the ability to identify which disparities are essentially impossible often depends heavily upon the neuropsychologist's experience and clinical judgment.

This approach to identifying malingering could also be criticized for being opportunistic in selecting which particular tests to compare. In Mr. Johnson's case we selected his good score of 36 sec on Trails B to compare with his score of 90 errors on the Category Test. We did not mention that Mr. Johnson was able to complete 80 trials on tests of tactile finger localization and finger-tip number writing without making a single error. The inexperienced neuropsychologist might consider perfect scores on finger localization and finger-tip number writing more remarkable than a score of 36 sec on Trails B, but the experienced neuropsychologist would know that a subject is far more likely to demonstrate no errors on the 80 sensory-perceptual trials than to complete Trails B in 36 sec.

Conclusions based on inconsistencies among test scores obviously depend on demonstration of such inconsistencies. If the defense attorney were to propose that Mr. Johnson's test results were invalid because of certain inconsistencies, the plaintiff's neuropsychologist could respond by comparing each test score against every other test score. Such a comparison would almost certainly reveal much more consistency than inconsistency, since many of Mr. Johnson's scores reflected at least a mild degree of impairment. If the defense's neuropsychologist claimed that the plaintiff's scores were inconsistent, he or she could easily be accused of focusing on selected test scores rather than performing an overall evaluation of the consistency of performances. Although the testifying neuropsychologist might protest and point out that there were gross inconsistencies in the plaintiff's performances, the protest would still be based on clinical experience rather than documented evidence.

In conclusion, although it might be quite possible for an experienced neuropsychologist to correctly identify the invalidity of a subject's test protocol on the basis of inconsistencies among scores, there appear to be significant barriers to using this method in a fully convincing manner.

IDENTIFYING INVALID TEST RESULTS BY COMPARING TWO OR MORE TESTINGS

As noted above, most of the psychometric approaches used to detect malingering have evaluated test scores based on a single examination, with the results interpreted in terms of adequacy (or level) of performance. This method, which compares the subject's test scores to the rest of the population, has the disadvantage of battling the normal probability curve. Because malingerers are not the only subjects who perform poorly on neuropsychological tests, the level-of-performance approach has a serious inherent problem. Obviously, 50% of the normal population fall below the average level of performance, and severely impaired individuals often produce legitimately poor scores. Severe cognitive impairment may be associated with a degree of confusion that produces scores well below a chance level. It must be recognized that malingerers may earn relatively good scores on a test even though they are not expending their best effort and are performing below their optimal level. A level-of-performance approach would completely fail to identify such malingerers.

In a prior section of this paper, we illustrated the implicit value as well as the problems in identifying malingerers by using an approach based on an evaluation of intraindividual (as compared with interindividual) test scores. In some cases (such as Albert Johnson's), a subject's performance on one test as compared with other tests may be a dependable basis for questioning the validity of the entire set of test scores. There is no assurance, though, that this approach would identify every person who was malingering. As we pointed out, there are additional problems that concern the expertise of the neuropsychologist and use of clinical judgment in implementing this method.

However, intraindividual test score comparisons are not limited to comparing different tests administered at the same time. Another useful approach is to compare the subject's scores on the same test administered on two different occasions. This method also uses intraindividual comparisons of test scores (using the subject as his/her own control), and avoids the problems implicit in interindividual evaluations. We have been using this approach since the late 1970's to evaluate the validity of test scores produced by persons involved in litigation. We have frequently observed remarkable, and seemingly unbelievable, changes in test scores on the two examinations. These observations support the contention that subjects who are malingering or not putting forth their best possible effort (as might occur in persons involved in litigation) respond less consistently, on separate examinations using the same tests, than subjects who are not adversely influenced by circumstantial factors.

For example, a subject may not remember the response he or she gave on the first testing to an item on the Information or Vocabulary subtest of the Wechsler Scale, and on the second testing give a response that is inferior (or perhaps superior) to the answer given on the first testing. Alternatively, persons without ulterior motives influencing their performances might be presumed to show less variability on the two testings because each response represented their best possible effort. Thus, test-retest comparisons can be performed by comparing the score produced on the same test administered on two different occasions and by comparing and analyzing responses to individual test items.

Cullum, Heaton, and Grant (1991), researchers who used three cases to illustrate this approach, stated that they believed that this was a previously unstudied method for detecting invalid test results. These authors compared subjects' performances on an extensive battery of tests on serial examinations and found highly variable performances that exceeded the presumed range for normal or neurologically stable subjects. Cullum et al. stated that "examination of performance reliability across testings may be a powerful means by which the neuropsychologist can detect patients who are not consistently putting forth adequate effort on the examination" (p. 168).

We have used this method for more than 20 years and have often constructed charts to use during trial to illustrate the inconsistency of a plaintiff's responses. Information presented in this manner is quite understandable and convincing to jurors. For example, if a subject is able on the first testing to name the capital of Italy and on the second examination has no idea of the correct response, an explanation would seem to be necessary. If some type of traumatic event occurred that affected the litigant's memory, the explanation might be obvious. In the absence of such a traumatic event, a more likely possibility is that the litigant was not expressing his or her best effort on the second examination, particularly if the pattern of knowing and then not knowing the correct answer was displayed in a number of instances.

RESEARCH RESULTS: DEVELOPMENT OF SPECIFIC QUANTITATIVE PROCEDURES FOR DETECTING INVALIDITY OF NEUROPSYCHOLOGICAL TEST RESULTS

Few (if any) subjects admit that they have malingered. Although convincing evidence that a subject has malingered is discovered and actually documented in only a small number of cases, reasons often abound for suspecting that a subject has malingered or failed to put forth the best possible effort. Since a group of proved malingerers has never been available for study (and if they were, one would have to question the validity of the results they produced!) how can the manifestations of malingering be discerned? Where would we be today in our understanding of the effects of brain damage if we had never studied a single group of persons with unequivocally established brain damage? The problem of malingering or dissimulation is even more complex, because it is entirely possible that many people, given the stresses and circumstances under which they are tested, may not even realize that they are not putting forth their best possible effort during a neuropsychological examination.

Considering the nature of the problem, and realizing that a focal point of concern often centers on the test result of litigants, we decided that practical and pertinent information might be discerned by comparing the neuropsychological test results of head-injured litigants with the performances of head-injured non-litigants. Because many litigants are tested more than once before their case is finally settled, appropriate data are often available. We also had data from a research project involving serial testing of subjects who had never been involved in litigation because second-party liability was not an issue.

Our hypothesis was that there would be a significant advantage in comparing the subject's test results obtained on two testings rather than comparing the subject's scores with the rest of the population. If the subject performed to the best of his or her ability on both examinations, one would presume that the scores on the second testing would be at least comparable or possibly better (because of practice-effects and/or recovery). If the subject was not putting forth his or her best effort, the scores on the two testings would be more variable, and perhaps even worse on the second testing, because of the need to "prove" one's impairment to others, such as insurance investigators or a jury.

We published three studies (Reitan & Wolfson, 1995b, 1995c, 1995d) that compared the test results of two groups of adult head-injured subjects. One group was involved in litigation related to the head injury; the other group was not. The same groups were used in all three studies.

Study 1: Consistency of Test Scores: Development of the Re-Test Consistency Index

Participants: The non-litigation group was composed of 17 males and 3 females who had sustained a head injury but were not involved in litigation. All of these subjects had volunteered to participate in a research project. The litigation group consisted of 14 males and 6 females, all of whom were involved in litigation to recover damages allegedly resulting from a head injury. It was impossible to accurately compare the severity of the head injuries in the two groups, primarily because the records of the litigation group varied and the diagnostic procedures had been performed in various locations. This made it difficult to obtain detailed and consistent records.

Neither group of subjects had been included in any systematic cognitive rehabilitation program, although a few subjects in the litigation group had received sporadic training to improve attention, concentration, memory, or other cognitive functions.

The mean age was 29.65 years (SD = 14.91) for the non-litigants and 41.85 years (SD = 10.19) for the litigants. The mean education was 12.30 years (SD = 2.23) for the non-litigants and 13.95 years (SD = 2.84) for the litigants. Comparisons of the distributions to evaluate age and education differences yielded t ratios of 3.02 ($p < .01$) and 2.05 ($p = .05$), respectively. Because of the differences in age and education distributions between the two groups and the inadequate comparative information about the severity of the subjects' head injuries, no direct comparisons were made of mean achievement (or error) scores on the various tests. Statistical analyses were based only on intraindividual difference scores that compared each subject's test scores obtained on two examinations which, since they were comparing the subjects against themselves, should not have been influenced to any great extent by differences in the age or education distributions.

The mean time between the two examinations was 12.00 months for the non-litigants and 14.45 months for the litigants. The intergroup difference was not statistically significant ($p < .20$). However, the non-litigants were initially tested soon after the head injury was sustained, whereas the litigants were initially tested at variable times following head injury.

An intergroup difference that may have been of significance derives from the fact that all of the non-litigants were examined on a strict schedule (they were initially tested within several weeks of the injury and retested 12 months later), whereas the litigants were initially tested at varying intervals following their head injuries. Thus, the non-litigation group may have had a somewhat greater potential for demonstrating spontaneous recovery.

Another factor that may have had an influence on the results of this study was that all of the non-litigants were tested by technicians who had been trained by and were directly responsible to one of the authors (RMR). These technicians were schooled in precise and objective test administration, and specifically in methods for obtaining the best possible performances on tests that permitted such examiner-patient interactions. Subjects in the litigation group had usually been tested by opposing representatives of an adversarial procedure, hired by either the plaintiff or the defense. In 12 cases, Testing I was done by the plaintiff's psychologist and Testing II was performed by the defense psychologist; in 5 cases, Testing I and Testing II were done by different psychologists hired by the plaintiff; in 2 cases, Testing I was done for clinical purposes and Testing II was done by the plaintiff's psychologist; and in 1 case, Testing I was done by the plaintiff's psychologist and Testing II was performed by a neutral psychologist.

One might presume that examiner bias, if it existed in the litigation group, would be in the direction of finding less impairment by the defense psychologist, leading to a trend for better scores on the second testing.

Method. This study used intraindividual differences in test scores on the two testing for comparison of the two groups.

Procedure. Study 1, concerned with consistency of test scores, focused on tests that traditionally have been demonstrated to be relatively insensitive to brain damage (taken from the Wechsler Scale) and tests that have been shown to be particularly sensitive to brain damage (taken from the Wechsler Scale and the Halstead-Reitan Battery). The postulate was that head-injured subjects involved in litigation would perform more poorly on the second examination than on the first, and head-injured subjects not in litigation would show improvement on the second examination (due to positive practice effects as well as spontaneous recovery). Thus, in accordance with the principle demonstrated by Reitan and Wolfson (1988) in their study of spontaneous recovery after head injury, we expected the greatest degree of improvement to occur on the tests that are most sensitive to brain damage.

The tests believed to be less sensitive measures were the Information, Comprehension, Arithmetic, Similarities, and Vocabulary subtests from either the WAIS or the WAIS-R. The more sensitive measures were the Picture Arrangement, Block Design, and Digit Symbol subtests from either the WAIS or WAIS-R, and the Category Test, Part B of the Trail Making Test, and the Localization component of the Tactual Performance Test (TPT-Localization) from the Halstead-Reitan Battery.

Mean scores and standard deviations were calculated for each variable in each group. Mean changes between Testing I and Testing II were compared in each group by evaluating difference score distributions for each variable using *t* tests.

Only the tests that achieved a probability level of .025 or less were used to compute the Retest Consistency Index. Six tests reached the specified level of significance in differentiating the two groups: Comprehension, Picture Arrangement, Digit Symbol, the Category Test, Part B of the Trail Making Test, and TPT-Localization. Difference scores on these tests for the combined litigation and non-litigation groups were transformed to a 5-point scale to reflect the degree of inconsistency (a score of 5 indicated the greatest degree of inconsistency; a score of 1 reflected the least degree of inconsistency). Using *t* ratios, means for the two groups were compared for the total of the scaled scores for the six most sensitive tests (the Retest Consistency Index) as well as for the individual tests.

The distributions, based on the 5-point scale, were compared for the litigation group and the non-litigation group, and a cutoff point that best differentiated the two groups was determined for the Retest Consistency Index.

Results. Table 1 presents means, standard deviations, *t* ratios comparing results of the first and second testings within each group, probability levels, and the proportion of subjects in each group that earned better scores on the second testing.

The non-litigation group had improved mean values on each of the 11 tests, and on each test, more than 50% of these subjects had improved scores on Testing II. The improvement was statistically significant, however, only for Picture Arrangement, Digit Symbol, the Category Test, Part B of the Trail Making Test, and TPT-Localization. Conversely, on Testing II the litigation group had poorer means on each of the 11 tests. Less than 50% of the subjects in the litigation group

TABLE 1. Means and Standard Deviations on Testings I and II for Non-Litigation and Litigation Groups; Comparisons of Testing I and II for Each Group; Percentage of Each Group Showing Improved Scores on Testing II; and Comparison of Difference Score Distributions, Based on Testing I and II, for the Two Groups

Group			Inf	Comp	Arith	Simil	Vocab	PA	BD	Digit Symbol	Category	Trails B	TPT-Loc
Non-Litigation	Testing I	M	10.20	10.45	9.10	11.60	10.10	9.00	11.40	8.75	45.95	109.00	3.25
		SD	3.27	3.65	4.91	4.22	3.57	3.31	3.68	3.42	27.88	63.91	1.65
	Testing II	M	10.45	11.30	9.95	11.70	10.20	11.00	11.70	12.05	35.90	89.40	4.35
		SD	3.27	3.80	4.48	4.66	3.93	3.77	3.60	3.50	27.45	53.76	2.52
			1.05	1.93	1.47	0.27	0.37	3.20	0.75	3.89	3.47	2.51	2.34
		p <	.40	.10	.20	.90	.80	.005	.50	.001	.001	.025	.05
	% Improving on Testing II		55	62.5	60	55	52.5	72.5	62.5	100	80	72.5	77.5
Litigation	Testing I	M	9.75	9.65	8.10	9.25	10.20	9.00	7.55	7.15	65.80	118.85	2.60
		SD	2.07	2.70	2.77	2.84	2.42	2.38	2.16	2.25	27.13	64.55	1.90
	Testing II	M	8.85	8.70	7.65	8.35	9.20	7.50	7.15	5.20	80.20	153.50	1.75
		SD	2.50	2.39	3.30	2.62	2.14	2.74	2.80	1.58	33.57	79.94	1.25
		t	1.69	1.58	0.68	2.20	2.21	2.24	0.79	4.45	2.66	2.14	1.95
		p<	.20	.20	.50	.05	.05	.05	.50	.001	.02	.05	.10
	% Improving on Testing II		40	40	37.5	32.5	30	30	45	22.5	30	27.5	30

showed improvement on the second examination, with the changes reaching significance at less than the .05 level on Similarities, Vocabulary, Picture Arrangement, Digit Symbol, the Category Test, and Part B of the Trail Making Test.

Although it was apparent that the general direction of change on Testing II was different for the two groups on every variable, the significance of intergroup differences was tested directly by comparing difference score distributions for the two groups on Testing I and Testing II. Mean difference scores between Testing I and Testing II for each group and the significance of differences in the two groups are presented in Table 2.

As shown in Table 2, the probability levels on each test were equivalent to or less than the probability levels presented in Table 1 for the groups individually. This reflects the fact that the direction of change (better versus poorer scores on Testing II) was different for the two groups on each variable, consistently leading to larger inter- than intragroup differences.

The next step was to develop a 5-point scale for converting difference scores to scaled scores. We included only those measures that yielded probability estimates of .025 or less and on which the two groups showed clearly significant differences. The six tests that met these criteria (see Table 2) were Comprehension, Picture Arrangement, Digit Symbol, the Category Test, Part B of the Trail Making Test, and TPT-Localization. Distributions of difference scores for the combined groups were tallied, and a score of 5 was assigned to the eight subjects (20% of the combined groups) who had the most inconsistent retest scores. A score of 4 was assigned to the next 20%, and so on, to a score of 1 for the most consistent subjects. (Some tied scores made it impossible to do this perfectly, but the 20% categorization was followed as closely as possible.) Table 3 presents the chart for converting difference scores to scaled scores.

Difference scores between Testing I and Testing II for individual subjects were computed so that negative values corresponded with a poorer performance on the second examination, regardless of whether the test score represented an achievement score or an error score.

Finally, the distributions on this 5-point scale were compared in the litigation and non-litigation groups for each of the six tests that contribute to the Retest Consistency Index. As shown in Table 4, these scores were greater on each of the six measures for the litigation group than for the non-litigation group, and the differences between the groups were statistically significant in each comparison. Nevertheless, there was a

TABLE 2. Mean Difference Scores Based on Testing I and Testing II, t Tests Comparing the Difference Score Distributions for the Non-Litigation and Litigation Groups, and Probability Levels

Group		Inf	Comp	Arith	Simil	Vocab	PA	BD	Digit Symbol	Category	Trails B	TPT-Loc
Non-Litigation	Means of differences	.25	.85	.85	.10	.10	2.00	.30	3.30	10.05	19.60	1.10
Litigation	Mean of differences	−.90	−.95	−.45	−1.10	−1.00	−1.50	−.40	−1.95	−12.65	−34.65	−.85
	t	1.98	2.40	1.51	2.26	2.12	3.80	1.09	8.61	3.73	3.10	2.67
	p <	.10	.025	.20	.05	.05	.001	.30	.001	.001	.005	.02

TABLE 3. Scaled Score Conversion Table Based Upon Difference Scores for the Six Variables that Reached Significance Levels Beyond a Probability of .025

	Difference Scores (minus values equal poorer performances on Testing II)					
Scaled Score	Comp	PA	Digit Symbol	Category	Trails B	TPT-Localization
1	3 or more	4 or more	4 or more	16 or more	34 or more	2 or more
2	1 and 2	2 and 3	1, 2, and 3	4-15	8 to 33	1
3	0	0 and 1	0	3 to −1	7 to −7	0
4	−1	−1 and −2	−1 and −2	−2 to −16	−8 to −47	−1
5	−2 or less	−3 or less	−3 or less	−17 or less	−48 or less	−2 or less

TABLE 4. Means, Standard Deviations, t-Ratios, and Probability Levels Based on Scaled Scores Transformed from Difference Scores

		Comp	PA	Digit Symbol	Category	Trails B	TPT-Loc	Total
Non-Litigation	M	2.55	2.40	1.55	2.25	2.20	2.15	13.10
	SD	1.23	1.23	0.51	1.12	1.01	1.42	2.67
Litigation	M	3.55	3.85	4.00	3.70	3.75	3.65	22.50
	SD	1.39	1.18	0.92	1.38	1.37	1.27	4.12
	t	2.40	3.80	10.43	3.65	4.08	3.52	8.55
		.025	.001	.001	.001	.001	.005	.001
								16/17 cutoff

substantial degree of intergroup overlap in several of the distributions for individual tests. The Retest Consistency Index, which is the sum of the scaled scores for the six tests, was clearly a more stable measure than scores for any of the individual tests, as indicated by a *t* ratio (8.55) that was much larger than the *t* ratios for the individual tests.

An analysis of the Retest Consistency Index for the combined groups indicated that a cutoff score of 16/17 yielded the best separation of the two groups. Ninety percent of the litigants had a Retest Consistency Index of 17 or higher, and 95% of the non-litigants had a Retest Consistency Index of 16 or less.

Conclusions. The results of this study clearly indicated that head-injured subjects involved in litigation tended to demonstrate much less consistent scores on retesting than head-injured subjects not in litigation. The Retest Consistency Index, a new measure based on six tests, differentially classified 90% of the litigants and 95% of the non-litigants. Differentiation of the two groups was achieved at highly significant levels.

These results, which demonstrate that subjects involved in litigation are less likely to perform consistently on retesting, indicate that an approach based upon the consistency of retest scores is highly promising. Retest mean scores of the litigation group were always lower than the initial mean scores, and some of these changes were statistically significant. Considering the fact that the non-litigants had better mean values on every test on the second testing (although not always significantly better), it is apparent that a scale reflecting direction of change would differentiate strikingly between the two groups.

Study 2: Consistency of Responses to Test Items

In Study 1 (Reitan & Wolfson, 1995b), our approach to identifying malingerers was based on a comparison of a subject's test scores on two examinations (retest consistency). Study 2 (Reitan & Wolfson, 1995c) compared subjects' responses on individual test items on two examinations (response consistency). Again, our basic hypothesis was that a subject who is malingering or not putting forth the best possible effort (as might occur among persons involved in litigation) will respond less consistently than a subject who is not adversely influenced (as might be presumed of subjects not involved in litigation). In the present investigation of this hypothesis, however, the evaluation was based on responses to individual items, presuming that a subject who was not putting forth his or her best effort would not remember specific responses originally given and thus demonstrate inconsistency of responses on two testings.

The Retest Consistency Index (Reitan & Wolfson, 1995c) showed the most striking intergroup differences on tests that were particularly sensitive to cerebral damage, such as Digit Symbol, the Category Test, and Part B of the Trail Making Test. However, a measure that evaluates the consistency of responses on individual items on two testings would have to use tests that require much more specific responses (such as the verbal subtests of the Wechsler Scale).

Procedure. In Study 2 we analyzed performances on Information, Comprehension, Arithmetic, Similarities, and Vocabulary from either the WAIS or WAIS-R (whichever version had been administered). For each subject, the same version of the Wechsler Scale (WAIS or WAIS-R) was used for both testings.

A raw consistency score for each subtest was obtained by comparing scores for every item on the two testings. If the subject earned a better score on an item on the second testing, 1 point was assigned to that item. If the subject earned a poorer score on an item on the second testing, 2 points were assigned. If an unequal number of items had been administered on the two testings (as a result of reaching the criterion for discontinuation at different points), failure to qualify for an item yielded a score of 0 for that item. This system yielded a raw consistency score for each subtest for each subject.

The raw consistency scores were then tabulated for the combined groups on each subtest, and a 5-point scale was developed for each subtest. A score of 5 was assigned to the 20% of the combined groups (8 subjects) who demonstrated the least consistency, a score of 4 was assigned to the next 20%, and so on, to a score of 1 for the 8 subjects who had the greatest consistency on the two testings. Scaled scores on the five subtests were then summed for each subject to produce the Response Consistency Index.

Data Analysis. In each group, means and standard deviations were computed, and statistical comparisons of Testing I versus Testing II were performed. Intergroup comparisons of level of performance scores were not calculated because of the significant differences in age and education noted above between the two groups.

Next, difference score distributions between Testing I and Testing II in each of the two groups were compared, and the consistency scores generated by comparing the responses on individual items on the two testings were evaluated. The procedure described above was used to generate raw consistency scores.

The raw consistency scores for each subtest were converted to scaled scores using the 5-point scale shown in Table 7. These conversions allowed the scaled scores for the five subtests to be summed to obtain a Response Consistency Index for each subject. Means and standard deviations were calculated for the scaled scores for each of the five subtests as well as for their sum (Response Consistency Index), and intergroup comparisons were made by computing *t* ratios. Finally, a cutoff point that best discriminated the groups was determined by comparing the distributions of the Response Consistency Index for the two groups.

Results. Table 5 presents means and standard deviations, *t* ratios and probability levels comparing Testing I versus Testing II in each group, and comparisons of difference score distributions for the two groups

TABLE 5. Scaled Score Means and Standard Deviations for Testing I and Testing II for Head-Injured Groups Either Involved or Not Involved in Litigation, Together with Comparisons of Difference Score Distributions Between Testings for the Two Groups

Group 1			Inf	Comp	Anth	Simil	Vocab
Non-Litigation	Testing I	M	10.20	10.45	9.10	11.60	10.10
		SD	3.27	3.65	4.91	4.22	3.57
	Testing II	M	10.45	11.30	9.95	11.70	10.20
		SD	3.27	3.80	4.48	4.66	3.93
		t	1.05	1.93	1.47	0.27	0.37
		p <	.40	.10	.20	.90	.80
Litigation	Testing I	M	9.75	9.65	8.10	9.25	10.20
		SD	2.07	2.70	2.77	2.84	2.42
	Testing II	M	8.85	8.70	7.65	8.35	9.20
		SD	2.50	2.39	3.30	2.62	2.14
		t	1.69	1.58	0.68	2.20	2.21
		p <	.20	.20	.50	.05	.05
Mean Difference Score Comparisons							
Mean Intergroup Difference			1.15	1.80	1.30	1.00	1.10
		t	1.98	2.40	1.51	1.89	2.12
		p <	.10	.025	.20	.10	.05

based on the two testings. (Table 5 essentially recapitulates the data presented in Tables 1 and 2.)

Although mean values were generally within the normal range for each group on both testings, the direction of change from Testing I to Testing II indicates that the non-litigation group had higher means than the litigation group on each subtest, whereas the litigation group had lower means than the non-litigation group in each instance. However, most of these intragroup differences were not statistically significant. A comparison of the difference score distributions of the two groups showed significant differences only on Comprehension ($p < .025$) and Vocabulary ($p < .05$), despite the fact that the direction of change was different in each instance. It is apparent that a level-of-performance approach (comparisons based on how well the subjects performed) reveals little significant information about differences between the two groups.

A rather different picture emerged, however, when response consistency scores were analyzed. Table 6 presents means, standard deviations, and a comparison of the two groups for scores generated by comparing responses to individual items on the two testings.

For every subtest except Information, the raw consistency mean score for the litigation group was more than twice as large as the score for the non-litigation group. For each subtest individually considered, the litigation group was less consistent than the non-litigation group at highly significant levels.

The next step was to use a 5-point scale to convert the raw consistency scores for each subtest to scaled scores. This conversion scale is presented in Table 7.

Table 8 presents means and standard deviations based on the 5-point scaled score distributions for each subtest and for the Response Consistency Index (which represents the sum of the scaled scores for each subject) together with intergroup comparisons.

Each intergroup comparison yielded highly significant differences, with the litigation group demonstrating less consistency in responses between Testing I and Testing II in every instance. As would be expected considering the greater degree of stability that tends to characterize summary measures, comparisons based on the Response Consistency Index yielded the largest *t* ratio.

The Response Consistency Index scores for individual subjects ranged from 6 (most consistent) to 25 (least consistent). The best cutoff score for differentiating the two groups was 15/16, with 100% of the non-litigation group having scores of 15 or less and 90% of the litigation group earning scores of 16 or more.

TABLE 6. Means and Standard Deviations Representing Consistency Raw Scores (0 for the Same Score, 1 for a Higher Score, and 2 for a Lower Score) on Testing II as Compared with Testing I for Head-Injured Groups Involved and Not Involved in Litigation.

Group		Inf	Comp	Arith	Simil	Vocab
Non-Litigation	M	4.50	4.55	2.00	4.05	8.00
	SD	1.85	2.13	1.49	3.07	3.80
Litigation	M	8.80	10.15	5.45	8.35	18.20
	SD	5.45	4.48	3.89	2.37	5.98
	t	3.33	5.00	3.71	6.09	6.46
	p <	.005	.001	.001	.001	.001

TABLE 7. Conversion of Raw Consistency Scores to Scaled Scores Based on a 5-Point Scale (a Score of 1 Equals the Most Consistent Performance and a Score of 5 Equals the Least Consistent Performance)

Scaled Score	Information	Comprehension	Arithmetic	Similarities	Vocabulary
1	3 or less	4 or less	0-1	2 or less	6 or less
2	4-5	5	2	3-5	7-10
3	6	6-7	3	6-7	11-14
4	7-8	8-10	4-5	8-9	15-19
5	9 or more	11 or more	6 or more	10 or more	20 or more

TABLE 8. Means, Standard Deviations and Probability Levels Based on a 5-Point Scale for Individual Tests and the Response Consistency Index (Total Score) for Head-Injured Groups Involved and Not Involved in Litigation

Group		Inf	Comp	Arith	Simil	Vocab	Response Consistency Index
Non-Litigation	M	2.15	2.05	2.10	2.15	1.95	10.40
	SD	0.93	0.94	1.17	1.23	0.89	2.62
Litigation	M	3.55	4.10	4.05	3.75	4.10	19.55
	SD	1.23	0.91	1.23	0.85	1.02	2.82
	t	4.05	6.97	4.88	4.80	7.12	10.64
	p <	.001	.001	.001	.001	.001	.001

Conclusions. The results of this study indicated that subjects involved in litigation were much less consistent between two testings in their responses to individual items on the Information, Comprehension, Arithmetic, Similarities, and Vocabulary subtests than were subjects not involved in litigation. A summary score that represented the sum of scaled scores for the individual subtests (the Response Consistency Index) correctly classified 100% of the non-litigants and 90% of the litigants. There seems to be little doubt that the groups differ strikingly.

The differences between the litigation group and the non-litigation group were derived from comparisons of performances on two testings (intraindividual comparisons that in effect used each subject as his/her own control) rather than from intergroup comparisons. The results suggested that level of performance, as evaluated with relation to normative distributions, would have been far less productive of differences between the groups than the evaluation of intragroup changes (the procedure used in this study).

Study 3: The Dissimulation Index

Although Study 1 and Study 2 used the same groups of subjects, completely separate data were used in each study. Both studies utilized intraindividual differences based on the scores of the same tests administered at different times. Study 1 was based on scores for six tests, and Study 2 was based upon consistency of responses to individual test items using five tests. Except for the Comprehension subtest, the tests used in Study 1 and Study 2 did not overlap. It appears that the Retest Consistency Index (Study 1) and the Response Consistency Index (Study 2) were essentially independent measures in terms of procedural considerations. Nevertheless, both measures were remarkably effective in differentiating litigants from non-litigants.

Under these circumstances, it seemed advisable to combine these two indexes and exploit their possible complementary effect. This combination was done in Study 3 and produced the Dissimulation Index (Reitan & Wolfson, 1995d).

Procedure. The Dissimulation Index, obtained by adding the scores for the Retest Consistency Index and the Response Consistency Index, represented the sum of 11 scores, with the range for each score extending from 1 to 5. Therefore, a subject who was inconsistent on each test of the two testings could receive a maximal score of 55. A subject who performed consistently could obtain a score of 11 (the most consistent score possible).

The Dissimulation Index was computed for each of the 40 subjects. Means and standard deviations were determined for each group, and *t* ratios were computed to compare the distributions. The degree of overlap of the distributions was used to determine the best cutoff scores.

Results. The mean Dissimulation Index was 42.05 ($SD = 6.14$) for the litigation group and 23.50 ($SD = 3.00$) for the non-litigation group, yielding a *t* ratio of 12.13 ($p < .001$). These results indicate that inconsistencies between the first and second testings were far more likely to be demonstrated by litigants than by non-litigants.

The distributions of the two groups showed that the scores ranged from 33 to 55 for the litigation group and from 18 to 29 for the non-litigation group. The frequency distributions are presented in Table 9.

Scores for the two groups did not overlap; in fact, none of the 40 subjects received scores of 30, 31, or 32, thus revealing a gap between the two distributions. On the basis of these samples, we judged that the best cutoff point would be 31/32.

TABLE 9. Distributions of Dissimulation Indexes for Two Head-Injured Groups, One Involved in Litigation and the Other Not Involved in Litigation

Dissimulation Index	16-20	21-25	26-30	31-35	36-40	41-45	46-50	51-55
Non-Litigation Group	4	11	5	0	0	0	0	0
Litigation Group	0	0	0	3	4	8	4	1

Conclusions. The results of this study demonstrated that retest performances were far less consistent in litigants than in non-litigants. As noted, there was a gap in the scores between the two distributions of Dissimulation Indexes. A cutoff point that separated the groups perfectly was identified, although this study, as with any first report, requires cross-validation. It should also be noted that different characteristics of litigants associated with consistency of test-retest performances may eventually be identified. In addition, the method of test-retest consistency should be studied among other groups in which the possibility of malingering may be likely. In any case, the results of this study strongly suggest that using the subject as his/her own control has significant advantages over interpreting the subject's scores with relation to the rest of the population.

The approach used to develop the Dissimulation Index has the advantage of generally bearing little or no direct relation to the subject's level of performance. Of course, if a subject scored 0 on every item, there would be no evidence of inconsistency. Consistently poor performances might also lower the Dissimulation Index. However, subjects in litigation appear generally to earn fairly adequate scores, with means that are not consistently significantly lower than the means earned by subjects not in litigation (Reitan & Wolfson, 1995b), even though in this study the Dissimulation Index perfectly differentiated the litigants from the non-litigants.

It should be noted that this study was not directly concerned with malingering; it compared persons involved in litigation with persons not involved in litigation. We knew of no reason why the non-litigation subjects would not put forth their best effort when taking the tests. It is possible, though, that litigants might deliberately, or because of the stress and pressure of the existing circumstances, fail to do their best on a second examination. In any case, the results of this study suggest that these two groups represent quite different samples in terms of the Dissimulation Index, and raise the probability of eventually identifying test results that are not completely valid.

Inspection of test results of the individual litigants in our series suggests that many tests, over and beyond those that contribute to the Dissimulation Index, often show very inconsistent results. Some of these subjects perform very poorly and inconsistently on the Tactual Performance Test as well as other measures. Further research might reveal that additional tests could profitably be added to the Dissimulation Index.

Finally, the limitations of these studies must be noted. The number of subjects was small, and cross-validation of the results necessary. Even if the sensitivity of these Indexes is confirmed, many additional details, concerned with specificity, will need to be explored. Do different results occur among litigants of different age ranges, male or female gender, with different socioeconomic or education statuses, with different prelitigation histories and neuropsychological or psychiatric status, and so on? What are the time limits between testings that may cause non-litigants to begin to show a greater degree of inconsistency? Every practical question concerned with human behavior is complex in terms of determinants of the answer, and detection of malingering, dissimulation, or invalid test scores is no exception.

CLINICAL APPLICATION OF RESEARCH RESULTS ON THE RETEST CONSISTENCY INDEX, THE RESPONSE CONSISTENCY INDEX, AND THE DISSIMULATION INDEX

In our experience, 40 years ago, nearly every plaintiff who was suing to collect damages for head and brain injuries had sustained significant damage, and the neuropsychologist's role was to document the impairment using objective methods. The opposing expert was usually a physician whose examination had produced results within normal limits. At least 15 years passed before we were even opposed by another expert neuropsychologist, and even then the two neuropsychologists were usually more in agreement than disagreement.

As we all know, this is rarely the situation today. There are, of course, many reasons for these changes, but we believe that a major reason stems from the growing sophistication of plaintiffs and their inclination to sue even when the head injury has been only very minor. We suspect that many plaintiffs now recognize the types of tests on which errors are to be expected and on which speed of performance is a factor, and in some instances, they may make unnecessary errors or perform poorly without a conscious or deliberate decision to malinger. In addition, both plaintiffs and lawyers have recognized the potential for substantial monetary gain, supported in part by the growing acceptance of expert neuropsychological testimony, even in cases of minor head injury. Obviously, an interpretation of neuropsychological test data, on the basis of level of performance alone, is in jeopardy of error.

Although we all favor compensation when the injury has been real, none of us feels, in principle, that compensation should exceed the damages. The problem is one of truly assessing the damages when the adversarial system promotes a tendency by one side to exaggerate and the other side to minimize the degree, nature, and effects of the damage. Certainly, there are plaintiffs who describe their symptoms as accurately and as honestly as possible and who also put forth their best possible efforts on neuropsychological tests; and with equal certainty we can propose just the opposite among other plaintiffs. Our question, as expert neuropsychologists, is how can we tell the difference?

We recently were involved in a case that exemplifies this problem. Ms. P. was a passenger in a car that was rear-ended by another vehicle. She reported that her head was shaken violently although she had no loss of consciousness and was not taken to the hospital. She was subsequently examined by a large number of medical professionals, and while no objective evidence of brain injury was found, she complained of the following: memory impairment; headaches; dizziness; confusion; depression; fatigue; irritability; edginess; being short-fused; tingling in her hands; pain involving her neck, left arm, and left shoulder; pain and spasms in the right side of her back; and occasional numbness and stiffness of her feet. All of these complaints had their onset following the accident. Mrs. P.'s husband and mother-in-law, who were in daily contact with her, were deposed and testified that these complaints were real and began only after the accident.

The plaintiff's attorney then had neuropsychological testing performed, consisting of the Wechsler Adult Intelligence Scale-Revised (WAIS-R), the Halstead-Reitan Battery (HRB), the Wide Range Achievement Test-3 (WRAT-3), the Minnesota Multiphasic Personality Inventory (MMPI), and a number of additional neuropsychological tests. The results were interpreted by the plaintiff's neuropsychologist as showing significant impairment of brain functions.

One of us (RMR) had an opportunity to review the test results prior to gaining any knowledge of the client's history or the circumstances surrounding the case and concluded that while Ms. P. had relatively average WAIS-R scores, was average or above on the WRAT-3, and had an

MMPI profile that suggested concern about bodily functions, anxiety, and feelings of frustration and tenseness, the neuropsychological tests demonstrated a broad range of scores, with some tests being done very poorly and others falling well within the normal range. While variability of this type might in some instances be a consequence of selective impairment due to brain damage, in this case, the tests done poorly tended to be ones that required the deliberate and concentrated effort of the subject (and without deliberate effort might well be done poorly).

Even more striking disparities were reflected by Mrs. P.'s almost total inability to perform the Tactual Performance Test with the right hand, even though finger tapping speed, grip strength, and tactile perceptual skills with the right hand were mainly within normal limits and certainly showed no special impairment on the right side. Inconsistencies of this kind raised a question of whether Ms. P. had been exerting her best effort on all of the tests, and suggested that the poor scores may, at least in part, have been due to diminished effort. These findings demonstrated the importance of using a battery that is designed to permit expression of inconsistencies among tests not only in terms of level of performance but also with respect to patterns of performance and comparative skills on the two sides of the body.

Nevertheless, the case had reduced itself to a situation in which (1) the severity of the injury was not consistent with the severity of the symptoms and complaints, (2) medical opinions varied concerning the validity of the symptoms and complaints, (3) one neuropsychologist felt strongly that the plaintiff was significantly impaired, and (4) the other neuropsychologist felt that inconsistencies in the test results suggested that the indications of neuropsychological impairment might well be exaggerated, if not invalid. How can this type of situation be resolved?

In this case, the neuropsychologist working for the defense requested that additional neuropsychological testing be done (inasmuch as the defense had done no testing at all) and the judge granted this request. Without mentioning that the requested tests were the ones needed to compute the Retest Consistency Index, the Response Consistency Index, and the Dissimulation Index (Reitan & Wolfson, 1998), the additional tests were given by a third neuropsychologist. Although the purpose of this additional testing was explained to the defense lawyer, he seemed to fail to understand the purpose until well after the testing was done, being committed to the notion that poor scores invariably indicated neuropsychological impairment. In fact, the results of the second testing yielded scores that did indeed reflect poor performances with relation to the initial test scores, prompting the defense attorney to bemoan the fact that the additional testing seemed only to confirm the impairment indicated by the original test findings.

After repeated explanations that the two testings provided the opportunity for evaluating intraindividual (as contrasted with interindividual) test scores, and that the scale for evaluation of intraindividual variations in test scores was based on comparisons of head-injured persons *who were not in litigation* with head-injured persons *who were in litigation,* the defense attorney finally did understand the nature and purpose of the additional testing. In fact, Ms. P.'s performances on the additional testing clearly deviated from the range of scores shown by head-injured persons who were not in litigation, demonstrating the inconsistency, and apparent invalidity, of her two sets of test scores. Her test scores produced a Dissimulation Index of 40, well above the cutoff of 31/32. When presented with this objective evidence of apparent malingering, Ms. P.'s lawyer decided not to try the case and, much to the anger of the plaintiff, urged her to accept a minimal settlement amount, which she finally did.

In summary, it is important to recognize that while existing tests for malingering sometimes produce accurate and helpful results, they are essentially based on a level-of-performance model that compares the client's performance with the population (or population sample). Most of these tests for malingering presume that a malingering client will perform poorly on a task that is presented as being difficult but actually is rather easy. When the client performs poorly on this supposedly easy task, it is presumed that the poor performance is due to malingering. This model fails to consider the fact that an individual may, in many instances, do poorly even on tasks thought to be easy for reasons other than malingering, and this would seem to be a factor which has led to conflicting reports in the literature. We attempted to avoid such problems by bypassing entirely a level-of-performance model. The procedure for developing and scoring the Retest Consistency Index, the Response Consistency Index, and the Dissimulation Index is *not* based on level of performance (or how well the client scores), but instead upon intraindividual difference scores, represented by the consistency of scores and responses on two separate testings. This difference in procedure would appear to have a substantial effect on the results obtained.

THE DAUBERT ISSUE AND SCIENTIFIC ADMISSIBILITY

The United States Supreme Court identified four considerations for trial judges to use in evaluating expert testimony, or in some cases, in deciding whether to admit expert testimony. Briefly, these include the following:

1. Has the method been tested?
2. Has the method been subjected to peer review and publication?
3. What is the error rate in applying the method?
4. To what extent has the method received general acceptance in the relevant scientific community?

In our experience, trial judges and lawyers gradually are giving increased consideration to these guidelines, and are giving serious consideration to the admissibility of testimony based on whether these guidelines have been met. In the main, concerns have centered around (3) and (4) above; namely, the error rate and the question of general acceptance.

It would seem perfectly legitimate, and even necessary, to know how accurate a method is in achieving its purpose. Acceptance in the scientific community, however, would carry with it a time factor, inasmuch as newer methods would need time to be incorporated into the knowledge, experience, and practical testing that might be required for acceptance. Neuropsychological tests and procedures, which have been subject to peer review and publication in acceptable outlets, however, might well be viewed as having appropriate acceptance by the scientific community.

Our recent experiences have mainly concerned (3) above–the error rate. The error rate is quite a different matter than the statistical probability of accepting the null hypothesis (or a chance effect), which some neuropsychologists have referred to in responding to this requirement. Even supplying a probability statement for multiple tests is hardly an answer, inasmuch as the independence of the tests is unknown and, in any case, this kind of information says nothing about the rate of errors in conclusions about the individual person. In legal matters concerning personal injury, data relating to the probability that groups of subjects are, or are not, drawn from the same population are essentially irrelevant, because the matter concerns the person rather than inferential statistics based on group comparisons.

In fact, the customary models of statistical analyses–the ones we all learned in school and are usually required to meet publication standards–have limited meaning when judgments, diagnoses, and conclusions must be made about the individual person. We often offer "more probable than not" statements with little or no hard evidence to support these conclusions. If knowledge of the error rate concerning the question of brain damage or impairment was actually required to permit one to testify as an expert, not many of us would be allowed to testify. Few of our studies on individual tests, or even conclusions based on batteries of tests, even report the number of false-positives and false-negatives. Such data are published for other diagnostic methods that require conclusions about the individual person (such as computed tomography and magnetic resonance imaging), and questions of accuracy were among the first issues studied when these procedures were developed and became available. Why have psychologists failed to produce such data, when they clearly are so necessary as a basis for giving neuropsychological methods a degree of credence? There are a number of possible answers to this question, a principal one being that, to produce such data, a specified procedure or set of tests is required, applied to each subject in a precise and standardized manner, in order to evaluate accuracy, or concurrence with independent criterion information. Neuropsychologists appear to be shying away from such specified and standardized procedures to an increasing extent, apparently wanting (or needing) to give whatever tests they wish and to thereby gain the right to draw whatever conclusions they wish (or that may be requisite in terms of the role they have accepted and the conclusions they have committed themselves to support).

In a recent case, a federal judge was asked to dismiss the testimony of a prominent neuropsychologist who was testifying on behalf of a plaintiff who had sustained a head injury. In many prior instances, both in his publications and sworn testimony, this neuropsychologist had supported the use of neuropsychological tests in evaluating individual persons. In this case, however, scores produced by an extensive set of tests that had been administered under his direct supervision fell essentially in the normal range. He admitted that the test findings were essentially normal, and, in fact, this conclusion was readily subject to documentation. However, he insisted that the plaintiff had sustained significant and serious impairment. There was strong evidence against this conclusion, such as the plaintiff having earned more income the year after the injury than the year before the injury. However, this prominent neuropsychologist pointed out that he had interviewed the plaintiff, his relatives, and a few friends, all of whom cited a host of complaints and problems that they attributed to the injury. When asked about the disparity between his conclusions and the normal neuropsychological test results, the neuropsychologist replied that neuropsychological tests contributed no more than 10% to his conclusions and that his clinical impressions were the primary basis for his testimony. The opposing attorney then appealed to the judge to exclude the neuropsychologist's testimony on the grounds that his methodology had not been adequately tested, had not been subjected to peer review, the error rate was unknown, and the neuropsychological community would disagree that neuropsychological tests should count for 10% and clinical impressions for 90%. The defense attorney said that, in his opinion, the judge "came very close to excluding the neuropsychologist's testimony, but in the end felt that he did not have enough information about prevailing practices in neuropsychology to make such a decision." Another consideration may have been that the judge was reluctant to make a ruling that would have devastated the plaintiff's case since, aside from the neuropsychologist's opinion, there was little additional credible evidence of brain impairment.

It seems clear that the time has come when we need to support our conclusions with hard evidence. We can hardly be proud that it is the legal processes that are forcing us in this direction rather than a feeling of clinical responsibility to our clients and patients.

With regard to the Indexes described in this article, the methodology has been subjected to peer review, the method has been tested as described in publications (Reitan & Wolfson, 1995b, 1995c, 1995d), and the error rate has been stated in these publications. Since it is a new method, cross validation is certainly called for, as was noted in the published papers. The extent to which the methodology has received acceptance in the neuropsychological community is difficult to judge because of the recency of development and publication, together with likely problems in replication arising from possible difficulties in providing the necessary data (repeated examinations not only of head-injured litigants, but especially of head-injured persons not involved in litigation).

Finally, the problem of testing the accuracy of neuropsychological test data must receive much more critical consideration than it has up to this point. One approach might be to make predictive judgments using whatever test data were available for each subject, and checking the accuracy of these predictions against criterion information. The problem with this approach would lie in the fact that there would be no clear definition of the test data used for making the predictions, inasmuch as the tests administered would surely vary from one subject to another. Neuropsychologists who use so-called flexible batteries would face exactly this problem, because their test batteries, designed according to the supposed complaints or deficits of the client, necessarily vary from one client to another. In fact, a procedure that first discerns the client's area of possible deficit via history information, relatives' observations of the client, or interview information, and then seeks to confirm or refute such hypotheses through selection of a range of tests judged to be appropriate, is clearly circular and can only be considered to be relevant to the complaints initially deemed to be significant. Under these circumstances, there can be no assurance that the battery of tests selected for each client represents a comprehensive, balanced, and validated set of measures of brain function or dysfunction. Of course, if *each* of these many symptom-oriented batteries had been checked for accuracy in correlating with and identifying brain lesions of a diffuse and/or focal nature, in varying locations of the brain, representing the full range of types of brain disease and injury in identifying both chronic and stabilized brain lesions versus acute and progressive brain conditions and effectively differentiating this entire cadre of people with brain involvement from non-brain-damaged people, there would be no problem. The field of *neuro*-psychology (the discipline based on establishing brain-behavior relationships) would be secure. It is obvious, however, that there is no likely prospect that *multiple* test batteries can be checked out in the detail necessary to establish their relationships to the broad range of conditions that, in total, represent brain damage. Yet, unless evidence is available that all the categories of brain damage are reflected by a particular neuropsychological battery (or that the battery validly differentiates between brain-damaged persons and non-brain-damaged persons regardless of all of the variations that occur under the rubric of brain damage), one cannot presume that the battery validly reflects brain pathology. In the absence of evidence supporting this presumption, we clearly lose the claim that identifies the essential nature of our field–the area of psychology that relates behavioral measurement to the biological status of the brain. Without a firm anchor to the brain, we become clinical psychologists, school psychologists, consulting psychologists, educational psychologists, or whatever type of psychologist appropriate to our particular interest. Of course, we will also find ourselves failing to compare favorably to the experts in each of these areas.

It is apparent that we cannot have it both ways. We either have to respect the brain as the basis for behavior, and validate our measures in accordance with the many conditions that can adversely affect the brain, or recognize that the *neuro* part of neuropsychology is added for respectability alone. If we are unable to document our valid relationship to brain status, in terms of our scientific methods and procedures, as individuals we should at least admit that the Supreme Court was quite reasonable and correct in requiring that the error rate in *neuro*psychology be specified with respect to individual subjects. Such an admission, of course, would also verify our inadequacy to function as expert witnesses.

One way out of this dilemma would be to use a neuropsychological test battery for which published evidence is available that meets the four criteria identified by the Supreme Court as necessary for admission as an expert witness. The Halstead-Reitan Neuropsychological Test Battery meets these four criteria (see Reitan & Wolfson, 1993), but competent interpretation (which, in the individual case, can be judged by a large and long paper trail) is required over and beyond training in test administration. Fortunately, detailed information is available for both administration and interpretation of these batteries of neuropsychological tests for adults, older children, and young children (Reitan & Wolfson, 1990, 1992, 1993).

REFERENCES

American Psychiatric Association. (1994). *Diagnostic and Statistical Manual for Mental Disorders* (4th ed.). Washington, DC: American Psychiatric Association.

Babcock, H. (1930). An experiment in the measurement of mental deterioration. *Archives of Psychology, 18*, 5-105.

Binder, L. M. (1990). Malingering following minor head trauma. *The Clinical Neuropsychologist, 4*, 25-36.

Cullum, C., Heaton, R. K., & Grant, I. (1991). Psychogenic factors influencing neuropsychological performance: Somatoform disorders, factitious disorders, and malingering. In H. O. Doerr & A. S. Carlin (Eds.), *Forensic neuropsychology: Legal and scientific bases* (pp. 141-171). New York: Guilford.

Faust, D., Ziskin, J., & Hiers, J. B. (1991). *Brain Damage Claims: Coping with Neuropsychological Evidence. Vol. I. The Scientific and Professional Literature.* Los Angeles: Law and Psychology Press.

Franzen, M. D., Iverson, G. I., & McCracken, L. M. (1990). The detection of malingering in neuropsychological assessment. *Neuropsychology Review, 1*, 247-279.

Goebel, R. A. (1983). Detection of faking on the Halstead-Reitan Neuropsychological Test Battery. *Journal of Clinical Psychology, 39*, 731-742.

Hunt, H. F. (1943). A practical clinical test for organic brain damage. *Journal of Applied Psychology, 27*, 375-386.

Nies, K. J., & Sweet, J. J. (1994). Neuropsychological assessment and malingering: A critical review of past and present strategies. *Archives of Clinical Neuropsychology, 9*, 501-552.

Reitan, R. M. (1955). Affective disturbances in brain-damaged patients: Measurements with the Minnesota Multiphasic Personality Inventory. *AMA Archives of Neurology and Psychiatry, 73*, 530-532.

Reitan, R. M. (1967). Psychological assessment of deficits associated with brain lesions in subjects with normal and subnormal intelligence. In J.L. Khanna (Ed), *Brain Damage and Mental Retardation: A Psychological Evaluation* (pp. 137-159). Springfield, IL: Charles C. Thomas.

Reitan, R. M., & Wolfson, D. (1988). *Traumatic Brain Injury. Vol. II. Recovery and Rehabilitation*. Tucson, AZ: Neuropsychology Press.

Reitan, R. M., & Wolfson, D. (1989). The Seashore Rhythm Test and brain functions. *The Clinical Neuropsychologist, 3*, 70-77.

Reitan, R. M., & Wolfson, D. (1990). *Neuropsychological Evaluation of Young Children. Manual*. Tucson, AZ: Neuropsychology Press.

Reitan, R. M., & Wolfson, D. (1992). *Neuropsychological Evaluation of Older Children*. Tucson, AZ: Neuropsychology Press.

Reitan, R. M., & Wolfson, D. (1993). *The Halstead-Reitan Neuropsychological Test Battery: Theory and Clinical Interpretation* (2nd ed). Tucson: Neuropsychology Press.

Reitan, R. M., & Wolfson, D. (1995a). The Category Test and the Trail Making Test as measures of frontal lobe functions. *The Clinical Neuropsychologist, 9*, 50-56.

Reitan, R. M., & Wolfson, D. (1995b). Consistency of neuropsychological test scores of head-injured subjects involved in litigation compared with head-injured subjects not involved in litigation: Development of the Retest Consistency Index. *The Clinical Neuropsychologist, 11*, 69-76.

Reitan, R. M., & Wolfson, D. (1995c). Consistency of responses on retesting among head-injured subjects in litigation versus head-injured subjects not in litigation. *Applied Neuropsychology, 2*, 67-71.

Reitan, R. M., & Wolfson, D. (1995d). The question of validity of neuropsychological test scores among head-injured litigants: Development of a Dissimulation Index. *Archives of Clinical Neuropsychology, 11*, 573-580.

Reynolds, C. R. (1998). *Detection of Malingering During Head Injury Litigation*. New York: Plenum Press.

Wechsler, D. (1955). *Manual for the Wechsler Adult Intelligence Scale*. New York: The Psychological Corporation.

Index

© 2002 by The Haworth Press, Inc. All rights reserved.

SPECIAL 25%-OFF DISCOUNT!

Order a copy of this book with this form or online at:
http://www.haworthpress.com/store/product.asp?sku=4858
Use Sale Code BOF25 in the online bookshop to receive 25% off!

Detection of Response Bias in Forensic Neuropsychology

___ in softbound at $29.96 (regularly $39.95) (ISBN: 0-7890-2061-0)
___ in hardbound at $44.96 (regularly $59.95) (ISBN: 0-7890-2060-2)

COST OF BOOKS ______
Outside USA/ Canada/ Mexico: Add 20% ______

POSTAGE & HANDLING ______
(US: $4.00 for first book & $1.50 for each additional book)
Outside US: $5.00 for first book & $2.00 for each additional book)

SUBTOTAL ______
in Canada: add 7% GST ______

STATE TAX ______
(NY, OH, & MIN residents please add appropriate local sales tax

FINAL TOTAL ______
(if paying in Canadian funds, convert using the current exchange rate, UNESCO coupons welcome)

❑ **BILL ME LATER:** ($5 service charge will be added)
(Bill-me option is good on US/Canada/ Mexico orders only; not good to jobbers, wholesalers, or subscription agencies.)

❑ **Signature** ______

❑ **Payment Enclosed: $** ______

❑ **PLEASE CHARGE TO MY CREDIT CARD:**

❑ Visa ❑ MasterCard ❑ AmEx ❑ Discover
❑ Diner's Club ❑ Eurocard ❑ JCB

Account # ______

Exp Date ______

Signature ______

(Prices in US dollars and subject to change without notice.)

PLEASE PRINT ALL INFORMATION OR ATTACH YOUR BUSINESS CARD

Name ______

Address ______

City ______ State/Province ______ Zip/Postal Code ______

Country ______

Tel ______ Fax ______

E-Mail ______

May we use your e-mail address for confirmations and other types of information? ❑Yes ❑No
We appreciate receiving your e-mail address and fax number. Haworth would like to e-mail or fax special discount offers to you, as a preferred customer. **We will never share, rent, or exhange your e-mail address or fax number.** We regard such actions as an invasion of your privacy.

Order From Your Local Bookstore or Directly From
The Haworth Press, Inc.
10 Alice Street, Binghamton, New York 13904-1580 • USA
Call Our toll-free number (1-800-429-6784) / Outside US/Canada: (607) 722-5857
Fax: 1-800-895-0582 / Outside US/Canada: (607) 771-0012
E-Mail your order to us: Orders@haworthpress.com

Please Photocopy this form for your personal use.
www.HaworthPress.com

BOF03